It has been known for some time that certain types of cell, including those in reproductive tissues, produce substances that act by autocrine and paracrine means to control cellular functions, including promotion and inhibition of cell growth. This volume is based on a symposium held under the sponsorship of the World Health Organization and the US National Institutes of Health to review the possible involvement of the many newly recognized growth factors in the control of physiological functions of the reproductive tract.

Growth factors may influence the reproductive tract in a local, self-regulatory manner, or via feedback loops, and chapters are devoted to the mechanisms involved in each case. Consideration is also given to the influence on reproductive function of proteins such as the interleukins, angiotensin and lymphokines. The authors generally agree that tools developed in endocrinology are suitable for the examination of the effects of growth factors on cells.

The book will serve reproductive biologists, as well as the wider community of molecular and cell biologists, as a source of information and ideas. It offers new insights into the functioning of the reproductive tract, examining many basic physiological and molecular mechanisms with potential for the development of new approaches to fertility regulation. Promising areas for further research are identified, and new systems for *in vitro* study of growth factors discussed.

SCIENTIFIC BASIS OF FERTILITY REGULATION

Growth factors in fertility regulation

SCIENTIFIC BASIS OF FERTILITY REGULATION

Books in this series contain the edited proceedings of symposia arranged by the WHO Special Programme of Research, Development and Research Training in Human Reproduction. The purpose of the series is to explore current knowledge in areas of biomedical science which have potential in the development of improved methods of fertility regulation. Containing invited and uniformly edited contributions from scientists in molecular and cell biology, and from leading clinicians, the series will find a wide audience among all those involved with reproductive biology and fertility control.

Already published
Safety requirements for contraceptive steroids
Edited by F. Michal

Cellular and molecular events in spermiogenesis
Edited by D.W. Hamilton and G.M.H. Waites

Contraception and mechanisms of endometrial bleeding
Edited by C. d'Arcangues, I.S. Fraser, J.R. Newton and V. Odlind

Forthcoming
Vaccines for fertility regulation: the assessment of their safety and efficacy
Edited by P.D. Griffin and G.L. Ada

SCIENTIFIC BASIS OF FERTILITY REGULATION

Growth factors in fertility regulation

Proceedings of the Symposium on Potential of Molecular Biology in Fertility Regulation: Growth Regulatory Factors, jointly sponsored by the World Health Organization and the National Institute of Child Health and Human Development and held at the National Institutes of Health, Bethesda, Maryland, on September 22–24, 1988.

EDITED BY

FLORENCE P. HASELTINE
Center for Population Research, National Institute of Child Health and Human Development, National Institutes of Health, Bethesda, Maryland, USA

JOCK K. FINDLAY
Prince Henry's Institute of Medical Research, Melbourne, Australia

The right of the University of Cambridge to print and sell all manner of books was granted by Henry VIII in 1534. The University has printed and published continuously since 1584.

Published on behalf of the World Health Organization

CAMBRIDGE UNIVERSITY PRESS
CAMBRIDGE
NEW YORK PORT CHESTER
MELBOURNE SYDNEY

Published by the Press Syndicate of the University of Cambridge
The Pitt Building, Trumpington Street, Cambridge CB2 1RP
40 West 20th Street, New York, NY 10011–4211, USA
10 Stamford Road, Oakleigh, Melbourne 3166, Australia

First published 1991

Printed in Great Britain at the University Press, Cambridge

British Library cataloguing in publication data

Symposium on Potential of Molecular Biology in Fertility
Regulation : Growth Regulatory Factors (1988 ; Betheseda,
Md.)
Growth factors in fertility regulation.
1. Man. Fertility. Regulation
I. Title II. Haseltine, Florence P. III. Findlay, Jock
K. IV. World Health Organization
612.6

Library of Congress cataloguing in publication data

Symposium on Potential of Molecular Biology in Fertility Regulation:
Growth Regulatory Factors (1988 : National Institutes of Health)
Growth factors in fertility regulation / edited by Florence P.
Haseltine, Jock K. Findlay.
p. cm. — (Scientific basis of fertility regulation)
"Proceedings of the Symposium on Potential of Molecular Biology in
Fertility Regulation: Growth Regulatory Factors, jointly sponsored
by the World Health Organization and the National Institute of Child
Health and Human Development and held at the National Institutes of
Health, Bethesda, Maryland, on September 22–24, 1988."
"Published on behalf of the World Health Organization."
Includes index.
ISBN 0 521 39026 5
1. Growth factors—Physiological effect—Congresses.
2. Fertility—Congresses. I. Haseltine, Florence, P. II. Findlay,
Jock K. III. World Health Organization. IV. National Institute of
Child Health and Human Development (U.S.) V. Title. VI. Series.
QP552.G76S96 1991
599.01′6—dc20 90-42848-CIP

ISBN 0 521 39026 5 hardback

SE

Dedication

To my daughters, Anna and Elizabeth, to whom these growth factors will be constant companions.

FLORENCE P. HASELTINE

Contents

Contributors

Dr Eli Adashi, University of Maryland, 655 W. Baltimore Street, Baltimore, MD 21201, USA.

Dr C. Wayne Bardin, Center for Biomedical Research, 1230 York Avenue, New York, NY 10021, USA.

Dr Etienne E. Baulieu, Laboratorie Hormones, INSERM U33 and Faculté de Médecine, 94270 Bicêtre, France.

Dr Mohamed Benahmed, Laboratoire de Biochimie, pav. 4 l'Hopital Sainte Eugenie, Centre Hospitalier Lyon-Sud, 69310 Pierre-Bénite, France.

Dr Eduardo Bustos-Obregón, Universidad de Chile, P.O. Box 70061, Santiago 7, Chile.

Dr Anne G. Byskov, Laboratory of Reproductive Biology, Department of Obstetrics and Gynecology, Rigshospitalat, University Hospital of Copenhagen, Blegdamsvej 9, DK-2100 Copenhagen, Denmark.

Dr Geoffrey Cooper, Dana-Farber Cancer Institute, 44 Binney Street, Boston, MA 02115, USA.

Dr Nava Dekel, Department of Hormone Research, The Weizmann Institute of Science, Rehovot 76100, Israel.

Dr Egon Diczfalusy, Rooningevagen 21, 14400 Ronninge, Sweden.

Dr Jock Findlay, Medical Research Centre, Prince Henry's Campus, Monash Medical Centre, St Kilda Road, Melbourne, Victoria 3004, Australia.

Dr Jack Gorski, Departments of Biochemistry and Animal Sciences, College of Agricultural and Life Sciences, University of Wisconsin, Madison, WI 53706, USA.

Dr Jouko Halme, Department of Obstetrics and Gynecology, UCLA School of Medicine, Center for the Health Sciences, Room 22177, 10833 LeConte, Los Angeles CA 90024-1740, USA.

Dr Shafiq A. Khan, Max Planck Clinical Research Unit for Reproductive Medicine, Steinfurter Strasse 107, D-4400 Munster, Federal Republic of Germany.

Dr Robert D. Koos, Department of Physiology, University of Maryland, Room 5-032, 655 West Baltimore Street, Baltimore, MD 21201, USA.

Dr David de Kretser, Department of Anatomy, Monash University, Clayton, Victoria 3168, Australia.

Dr Nicholas Ling, Laboratories for Neuroendocrinology, The Salk Institute, 10010 N. Torrey Pines Road, La Jolla, CA 92037, USA.

Dr Frederick Naftolin, Department of Obstetrics and Gynecology, Yale University School of Medicine, 333 Cedar Street, Box 3333, New Haven, CT 06510, USA.

Dr Martti Parvinen, Institute of Biomedicine, University of Turku, Kiinamyllynkatu 10, SF-20520 Turku, Finland.

Dr Mary Lake Polan, Department of Obstetrics and Gynecology, Section of Reproductive Endocrinology, Yale University School of Medicine, 333 Cedar Street, Box 3333, New Haven, CT 06510, USA.

Dr Joanne S. Richards, Department of Cell Biology, Baylor College of Medicine, One Baylor Plaza, Houston, TX 77030, USA.

Dr Focko F.G. Rommerts, Department of Biochemistry, Erasmus Universiteit Rotterdam, Postbus 1738, 3000 DR Rotterdam, The Netherlands.

Dr Anil Sheth, Institute for Research in Reproduction, Indian Council of Medical Research, Jehangir Merwanji Street, Parel Bombay 400 012, India.

Dr Marianne K. Steele, Department of Physiology, University of California, S-762 San Francisco, CA 97143, USA.

Dr Anna Steinberger, Department of Obstetrics, Gynecology, and Reproductive Sciences, University of Texas Medical School at Houston, 6431 Fannin, Suite 3.204, Houston, TX 77030, USA.

Dr Lars Grabow Westergaard, Department of Obstetrics and Gynecology, G 114, Herlev Hospital, University of Copenhagen, Herlev Ringvej, DK-2730 Herlev, Denmark.

Dr Debra Wolgemuth, Department of Genetics and Development, College of Physicians and Surgeons, Columbia University, 630 West 168 Street, New York, NY 10032, USA.

Dr Wang Han-Zhen, Shanghai Institute of Planned Parenthood Research, 2200-4 Xie Tu Road, Shanghai 200030, People's Republic of China.

Foreword

In 1987 the Special Programme launched a series of Basic Science Symposia with the aim of promoting biomedical research in areas that might yield new leads for fertility regulation and for the treatment of infertility. Potentials of Molecular Biology in Fertility Regulation: Growth Regulatory Factors was the second symposium in the series and it was organized by the Special Programme in collaboration with the Center for Population Research of the National Institute of Child Health and Human Development, Bethesda, MD, USA.

It has been known for some time that certain types of cell, including those in reproductive tissues, produce substances that act by autocrine and paracrine means to control cellular functions, including promotion and inhibition of the growth of cells. The main aim of the symposium was to review what is currently known about these substances, in particular their role in human reproduction.

Apart from bringing together a large amount of knowledge on the topic of growth factors, the symposium identified a number of areas where further research might produce new leads for developing fertility regulation methods. One such area related to the factor produced as a result of the expression of the *c-mos* proto-oncogene, which appears to be unique to meiosis. A second possibility was interfering with growth factor(s) that appear to control angiogenesis in the ovary and the receptors of growth factors and other hormones with a future aim of synthesizing compounds that can selectively block the receptors without producing any other biological effects. A final area where further research was suggested relates to the interaction between the reproductive and immune systems. The rationale for this is that substances such as interleukins exert effects on both the immune and reproductive systems; in the case of the latter, for example, interleukin-1 is known to be capable of inducing the production of prostaglandins.

The chapters included in this volume present data from research taking place at the frontiers of biomedical science. The rapid developments occurring in this field are encouraging for the possibility of developing a new generation of agents for the regulation of fertility and treatment of infertility.

Dr M.F. Fathalla

Director, Special Programme of Research, Development and Research Training in Human Reproduction

Preface

The purpose of the symposium was to provide a forum at which physicians and scientists would discuss the interactions of the many newly recognized growth factors that are involved in the control of physiological functions of the reproductive tract which are so important to our everyday health. In addition, the changing needs of the population in terms of fertility regulation and possible new factors that could help improve reproductive health are of great interest to us.

The field of endocrinology has expanded and changed. No longer are explanations of the responses by end organs to hormones purely descriptive. No longer are scientists willing simply to refine feedback loops. The basic tools of the endocrinologists are now being used to look at extremely detailed mechanisms of cellular control. Growth factors have been of interest for a number of years and many such factors have been discovered as a result of their enhancement of the growth of cells in culture. These same substances have often been shown subsequently to be inhibitors of growth in other cell systems. The ability of many of these factors to stimulate growth in one system and to inhibit growth in another system has forced us to examine the details of the mechanisms by which they work. The ability of many growth factors to exert autocrine, paracrine and endocrine effects has further demonstrated their multiple regulatory functions. Several such factors influence the reproductive tract both in a local, self-regulatory manner and at more distal sites in beautifully integrated feedback loops.

The gonads provide an example of the interaction between the systematic growth factors and the intercellular interactions that must occur to promote gamete development. The ovary and the testis not only respond to signals from the pituitary but also act as autocrine organs. Gonadotropins have the primary task of regulating gonadal function but their actions are influenced by growth factors. Some of the chapters in this volume focus on the role of the extracellular matrix and intercellular communications as facilitators of the activity of growth factors. Inhibin, activin, and transforming growth factor-β(TGF-β), members of the inhibin/TGF-β family of genes, act as local regulators within the gonads but they also have endocrine functions and modulate the gonadal–hypothalamic–pituitary loop. Speculation as to how these proteins work as growth factors, via regulation of multiple and, frequently, very different functions of cells, led to a discussion of the receptors for these molecules and to the proto-oncogenes that may mediate their responses.

The topic of growth factors is quite general, and the participants discussed factors that were not considered originally to be a part of the reproductive system or to have the potential to alter growth of gonadal cells. Such systemic and neuroactive proteins (interleukins and angiotensin) were discussed in terms of their activity in the reproductive tract. The lymphokine system was discussed in terms of growth factors that affect the reproductive tract. Moreover, even the immunologic system is considered to interact with the endocrine system.

At the time of this workshop, it was not possible to define which system would provide the most insight into cellular responses. The investigators discussed many different areas and the puzzle is nowhere near complete. Demonstration was ample, however, that the reproductive endocrine system is a valuable tool with which to examine the way in which growth factors influence cells.

The work presented at the symposium offers expanded insight into the functioning of the reproductive tract. It is clear that studies of the reproductive tract, with the many regulatory loops and fine-tuning of function, are rewarding because of the exciting, basic physiological and molecular questions that can be answered using this system. Studies of the subtle signals involved in fertility will be vigorously continued as we search for more clues to the control of reproductive health and try to learn more about the way cells grow and carry out their predestined functions.

We would like to thank Mr J. Khanna, Dr Ann Korner and Margie Perikles for their help in editing, typing and assembling the manuscripts.

Florence P. Haseltine
Jock K. Findlay

Abbreviations

This list is not an exhaustive list of all the abbreviations in the text. It includes all the common abbreviations used throughout this volume. Other abbreviations are defined operationally within the text where they appear.

3-β-HSD	3β-Hydroxysteroid dehydrogenase
20α-DHP	20α-Dihydroxyprogesterone
A	Androgen or Androstenedione
AII	Angiotensin II
ABP	Androgen-binding protein
AC	Adenylate cyclase
ACE	Angiotensin-converting enzyme
aCSF	Artificial cerebrospinal fluid
ACTH	Adrenocorticotropic hormone
aFGF	Acidic fibroblast growth factor
AMH	Anti-Mullerian hormone
ANP	Atrial natriuretic peptide
bFGF	Basic fibroblast growth factor
C	Catalytic subunit of protein kinase C
$[Ca^{2+}]$out	Concentration of Ca^{2+} in medium
cAMP	Cyclic AMP, i.e. cyclic adenosine 3',5'-monophosphate
cDNA	Complementary DNA
CHAPS	3-[(3-cholamidopropyl)-dimethylammonio]-1-propanesulfonate
Con A	Concanavalin A
CRE	cAMP regulatory element
DBD	DNA-binding domain
DDC	Diethyldithiocarbamate
DES	Diethylstilbestrol
DHEA	Dehydroepiandrosterone
DMEM	Dulbecco's modified Eagle's medium

E	Estradiol or Estrogen
ECM	Extracellular matrix
EDS	Ethylene dimethane sulphonate
EGF	Epidermal growth factor
ERE	Estrogen response element
ET	Embryo transfer
FBS	Fetal bovine serum
FF	Follicular fluid
FGF	Fibroblast growth factor
FSH	Follicle-stimulating hormone
G	Glucocorticosteroid
GCCM	Granulosa cell-conditioned medium
GH	Growth hormone
GnRH	Gonadotropin-releasing hormone
GnRHa	Agonist analog of gonadotropin-releasing hormone
GV	Germinal vesicle
GVB/GVBD	Germinal vesicle breakdown
hCG	Human chorionic gonadotropin
HDL	High-density lipoprotein
hFF	Human ovarian follicular fluid
hMG	Human menopausal gonadotropin
hMG-CoA	3-Hydroxy-3-methylglutaryl coenzyme A reductase
HMWGF	High-molecular-weight growth factor
HPLC	High-performance liquid chromatography
H–R	Hormone–receptor complex
HRE	Hormone-response element
hsp90	Heat-shock protein 90
hst70	Transcript related to heat-shock protein 70
i	Immunoreactive
ICSA	Interstitial-cell stimulatory activity
ICV	Intracerebroventricular
IFN-α	Interferon-α
IGF	Insulin-like growth factor
iIGF-1	Immunoreactive IGF-1
IL	Interleukin
IL-1	Interleukin 1
IVF	In-vitro fertilization
IVF-ET	In-vitro fertilization embryo transfer therapy

LBD	Ligand-binding domain
LDL	Low-density lipoprotein
LH	Luteinizing hormone
LHRH	Luteinizing hormone-releasing hormone
LMWGF	Low-molecular-weight growth factors
M	Mineralocorticosteroid
MIS	Mullerian inhibiting substance
MPF	Maturation-promoting factor (also, meiosis-promoting factor)
MPOA	Medial preoptic area
MSH	Melanin-stimulating hormone
NE	Norepinephrine
NRK	Normal rat kidney (fibroblasts)
OMI	Oocyte meiosis inhibitor
OVRAS	Ovarian angiotensin II-generating system
$P450_{arom}$	Aromatase cytochrome P450
$P450_{17\alpha}$	17α-Hydroxylase cytochrome P450
$P450_{scc}$	Cholesterol side-chain cleavage cytochrome
P450	Cytochrome P450
P	Progestin
PA	Plasminogen activator
PAGE	Polyacrylamide gel electrophoresis
Pc	Peritubular myoid cells
PDE	Cyclic nucleotide phosphodicsterase
PDGF	Platelet-derived growth factor
pFF	Porcine follicular fluid
PGE	Prostaglandin E
PGS	Prostaglandin endoperoxidase synthase
PKC	Protein kinase C
PKI	Protein kinase inhibitor
PMSG	Pregnant mare's serum gonadotropin
PO	Preovulatory follicle
POMC	Pro-opiomelanocortin
PRL	Prolactin
QCT	Quantitative computerized tomography
R	Receptor or regulatory subunit of protein kinase
RIIβ	Regulatory subunit of cAMP-dependent protein kinase type II

RAS	Renin–angiotensin system
RIA	Radioimmunoassay
RNP	Ribonuclear protein
rPL	Rat placental lactogen
SA	Small antral (follicle)
SAR	Saralasin
Sc	Sertoli cells
T	Testosterone
T.E.	Testicular extract
TGF	Transforming growth factor
TIF	Testicular interstitial fluid
TNF	Tumor necrosis factor
tPA	Tissue plasminogen activator
Trf	Transferrin
TSH	Thyroid-stimulating hormone
uPA	Urokinase plasminogen activator

I Control of germ cell proliferation and differentiation

Differentiation, growth and maturation of oocytes

A.G. BYSKOV, P. BAGGER, C.Y. ANDERSEN, C. WILKEN-JENSEN AND L. WESTERGAARD

Laboratory of Reproductive Biology, Department of Obstetrics and Gynecology, Rigshospitalet, University Hospital of Copenhagen, Blegdamsvej 9, 2100 Copenhagen, Denmark.

Keywords

Meiosis, folliculogenesis, oocyte maturation.

Introduction

The ontogeny of the oocyte involves a series of unique events in terms of patterns of cell division and growth. The transformation of the mitotically dividing oogonium to a meiotic oocyte begins early in life, often during fetal life, when the germ cell enters the premeiotic phase of DNA synthesis.

The meiotic prophase itself consists of four consecutive stages: leptonema, zygonema, pachynema, and diplonema. Diplonema, or the diplotene stage, lasts for a long time – sometimes as long as a whole life span. The meiotic prophase is not finished until the oocyte 'resumes meiosis', i.e. when the meiotic prophase proceeds and the oocyte enters metaphase. These events do not occur until shortly before ovulation in the mature animal.

In leptonema, the condensation of chromosomes begins at a time when the premeiotic synthesis of DNA is still in progress. During zygonema the homologous sister chromatids pair and form the synaptonemal complexes. The maximal extent of condensation of chromosomes is reached in pachynema, and in diplonema the exchange of genes between the maternal and the paternal chromatids takes place. During the early diplotene stage the chromosomes of the oocyte decondense.

As soon as the diplotene oocyte is formed, it becomes surrounded by presumptive granulosa cells which enclose themselves and the oocyte with a basal lamina, thereby creating a small follicle. A small follicle may at a certain time start to grow, which means that the granulosa cells multiply and the oocyte grows in size. As long as a pool of small, resting follicles remains, the ovary may produce growing and ovulating follicles.

When the oocyte resumes meiosis at the time of ovulation, it continues through the first meiotic division, the DNA being reduced to 2c and the chromosome number still being 2n. During the second meiotic division, which begins immediately after fertilization, the amount of DNA is halved and the DNA content of the oocyte is now 1c and the chromosomal complement is 1n. The mechanisms that control these crucial events are almost unknown.

Initiation of meiosis

In the female, meiosis in mammalian germ cells starts in fetal life or shortly after birth with synthesis of the premeiotic oocyte DNA (Peters *et al.*, 1965). Even before DNA synthesis is finished, the chromosomes begin to condense in the leptotene phase of the meiotic prophase, a phenomenon which is not seen in somatic cell cycles (Larsen *et al.*, 1986).

The mechanisms responsible for the onset of meiosis are not understood. Meiosis in all species studied starts in close association with the invasion by rete cells, an observation responsible for the idea that the rete system exerts a meiosis-inducing effect (Byskov, 1979). Different experiments have shown that not only the rete system but also the gonads in which meiosis is occurring do actually contain and secrete a meiosis-inducing substance (for review, see Byskov, 1986).

It has been proposed that meiosis-inducing substance triggers meiosis in the female as well as in the male germ cells (Byskov & Saxen, 1976). A series of experiments showed that meiosis-inducing substance, derived from adult testes or from preovulatory follicular fluids, triggers meiosis in fetal mouse testes, *in vitro* (Westergaard, 1988). We recently showed that receptors for meiosis-inducing substance exist, and that triggering and progression through the various stages of meiosis depend on the second messenger systems of cyclic nucleotides and phospholipids (Byskov *et al.*, unpublished observations).

The dramatic conformational changes of the chromosomes which occur during the transitory stages of the meiotic prophase are mirrored in the changes in volume of the oocyte nucleus. We have measured the volumes of nuclei in oogonia and oocytes in 2-μm thick sections of plastic-embedded ovaries from mice of fetal age 16 days, from newborn mice and from mice 7 days after birth. The method employed for the measurements, using the nucleator, is described by Gundersen (1988). We found that the volume of the oogonium nucleus is about 160 μm^3, while at leptonema it is almost 600 μm^3, which is almost three times larger than the nuclear volume at pachynema. The nuclear volume at the early diplotene stage is about 400 μm^3 and remains unchanged even when the oocyte becomes enclosed in a small follicle (Bagger *et al.*, unpublished results).

Folliculogenesis

A follicle is formed when the presumptive granulosa cells and the oocyte are enclosed by an intact basal lamina. The formation of follicles occurs early in life, shortly after the oocyte has reached the diplotene stage (Peters, 1978). The survival of the diplotene oocyte seems to depend on its enclosure in a follicle, which provides a unique environment for its growth and maturation. Sometimes more than one oocyte is confined in a follicle, but it seems that only one of these ever reaches maturity (Al-Mufti *et al.*, 1988).

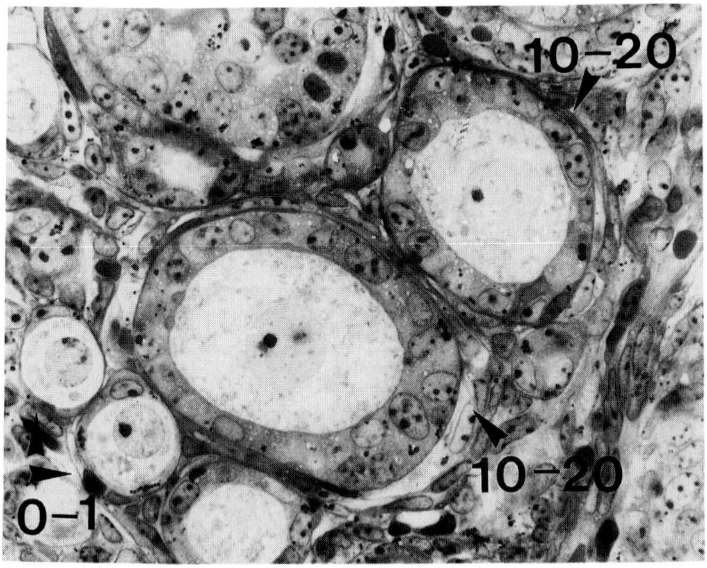

Fig. 1 Part of the ovary of a 7-day-old mouse showing two small, non-growing follicles, in each of which only one granulosa cell is seen, and two small, growing follicles with between 10 and 20 granulosa cells each. Plastic section, 2 μm (x4200).

Follicular development always begins in the inner part of the ovary, around the first diplotene oocytes. In early ovarian development the presumptive granulosa cells of these follicles are connected to the intraovarian rete cords or tubules which originate in the mesonephros. This connection prompted the hypothesis that granulosa cells are derived from mesonephric cells (Byskov & Lintern-Moore, 1973; Zamboni *et al.*, 1980). Moreover, experiments *in vitro* with fetal mouse ovaries have shown that early follicular development is impaired or completely inhibited if the ovarian anlage is depleted of mesonephric tissue (Byskov *et al.*, 1977).

Onset of the growth of follicle and oocyte

As long as a pool of small follicles exists, a certain number of these will, over time, escape from the resting phase and begin to grow (Krarup *et al.*, 1969). It is not known whether the oocyte, the granulosa cells, or both in combination are responsive to the trigger for growth.

The nature of the trigger for follicular growth is obscure. It may be a substance(s) of local or extraovarian origin. The trigger may only function in certain areas of the ovary, so that its activity is controlled by intraovarian mechanisms.

A few experiments have provided clues as to the mechanisms that may be

Table 1. *Volumes of oocyte nuclei, oocytes and follicles in the 7-day-old mouse*[a]

No. of granulosa cells in largest cross section	No. of follicles investigated	Volume (μm^3 x 10^2)		
		Oocyte nucleus	Oocyte	Follicle
0–1	35	4	27	45
2–3	40	5	33	61
4–6	19	9	59	128
7–9	20	10	91	253
10–20	24	12	165	511
1–2 layers	37	32	474	2385
2–3 layers	7	36	633	3848

[a]Volumes of oocyte nuclei, oocytes and follicles with different numbers of granulosa cells in the largest cross section of 2-μm-thick plastic sections.

involved in the triggering of follicular growth. In small mouse oocytes, an increased activity of the nucleolar RNA polymerase has been shown to develop concomitant with the beginning of growth of the oocyte and with increasing numbers of granulosa cells within the follicular compartment (Lintern-Moore and Moore, 1979). At that stage, the follicle is made up of nine granulosa cells, whereas the non-growing oocyte is surrounded by four or fewer granulosa cells, as measured in the widest cross-section of 8-μm-thick sections. These observations suggest that follicular growth may begin with an increase in the number of granulosa cells.

Using the nucleator method referred to above for measuring the volume of the oocyte nucleus and of granulosa cells in 2-μm-thick, plastic-embedded sections, we found that the rate of increase in the nuclear volume was greater than that of the cytoplasm and granulosa cell volumes when the number of granulosa cells began to increase (Table 1). This difference may be indicative of the importance of nuclear activity in the oocyte for the onset of its growth.

The centrally placed follicles which are first formed during early ovarian development seem to differ with respect to growth and differentiation from subsequently formed follicles. These early follicles often remain connected to the rete system and eventually degenerate (Hoyer & Byskov, 1981).

Various experiments have been performed to study the mechanisms that trigger the recruitment of growing follicles from the pool of small, resting follicles. In the newborn mouse, exogenous gonadotrophins have been reported to stimulate follicular growth (Lintern-Moore, 1977). In contrast, injections of crude preparations of epidermal growth factor (EGF) from the submandibular gland resulted in inhibition of gain in body weight and of onset of follicular growth (Lintern-Moore *et al.*, 1981).

In our laboratory, Wilken-Jensen and co-workers are studying the effect of pure EGF on recruitment of growing follicles in newborn mice. Their

Table 2. *Follicular recruitment by EGF in vivo*[a]

Follicles	Control Follicles/ovary	Test (EGF-treated) Follicles/ovary	Statistical difference
Total	964 (100%)	1030 (100%)	$p \geqslant 0.10$
Class I granulosa cells ⩽ 4	826 (86%)	699 (75%)	$p \leqslant 0.05$
Class II granulosa cells 5–8	93 (9%)	188 (18%)	$p \leqslant 0.01$
Class III granulosa cells 9–20	36 (3%)	62 (7%)	$p \leqslant 0.01$
Class IV granulosa cells ⩾ 21	6 (0.7%) 0.6%	0 (0%)	

[a]Follicular growth in control and EGF-treated immature mice. Follicles were counted in every 10th section of 5-μm serially sectioned ovaries. The number of non-growing small follicles (class I) was lower in the EGF-treated mice, whereas the numbers of small growing class II and III follicles were larger. Class IV follicles were not present in the ovaries of EGF-treated mice.

preliminary results indicate that daily injections of EGF from day 1 to day 5 significantly stimulate the onset of follicular growth (Table 2), whereas increase in body weight is not affected (Wilken-Jensen *et al.*, unpublished observations). The discrepancy between the results of the study by Lintern-Moore *et al.* (1981) of the effects of EGF on follicular recruitment and ours may be due to unwanted effects of contaminants in the less pure preparation of EGF used in the former study, as reflected in the absence of sufficient gains in body weight. From our experiments we cannot tell whether EGF affects the germ cells, the somatic cells of the ovary, or whether the effect is indirectly mediated by other cell systems. However, our results represent the first time that a growth factor has been shown to stimulate the growth of ovarian follicules *in vivo*. Studies of the effects of EGF and other growth factors *in vitro* on follicular and oocyte growth are, therefore, crucial for characterization of the target cells for these various factors.

Advancing growth of follicle and oocyte

The growth of the oocyte and of the granulosa cells is already closely related from the very early stages of follicular development. In several mammalian species, the increase in diameter of an oocyte and its nucleus has been correlated with the number of granulosa cells in that follicle (for review, see Lintern-Moore *et al.*, 1974). With regard to this correlation, in 1928 Brambell found that the oocyte exhibited a biphasic pattern of growth in terms of the size of the follicle (as measured in the largest cross-section by the diameter and number of granulosa cells).

The apparently well-established fact that the oocyte grows fast during early stages of follicular development and remains almost constant in size during later stages is not valid if the time – and not the type of follicle – is the correlation unit. Arendsen de Wolff-Exalto and Groen-Clevant (1980) showed that, in the mouse ovary, the growth of the oocyte is linear with time. The simple explanation for the above-cited biphasic growth of the oocyte is that the small follicles grow very slowly whereas the larger ones grow rapidly (Pedersen, 1970).

When the oocyte has reached a certain size in the growing antral follicle, it gains the capacity to mature, i.e. to continue the meiotic prophase by entering metaphase of the first meiotic division (Erickson and Sorensen, 1974), although such oocytes have not yet reached their final, preovulatory size.

Thus, the oocytes of large, antral, non-preovulatory follicles seem to possess all the necessary equipment for completing the first meiotic division. Although the oocyte seems to be ready, ovulation does not occur until the rest of the follicle has matured.

Preovulatory maturation

As the ovarian follicle develops towards ovulation, it enlarges as the result of proliferation of the granulosa cells and accumulation of follicular fluid. During the later stages of antral development, increasing amounts of estradiol accumulate in the follicular fluid. It is well established that intrafollicular estradiol is the essential mitogen for granulosa cells at this stage of development (McNatty *et al.*, 1979). The intrafollicular stimuli for growth at earlier stages are not known. Estradiol does not accumulate in these small follicles (Westergaard, 1988).

Perhaps EGF and other growth factors may be essential stimulators of growth in these small antral follicles, just as EGF seems to stimulate the onset of follicular growth (see above). In the larger antral follicles, intrafollicular estradiol in synergy with follicle-stimulating hormone (FSH) stimulates formation of luteinizing hormone (LH) receptors on the granulosa cells and renders the follicle responsive to the LH surge (Uilenbrook and Richards, 1979). The LH surge induces, in the preovulatory follicle, luteinization of the granulosa cells, which is characterized by a decline in mitotic activity and a shift in the production of steroids from estradiol to progesterone. The LH surge also triggers the final maturation of the oocyte by inducing cytoplasmic and nuclear changes (resumption of meiosis), which prepare the oocyte for fertilization at the time of rupture of the follicle (Moor and Warnes, 1979). This effect of LH is probably indirect and mediated through local substances produced in the follicle.

A number of substances which have been detected in antral fluid, such as oocyte maturation inhibitor (OMI; Channing *et al.*, 1978), meiosis-inducing substance (Byskov, 1979), and hypoxanthine (Downs *et al.*, 1985) have been proposed to interfere with resumption of meiosis. One hypothesis is that resumption of meiosis is caused by a decline in the intrafollicular levels of OMI (Channing *et al.*, 1983) or hypoxanthine (Downs *et al.*, 1985). Another proposal is that meiosis-inducing substance, the amount of which increases in the follicle after the LH surge, exerts a direct stimulative effect on resumption of meiosis (Westergaard *et al.*, 1984).

Some studies of rat oocytes *in vitro* suggest that EGF may be involved in triggering resumption of meiosis (Dekel and Scherizly, 1985; Feng *et al.*, 1988). However, a recent study of EGF in human follicular fluid does not support the suggestion that EGF acts as a stimulator for the resumption of meiosis in the preovulatory follicle (Westergaard and Yding Andersen, 1989). Thus, our knowledge of the mechanism behind the regulation of meiosis in the preovulatory oocyte is still incomplete.

References

Al-Mufti, W., Bomsel-Helmreich, O. & Christides, J.P. (1988). Oocyte size and intrafollicular position in polyovular follicles in rabbits. **Journal of Reproduction and Fertility** 82:15–25.

Arendsen de Wolff-Exalto, E. & Groen-Clevant, D. (1980). Oocyte growth in the immature rat. **Journal of Reproduction and Fertility** 59:187–192.

Brambell, F.W.R. (1928). The development and morphology of the gonads of the mouse. Part III. The growth of the follicles. **Proceedings of the Royal Society**, B103:258–272.

Byskov, A.G. (1979). Regulation of meiosis in mammals. **Annals of Biology and Biochemical Biophysics** 19:1251–1261.

Byskov, A.G. (1986). Differentiation of mammalian embryonic gonad. **Physiology Review** 66(1):71–117.

Byskov, A.G. & Lintern-Moore, S. (1973). Follicle formation in the immature ovary: the role of the rete ovarii. **Journal of Anatomy** 116:207–217

Byskov, A.G. & Saxen, L. (1976). Induction of meiosis in foetal mouse testis *in vitro*. **Developmental Biology** 53:193–200.

Byskov, A.G., Skakkebaek, N.E., Stafanger, G. & Peters, H.(1977). Influence of ovarian surface epithelium and rete ovarii on follicle formation. **Journal of Anatomy** 123:77–86.

Catt, K.J. & Knecht, M. (1988). Transforming growth factor beta stimulates meiotic maturation of the rat oocyte. **Endocrinology** 122:181 186.

Channing, C.P., Chen-Quan, L., Seegar-Jones, G. & Jones, H. (1983). Decline of follicular oocyte maturation inhibitor coincident with maturation and achievement of fertilizability of oocytes recovered at midcycle of gonadotrophin-treated women. **Proceedings of the National Academy of Sciences, USA** 80:4184–4188.

Channing, C.P., Hillensjo, T. & Schaerf, F.W. (1978). Hormonal control of oocyte meiosis, ovulation and luteinization in mammals. **Clinical Endocrinology and Metabolism** 7:601–624.

Dekel, N. & Scherizly, I. (1985). Epidermal growth factor induces maturation of rat follicle-enclosed oocytes. **Endocrinology** 116:406–409.

Downs, S.M., Coleman, D.L., Ward-Bailey, P.F. & Eppig, J.J. (1985). Hypoxanthine is the principle inhibitor of murineoocyte maturation in a low molecular weight fraction of porcine follicular fluid. **Proceedings of the National Academy of Sciences, USA** 82:454–458.

Erickson, G.F. & Sorensen, R.A. (1974). *In vitro* maturation of mouse oocytes isolated from late, middle, and pre-antral Graafian follicles. **Journal of Experimental Zoology** 190:123–127.

Gundersen, H.-J. (1988). The nucleator. **Journal of Microscopy** 151:3–21.

Hoyer, P.E. & Byskov, A.G. (1981).Quantitative cytochemical study of 5-3-hydroxysteroid dehydrogenase activity in the rete system of the immature mouse ovary. In: Byskov, A.G. & Peters, H., eds. **Development and Function of Reproductive Organs**, Amsterdam, Excerpta Medica, pp.216–224.

Krarup, T., Pedersen, T. & Faber, M. (1969). Regulation of oocyte growth in the mouse ovary. **Nature** 224:187–188.

Larsen, K.J., Byskov, A.G. & Christensen, I.L. (1986). Flow cytometry and sorting of meiotic prophase cells of female rabbits. **Journal of Reproduction and Fertility** 76:587–596.

Lintern-Moore, S. (1977). Initiation of follicular growth in the infant mouse ovary by exogenous gonadotrophins. **Biology of Reproduction** 17:635–639.

Lintern-Moore, S. & Moore, G.P.M. (1979). The initiation of follicle and oocyte growth in the mouse ovary. **Biology of Reproduction** 20:773–778.

Lintern-Moore, S., Moore, G.P.M., Panaretto, B.A. & Robertson, D. (1981). Follicular development in the neonatal mouse ovary; effect of epidermal growth factor. **Acta Endocrinologica** 96:123–126.

Lintern-Moore, S., Peters, H., Moore, G.P.M. & Faber, M. (1974). Follicular development in the infant human ovary. **Journal of Reproduction and Fertility** 39:53–64.

McNatty, K.P., Moore Smith, D., Makris, A., Osathanondh, R. & Ryan, K. (1979). The microenvironment of the human antral follicle: interrelationships among the steroid levels in antral fluid, the population of granulosa cells and the status of the oocyte *in vivo* and *in vitro*. **Journal of Clinical Endocrinolgy and Metabolism** 49:851–860.

Moor, R.M. & Warnes, G.M. (1979). Regulation of meiosis in mammalian oocytes. **British Medical Bulletin** 35:99–103.

Pedersen, T. (1970). Determination of follicle growth rate in the ovary of the immature mouse. **Journal of Reproduction and Fertility** 21:81–93.

Peters, H. (1978). Folliculogenesis in mammals. In: Jones, R.E., ed. **The Vertebrate Ovary**, New York, Plenum Press, pp.121–144.

Peters, H., Levy, E. & Crone, M. (1965). DNA synthesis in oocytes of mouse embryos. **Nature** 195:915–916.

Uilenbrook, J.T.J. & Richards, J.S. (1979). Ovarian follicular development during the rat estrus cycle: gonadotrophin receptors and follicular responsiveness. **Biology of Reproduction** 20:1159–1165.

Westergaard, L.F. (1988). Intrafollicular factors regulating human ovarian follicular development and oocyte maturation. Thesis, Copenhagen University, Laegeforeningens Forlag, Copenhagen, pp.1–48.

Westergaard, L.G., Byskov, A.G., Yding Andersen, C.,Grinsted, J. & McNatty, K.P. (1984). Is resumption of meiosis in the human preovulatory oocyte triggered by ameiosis-inducing substance (MIS) in the follicular fluid? **Fertility and Sterility** 41:377–384.

Westergaard, L.G. & Yding Andersen, C. (1989). Epidermal growth factor in human preovulatory follicles. **Human Reproduction** 4:257–260.

Zamboni, L., Upadhyay, S., Bezard, J., Luciani, J.M. & Mauleon, P. (1980). The role of mesonephros in the development of the mammalian ovary. In: Tozzini, R.I.,Reeves, G. & Pineda, R.L., eds. **Endocrine Physiopathology of the Ovary**, Amsterdam, Elsevier/North-Holland, pp.3–42.

GnRH-induced maturation of rat oocytes: a calcium-dependent process

SARI GOREN, YORAM ORON[1] AND NAVA DEKEL

Department of Hormone Research, The Weizmann Institute of Science, Rehovot 76100, Israel;
[1]Department of Physiology and Pharmacology, Sackler Faculty of Medicine, Tel Aviv, Israel.

Keywords

GnRH, oocyte maturation, calcium.

Introduction

Resumption of meiosis (maturation) is an obligatory step in the preparation of oocytes for fertilization. Luteinizing hormone (LH) is the physiological signal for oocyte maturation in mammals *in vivo* (Lindner *et al.*, 1974). LH also induces maturation in follicle-enclosed oocytes *in vitro* (Tsafriri *et al.*, 1972). Maturation of mammalian oocytes also occurs spontaneously after separation of the oocyte from the ovarian follicle (Pincus and Enzmann, 1935; Edwards, 1965). Spontaneous maturation of isolated oocytes is prevented by membrane-permeable derivatives of cAMP and by inhibitors of phosphodiesterase activity (Cho *et al.*, 1974; Dekel and Beers, 1978).

Within the ovarian follicle, the oocyte is encapsulated by the cumulus and granulosa cells. It has been proposed that the action of LH, which involves the elevation of levels of cAMP in the surrounding follicular cells, leads to the disruption of cell-to-cell communication which is followed by a decrease in levels of cAMP in the oocyte. This decrease in levels of cAMP removes the putative tonic inhibition of oocyte maturation and is considered to be a sufficient signal for the resumption of meiosis (Dekel, 1986). Hence, the mechanical disruption of cell-to-cell communication by the removal of the oocyte from the follicle results in spontaneous maturation *in vitro* that is preceded by a decrease in levels of cAMP in the oocytes (Schultz *et al.*, 1983, Vivarelli *et al.*, 1983; Aberdam *et al.*, 1987).

It has recently been demonstrated that agonist analogs of gonadotropin-releasing hormone (GnRH) also induce maturation of mammalian oocytes both *in vivo* in hypophysectomized rats (Corbin and Bex, 1981; Ekholm *et al.*, 1981; Dekel *et al.*, 1985) and *in vitro* in isolated intact follicles (Hillensjo and LeMaire, 1980; Dekel *et al.*, 1983). GnRH-induced maturation in follicle-enclosed oocytes is not associated with elevation of follicular levels of cAMP (Dekel *et al.*, 1985). Although the mechanism of this effect of the analogs of GnRH is not known, it is clear that oocyte maturation can be induced via a pathway that does not involve changes in follicular levels of cAMP. Indeed, in the pituitary gonadotrophs, GnRH induces the release of LH via the phosphoinositide–Ca–protein kinase C cascade (Hirota *et al.*, 1985; Naor *et al.*, 1985; Harris *et al.*, 1985).

Calcium is an important participant in the transduction of numerous signals in various tissues and cell types (Berridge and Irvine, 1984), and the role of calcium in oocyte maturation has been studied in invertebrates and amphibians (Baulieu *et al.*, 1978; Masui and Clarke, 1979; Morrill and Kostellow, 1986) and less extensively in mammals. Recent reports (Robinson, 1985; Cicirelli and Smith, 1987; Cork *et al.*, 1987) challenge the direct involvement of calcium in the maturation of amphibian oocytes. In mammalian oocytes, the data are often contradictory (Tsafriri and Bar-Ami, 1978; Leibfried and First, 1979; Paleos and Powers, 1981; Jagiello *et al.*, 1982; Maruska *et al.*, 1984; Bae and Channing, 1985; Racowsky, 1986) and no clear picture has yet emerged of the role of calcium in this process.

Most of the studies cited above involved spontaneous, hormone-independent maturation *in vitro*. We have studied the role of calcium in the induction of maturation using a system of follicle-enclosed rat oocytes *in vitro*. In this system, meiotic arrest is fully maintained, allowing analysis of the role of calcium in the induction as well as the modulation of hormonally induced maturation. Follicles were incubated in the presence of an agonist analog of GnRH (GnRHa) alone or in combination with calcium-modulating agents. After various periods of incubation the follicles were incised and the oocytes were recovered and analyzed for maturation. Meiotically arrested oocytes are characterized by the presence of the germinal vesicle (GV). Upon re-initiation of meiosis the GV disappears. Resumption of meiosis in the individual oocytes is indicated by GV breakdown (GVB). The data presented here suggest the involvement of calcium in the GnRHa-induced maturation of oocytes.

Induction of oocyte maturation by calcium

Meiotic arrest of the follicle-enclosed oocytes is fully maintained at a $[Ca^{2+}]$out of 1.3 mmol/l, which is the routine concentration of Ca^{2+} in our incubation medium. Addition of GnRHa to the follicles incubated under these conditions results in resumption of meiosis (Dekel *et al.*, 1983). To study the possible involvement of calcium in hormonally induced maturation of oocytes, we initially examined whether elevation of levels of Ca^{2+} in the incubation medium could mimic the action of hormones. We found that increasing $[Ca^{2+}]$out up to 20 mmol/l induced resumption of meiosis in only 10% of the follicle-enclosed oocytes (Fig. 1). However, addition of divalent cation ionophores (A23187 or ionomycin), to enhance the rate of entry of calcium into the cytoplasm, resulted in a partial response that was further potentiated by increasing concentrations of calcium (Fig. 1).

Analysis of the kinetics of calcium-induced maturation of oocytes in the presence of ionomycin revealed that the maximal response was obtained

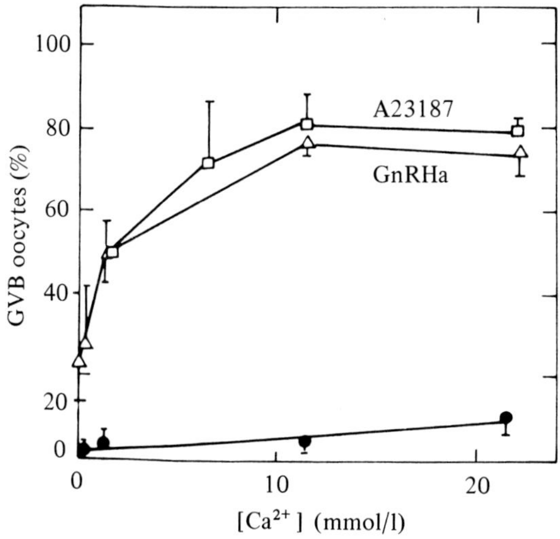

Fig. 1 Effects of calcium on GnRHa-induced and ionophore A23187-induced maturation of oocytes. Follicles were incubated in the presence of GnRHa (10^{-7} mol/l) or ionophore A23187 (10^{-6} mol/l) with the indicated concentrations of calcium ions. After 24 hours, the oocytes were recovered and examined for germinal vesicle breakdown (GVB). The pooled results of three experiments are presented with at least 90 oocytes examined at each experimental point (Dekel *et al.*, 1989, with permission).

within a 2-hour incubation. In the presence of the ionophore A23187, the response to calcium was somewhat slower (53% of the maximal response was obtained after 6 hours).

Involvement of calcium in GnRHa-induced maturation of oocytes

We tested the effect of calcium on the hormonally induced resumption of meiosis in follicle-enclosed oocytes incubated in the presence of submaximal concentrations of GnRHa. As shown in Figure 1, in the presence of elevated levels of Ca^{2+} in the medium, GnRHa-induced resumption of meiosis was markedly potentiated.

A full response of follicle-enclosed oocytes to GnRHa was obtained in incubation medium that contained 1.3 mmol/l calcium. Reduction of $[Ca^{2+}]$out to 0.6 mmol/l decreased the response of the follicle-enclosed oocytes to GnRHa by 65% (Table 1). Total elimination of calcium from the incubation medium by addition of EGTA (2 mmol/l), did not result in a further inhibition of hormone action (Table 1).

Table 1. *The effects of a reduced concentration of Ca^{2+} in the medium ($[Ca^{2+}]out$) on GnRHa-induced maturation of oocytes*

	GVB	
$[Ca^{2+}]$out (mmol/l)	Percentage ± SEM	Total number of oocytes examined
1.3	84 ± 7.5	70
0.6	28 ± 14	95
0	23 ± 9	43

Follicles were incubated with 10^{-7} mol/l GnRHa and the indicated concentrations of $CaCl_2$. After 6 h, the oocytes were recovered and examined for germinal vesicle breakdown (GVB).

The putative recruitment of calcium ions during oocyte maturation did not involve voltage-sensitive calcium channels. This conclusion is supported by the absence of any effect on the maturation process of antagonists of calcium channels (verapamil, nifedipine, diltiazem) (Fig. 2) or of an agonist (BAY-K 8644) (Fig. 3). Similarly, depolarization by 50 mmol/l KCl did not induce maturation (Fig. 4).

Activation of protein kinase C is thought to be biochemically dependent on calcium ions. From our earlier findings that activators of protein kinase C mimic hormone action by inducing oocyte maturation, we previously proposed that the action of GnRHa on the oocyte is mediated by the calcium-dependent protein kinase C second-messenger system (Aberdam and Dekel, 1985). The requirement for the activity of protein kinase C during the maturation process is also suggested in the present study by the partial inhibition of A23187-induced maturation (from 52 ± 9% to 32 ± 5%, n = 112 and 165 oocytes, respectively; $p < 0.05$) by 0.1 mmol/l H-7. Similar results were obtained when we examined the effects of H-7 or H-8 on ionomycin-induced maturation and on GnRHa-induced maturation. H-7 and H-8 are newly synthesized derivatives of isoquinoline-sulfonamide that bind with different affinities to a variety of protein kinases (Hidaka *et al.*, 1984). The relative inhibitory effects of these agents on GnRHa-induced maturation of oocytes corresponded directly to their Ki values for protein kinase C, suggesting that this kinase is indeed involved in oocyte maturation (Dekel *et al.*, 1989). The involvement of calmodulin in the induction of maturation appears unlikely since an inhibitor of Ca-calmodulin fluphenazine (at 30 μmol/l) did not affect GnRHa-induced or A23187-induced maturation.

The effect of dibutyryl cAMP on calcium-induced maturation of oocytes

Spontaneous maturation of isolated oocytes and hormonally induced maturation of follicle-enclosed oocytes are both blocked by the presence of

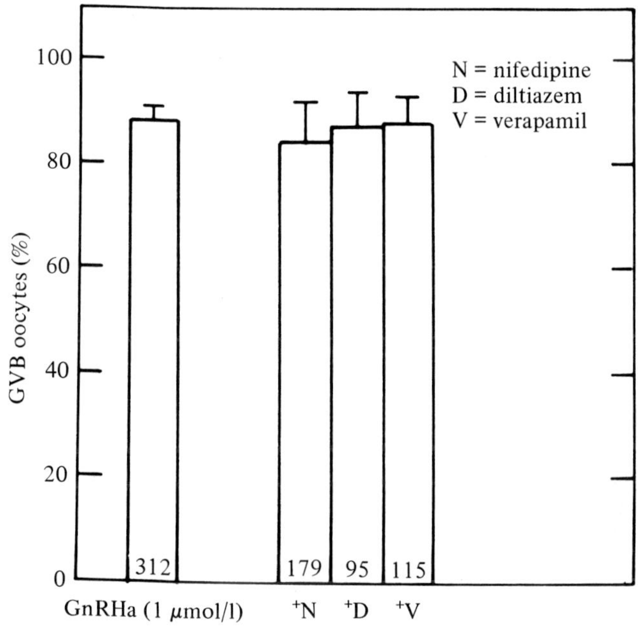

Fig. 2 GnRHa-induced maturation of oocytes in the presence of calcium channel blockers. Follicles were incubated with GnRHa in the presence or absence of 10^{-6} mol/l of the indicated blockers of calcium channels. After 6 hours, the oocytes were recovered and examined for GVB. The pooled results of three experiments are presented and the total number of oocytes examined at each experimental point is indicated at the bottom of each bar.

derivatives of cAMP in the culture medium (Cho *et al.*, 1974; Dekel and Beers, 1978; Dekel *et al.*, 1981). Moreover, oocyte maturation, both *in vivo* and *in vitro*, is preceded by a drop in intra-oocyte concentrations of cAMP (Shultz *et al.*, 1983; Vivarelli *et al.*, 1983; Aberdam *et al.*, 1987). To locate the relative sites of action of calcium and cAMP along the pathway that leads to oocyte maturation, we have examined the effects of dibutyryl cAMP on calcium-induced maturation of oocytes. As seen in Figure 5, 2 mmol/l dbcAMP blocked the calcium-induced maturation of follicle-enclosed oocytes, suggesting that the site of action of cAMP is distal to that of calcium ions.

Conclusions

The physiological signal for induction of oocyte maturation in mammals is provided by the pituitary gonadotropin, LH. It has been demonstrated that, in the rat, GnRHa can also induce oocyte maturation (Hillensjo and LeMaire,

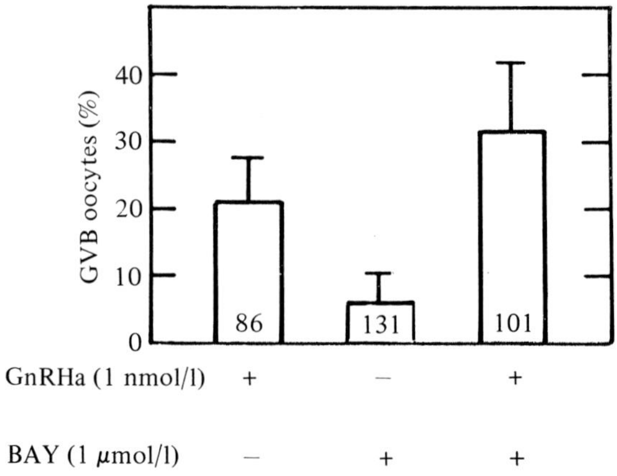

Fig. 3 Effects of BAY-K8644 on GnRHa-induced maturation of oocytes. Follicles were incubated with either GnRHa (10^{-9} mol/l), BAY-K8644 (10^{-6} mol/l) or a combination of the two. After 6 hours, the oocytes were recovered and examined for GVB. The total number of oocytes examined at each experimental point is indicated at the bottom of each bar.

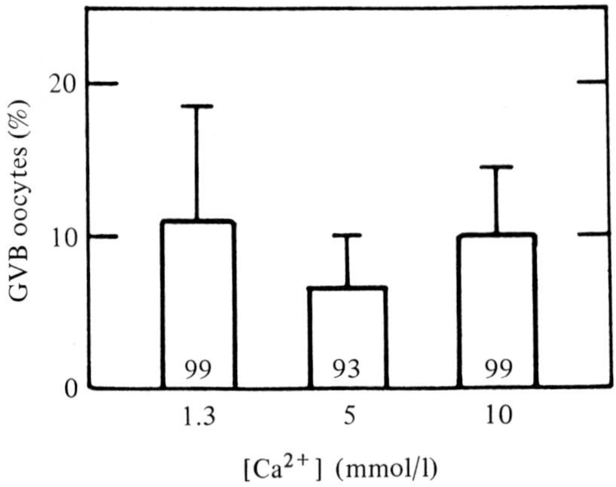

Fig. 4 Effect of depolarization by KCl on the maturation of follicle-enclosed oocytes. Follicles were incubated with 50 mmol/l KCl in the presence of the indicated concentrations of $CaCl_2$. After 6 hours, the oocytes were recovered and examined for GVB. The pooled results of three experiments are presented and the total number of oocytes examined at each experimental point is indicated at the bottom of each bar.

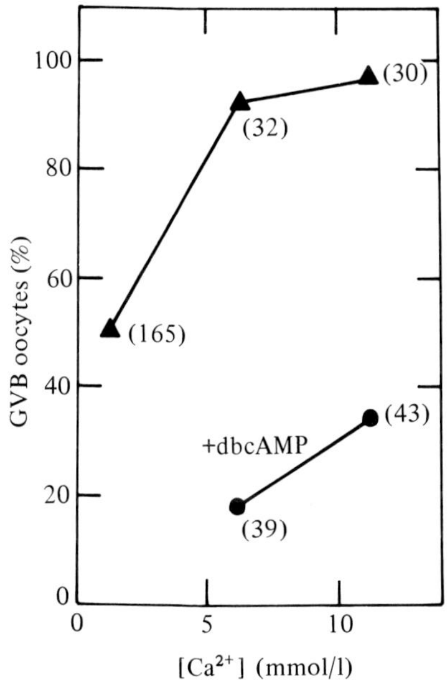

Fig. 5 Effect of dibutyryl cAMP on the calcium-induced maturation of oocytes. Follicles were incubated in the presence of the indicated concentrations of $CaCl_2$ and 10^{-6} mol/l of A23187, with or without 2 mmol/l dibutyryl cAMP (dbcAMP). After 20 hours, the oocytes were recovered and examined for GVB. The number of oocytes examined at each experimental point is indicated in parentheses.

1980; Corbin and Bex, 1981; Ekholm *et al.*, 1981; Dekel *et al.*, 1983, 1985). In this chapter, we have described some results that suggest that calcium ions are involved in this action of GnRHa.

Our present study was performed with follicle-enclosed oocytes. Unlike the isolated oocyte which undergoes spontaneous maturation, the intact follicle allows mechanistic studies on hormonally induced responses of the oocyte *in vitro*. However, being a complex structure composed of a heterogeneous population of cells, the follicle does not allow determination of the cellular target for the action of GnRHa. It is likely that the hormone acts on the granulosa/cumulus compartment, since specific receptors for GnRH on rat granulosa cells have been demonstrated (Clayton *et al.*, 1979; Jones *et al.*, 1980) and biological responses to the hormone, by both granulosa and cumulus cells, have been reported (Clark *et al.*, 1980; Hsueh and Jones, 1981; Dekel *et al.*, 1985). However, in view of our recent report that receptors for GnRH are also present on isolated rat oocytes (Dekel *et al.*, 1988), we cannot exclude the possibility of direct action of GnRHa on the female gamete. The data presented here strongly suggest that calcium participates in the mechanism of GnRHa-induced maturation. However, the target cell and the effector enzymes involved in this process are yet to be determined.

Acknowledgements

We acknowledge the secretarial assistance of Mrs R. Levin. This study was supported by grants from the United States–Israel Binational Science Foundation and from the Israel Academy of Sciences and Humanities.

References

Aberdam, E. & Dekel, N. (1985). Activators of protein kinase C stimulate meiotic maturation of rat oocytes. **Biochemical and Biophysical Research Communications** 132:570–574.

Aberdam, E., Hanski, E. & Dekel, N. (1987). Maintenance of meiotic arrest in isolated rat oocytes by the invasive adenylate cyclase of *Bordetella pertussis.* **Biology of Reproduction** 36:530–535.

Bae, I. & Channing, C.P. (1985). Effect of calcium ion on the maturation of cumulus-enclosed pig follicular oocytes isolated from medium-sized Graafian follicles. **Biology of Reproduction** 33:79–87.

Baulieu, E.E., Godeau, F., Schorderet, M. & Schorderet-Slatkine, S. (1978). Steroid-induced meiotic division in *Xenopus laevis* oocytes: surface and calcium. **Nature** 275:593–598.

Berridge, M.J. & Irvine, R.F. (1984). Inositol trisphosphate, a novel second messenger in cellular signal transduction. **Nature** 312: 315–321.

Cho, W.K., Stern, S. & Biggers, J.D. (1974). Inhibitory effect of dibutyryl cAMP on mouse oocyte maturation *in vitro.* **Journal of Experimental Zoology** 187:383–386.

Cicirelli, M.F. & Smith, L.D. (1987). Do calcium and calmodulin trigger maturation in amphibian oocytes? **Developmental Biology** 121:48–57.

Clark, M.R., Thibier, C., Marsh, M.R. & LeMaire, W.J. (1980). Stimulation of prostaglandin accumulation by luteinizing hormone-releasing hormone (LHRH) and LHRH analogs in rat granulosa cells *in vitro.* **Endocrinology** 107:17–23.

Clayton, R.N., Harwood, J.P. & Catt, K.J. (1979). Gonadotropin-releasing hormone analogue binds to luteal cells and inhibits progesterone production. **Nature** 282:90–92.

Corbin, A. & Bex, F.J. (1981). Luteinizing hormone-releasing hormone agonists induce ovulation in hypophysectomized proestrous rats: direct ovarian effect. **Life Sciences** 29:185–192.

Cork, R.J., Cicirelli, M.F. & Robinson, K.R. (1987). A rise in cytosolic calcium is not necessary for maturation of *Xenopus laevis* oocytes. **Developmental Biology** 121:41–47.

Dekel, N. (1986). Hormonal control of ovulation. In: Litwack, G., ed. **Biochemical Actions of Hormones**, Vol. 13, New York, Academic Press, pp.57–90.

Dekel, N., Aberdam, E., Goren, S., Feldman, B. & Shalgi, R. (1989). Mechanism of action of GnRH-induced oocyte maturation. **Journal of Reproduction and Fertility** Suppl. 37:319–327.

Dekel, N. & Beers, W.H. (1978). Rat oocyte maturation *in vitro*: relief of cyclic AMP inhibition by gonadotropins. **Proceedings of the National Academy of Sciences, USA** 75:4369–4373.

Dekel, N., Lawrence, T.S., Gilula, N.B. & Beers, W.H. (1981). Modulation of cell-to-cell communication in the cumulus–oocyte complex and the regulation of oocyte maturation by LH. **Developmental Biology** 86:356–362.

Dekel, N., Lewysohn, O., Ayalon, D. & Hazum, E. (1988). Receptors for gonadotropin-releasing hormone are present in rat oocytes. **Endocrinology** 123:1205–1207.

Dekel, N., Sherizly, I., Phillips, D.M., Nimrod, A., Zilberstein, M. & Naor, Z. (1985). Characterization of the maturational changes induced by a GnRH analogue in the rat ovarian follicle. **Journal of Reproduction and Fertility** 75:461–466.

Dekel, N., Sherizly, I., Tsafriri, A. & Naor, Z. (1983). A comparative study of the mechanism of action of luteinizing hormone and gonadotropin-releasing hormone analog on the ovary. **Biology of Reproduction** 28:161–166.

Edwards, R.G. (1965). Maturation *in vitro* of mouse, sheep, cow, pig, rhesus monkey and human ovarian oocytes. **Nature** 208:349–351.

Ekholm, C., Hillensjo, T. & Isaksson, O. (1981). Gonadotropin-releasing hormone agonists stimulate oocyte meiosis and ovulation in hypophysectomized rats. **Endocrinology** 108:2022–2024.

Harris, C.E., Staley, D. & Conn, P.M. (1985) Diacylglycerol and protein kinase C: potential amplifying mechanism for Ca^{2+}-mediated GnRH-stimulated LH release. **Molecular Pharmacology** 27:532–536.

Hidaka, H., Inagaki, M., Kawamoto, S. & Sasaki, Y. (1984). Isoquinolinesulfonamides, a novel and potent inhibitor of cyclic nucleotide-dependent protein kinase and protein kinase C. **Biochemistry** 23:5036–5041.

Hillensjo, T. & LeMaire, W.J. (1980). Gonadotropin-releasing hormone agonists stimulate meiotic maturation of follicle-enclosed rat oocytes *in vitro*. **Nature** 287:145–146.

Hirota, K., Hirota, T., Aguilera, G. & Catt, KJ (1985). Hormone-induced redistribution of calcium-activated phospholipid-dependent protein kinase in pituitary gonadotrophs. **Journal of Biological Chemistry** 260:3243–3246.

Hsueh, A.J.W. & Jones, P.B.C. (1981). Extrapituitary action of gonadotrophin-releasing hormone. **Endocrine Reviews** 2:437–461.

Jagiello, G., Ducayen, M.B., Downey, R. & Jonassen, A. (1982). Alterations of mammalian oocyte meiosis I with divalent cations and calmodulin. **Cell Calcium** 3:153–162.

Jones, P.B.C., Conn, P.M., Marian, J. & Hsueh, A.J.W. (1980). Binding of gonadotropin-releasing hormone agonist to rat ovarian granulosa cells. **Life Sciences** 27:2125–2132.

Leibfried, L. & First, N.L. (1979). Effects of divalent cations on *in vitro* maturation of bovine oocytes. **Journal of Experimental Zoology** 210:575–580.

Lindner, H.R., Tsafriri, A., Lieberman, M.E., Zor, U., Koch, Y., Bauminger, S. & Barnea, A. (1974). Gonadotrophin action on cultured Graafian follicles: induction of maturation division of the mammalian oocyte and differentiation of the luteal cell. **Recent Progress in Hormone Research** 30:79–138.

Maruska, D.V., Leibfried, M.L. & First, N.L. (1984). Role of calcium and the calcium–calmodulin complex in resumption of meiosis, cumulus expansion, viability and hyaluronidase sensitivity of bovine cumulus–oocyte complexes. **Biology of Reproduction** 31:1–6.

Masui, Y. & Clarke, H.J. (1979). Oocyte maturation. **International Review of Cytology** 7:185–282.

Morrill, G.A. & Kostellow, A.B. (1986) The role of calcium in meiosis. **Calcium and Cell Function** 6:209–252.

Naor, Z., Zer, J., Zakut, H. & Hermon, J. (1985). Characterization of pituitary calcium-activated, phospholipid-dependent protein kinase: redistribution by gonadotropin-releasing hormone. **Proceedings of the National Academy of Sciences, USA** 82:8203–8208.

Paleos, G.A. & Powers, R.D. (1981). The effect of calcium on the first meiotic division of the mammalian oocyte. **Journal of Experimental Zoology** 217:409–416.

Pincus, G. & Enzmann, E.V. (1935) The comparative behavior of mammalian eggs *in vivo* and *in vitro*. I. The activation of ovarian eggs. **Journal of Experimental Medicine** 62:665–675.

Racowsky, C. (1986) The releasing action of calcium upon cyclic AMP-dependent meiotic arrest in hamster oocytes. **Journal of Experimental Zoology** 239:263–275.

Robinson, K.R. (1985). Maturation of *Xenopus oocytes* is not accompanied by electrode-detectable calcium changes. **Developmental Biology** 109:504–508.

Schultz, R.M., Montgomery, R.R. & Belanoff, J.R. (1983). Regulation of mouse oocyte meiotic maturation: implication of a decrease in oocyte cAMP and protein dephosphorylation in commitment to resume meiosis. **Developmental Biology** 97:264–273.

Tsafriri, A. & Bar-Ami, S. (1978). Role of divalent cations in the resumption of meiosis of rat oocytes. **Journal of Experimental Zoology** 205:293–300.

Tsafriri, A., Lindner, H.R. & Zor, U. (1972). *In vitro* induction of meiotic division in follicle-enclosed rat oocytes by LH, cAMP and PGE_2. **Journal of Reproduction and Fertility** 31:39–50.

Vivarelli, E., Conti, M., De Felici, M. & Siracusa, G. (1983). Meiotic resumption and intracellular cAMP levels in mouse oocytes treated with compounds which act on cAMP metabolism. **Cell Differentiation** 12:271–276.

A G_1-specific spermatogonial chalone

E. BUSTOS-OBREGÓN, J. BALBONTIN AND P. ARENAS

Department of Cell Biology and Genetics, Unit of Biology of Reproduction, University of Chile Medical School, Santiago, Chile.

Keywords

Spermatogonial chalones, spermatogonial proliferation, kinetics of spermatogenesis, testicular cell proliferation and differentiation.

Introduction

The presence of tissue-specific inhibitors of cell proliferation, known as chalones, has been demonstrated for many different tissues (epidermis, lung, liver, melanocytes, kidney, granulocytes, lymphocytes, testis, erythrocytes, fibroblasts, lens, uterus, intestine, muscle, stomach, etc: see Finkler and Acker, 1978; Fremuth, 1984).

According to Iversen (1981), the following definitions apply: (a) chalones are naturally occurring, physiological inhibitors of cell proliferation; (b) chalones must be produced in and be present in the tissues (the cell lines) on which they selectively act, and they are probably mainly produced by the more mature cells of the series; (c) chalones are specific for given tissues or cell lines, but are not species specific; (d) the action of chalones is non-toxic and reversible and, hence, chalones do not injure cells or cell membranes; (e) chalones are water-soluble molecules, either small peptides or large glycoproteins, with molecular weights ranging from less than 2 kDa to more than 100 kDa; (f) chalones may act at the G_1/S phase of the cell cycle, delaying the flux of cells into DNA synthesis, or in the G_2 phase, delaying the flux of cells into mitosis.

Spermatogonial chalones

Clermont and Mauger (1974) demonstrated *in vivo* the G_1-specific chalone activity of a testicular extract, using adult rats previously irradiated to the scrotum. The same effect was found in young (33-day-old) rats, in which a decrease in uptake of [^{3}H]-thymidine into type A spermatogonia was noted (Clermont and Mauger, 1976). A G_2-specific spermatogonial chalone was found in the rat, also *in vivo*, by counting mitotic spermatogonia in whole-mounted seminiferous tubules (Irons and Clermont, 1979).

We have confirmed, both *in vivo* and *in vitro*, the G_1-specific activity of a chalone on spermatogonia in the irradiated rat and mouse (Thumann and Bustos-Obregón, 1978, 1982; Thumann *et al.*, 1981; Bustos-Obregón, 1984,

1986). The G_1-specific chalone can be lyophilized, thereby allowing a more standardized bioassay. It is heat labile, precipitable with ethanol, tissue specific but not species specific. Its inhibitory effect on DNA synthesis is compatible with the theory of occupation of cell (membrane) receptor sites. The bioeffect can be obtained with a steroid-free testicular extract and the active molecule is probably a glycoprotein with a molecular weight of less than 5 kDa. Ultrafiltration of a testicular extract through an Amicon membrane (YM5) with a retention limit of 5 kDa results in a more than 100-fold increase in specific (chalone) activity. The latter is defined for the G_1-specific chalone as the ratio (I.F.) of the proportional reduction in uptake of [^{3}H]thymidine (into testicular DNA) to the protein content of the sample.

Chalone activity and populations of testicular cells

No chalone activity is demonstrable in a testicular extract prepared from 'Sertoli-only rats'. These are adult male rats, born of females that were injected intraperitoneally with busulfan (10 mg/kg body weight), on the 13th day of pregnancy (Bustos-Obregón, 1984).

The G_1-specific spermatogonial chalone (both in rat and mouse) shares the general properties of chalones and its biological effect can be demonstrated *in vivo* and *in vitro* in young or postirradiated animals. The generative compartment of the spermatogenic series, by either type A_0 or the whole type A population of spermatogonia, is the target for the chalone, whereas the differentiated cells that produce the mitotic regulator range from primary spermatocytes to round spermatids (Bustos-Obregón, 1986).

There is a clear correlation between the activity of the spermatogonial chalone and the population of germ cells present in the seminiferous tubules of immature (non-irradiated) rats. Thus, no chalone activity is found in testicular extract (T.E.)* of 15-day-old rats, whereas the I.F. for testicular extracts of 20-, 25- and 40-day-old rats is 0.21, 0.26 and 0.40, respectively (Thumann and Bustos-Obregón, 1982).

The chalone receptor site may be demonstrable *in vitro* on seminiferous tubules of 20- and 25-day-old rats (I.F. values of 0.18 and 0.42). No chalone activity is apparent in extracts from non-irradiated animals by the time they are 40 days old, when the spermatogenic cell line is qualitatively (though not numerically) complete in the rat.

* Testicular extract was prepared by homogenizing testis without the tunica albuginea in 1.5 times the testicular volume of phosphate saline buffer, pH 7.2 at 4°C in a motor-driven Potter-Elvejhem at 2000 r.p.m. for 2 minutes. The homogenate was then centrifuged at 4°C for 10 minutes at 2500 g; the supernatant fluid was centrifuged at 20 000 g for another 10 minutes and finally for 2 hours at 105 000 g. The final supernatant was treated with activated charcoal, thus producing a steroid-free T.E. that was lyophilyzed and stored at −20°C until use.

Table 1. *Concentrations of cAMP in rat seminiferous tubules (ST) or testicular extracts (T.E.)*

Groups	Concentration of cAMP (x 10^{-7}mol/l)
1. ST of normal rats	11.9
2. ST of irradiated rats (IR)	1.4
3. ST of IR + BSA (control)	1.2
4. ST of IR + T.E.	4.9
5. T.E.	not detectable

Table 2. *Inhibition of uptake of [^3H]-thymidine by seminiferous tubules of irradiated rats elicited by dibutyryl-cAMP (dib-cAMP)*

Group	cpm/mg DNA (x + SD)	I.F.[a]	n	P
Control (BSA)	18.024 ± 1.629	—	4	—
Testicular extract	9.271 ± 1.392	0.49	5	⟨0.001
Theophyline (2 mmol/l)	13.203 ± 1.548	0.27	5	⟨0.001
dib-cAMP 10^{-6}mol/l + theoph. (2 mmol/l)	9.739 ± 1.383	0.46	5	⟨0.001
dib-cAMP 10^{-4} mol/l + theoph. (2 mmol/l)	8.162 ± 0.743	0.55	5	⟨0.001
dib-cAMP 10^{-2}mol/l + theoph. (2 mmol/l)	7.626 ± 1.199	0.58	5	⟨0.001

[a]IF is the ratio of the proportional reductions in uptake of [^{3}H]-thymidine (into testicular DNA) to the protein content of the sample.

Cell biology of the G_1-specific spermatogonial chalone

The chalone receptor described by Iversen (1969) could well be adenylate cyclase on the target cell membranes and, hence, an increase in intracellular cyclic AMP would be expected. In order to explore this possibility in our model, seminiferous tubules of rats irradiated to the scrotum with 300 r, 11 days before sacrifice, were incubated either in the presence of bovine serum albumin (control), testicular extract (T.E.) or different concentrations of dibutyryl cAMP. In addition, levels of cAMP were determined in control and chalone-treated seminiferous tubules (Tables 1 and 2).

It was found that incubation with T.E. raised the levels of cAMP as compared to those in the control seminiferous tubules (of irradiated rats). The latter have a low level of cAMP when compared to the seminiferous tubules of non-irradiated rats, thus accounting for the inverse relationship between levels of cAMP in tissues and their mitotic activity. Addition of dibutyryl cAMP restores the controlled growth of cells (Teel, 1972). As seen in Table 2, addition of T.E. elicits an I.F. of 40% and addition of dibutyryl-cAMP results in an I.F.

of up to 55%. These observations strongly support the view that cAMP is the second intracellular messenger involved in the effect of the spermatogonial chalone. Attallah (1976) proposed that chalones may contain two active sites, one site being specific for the cell membrane and the other site being non-specific and involved in stimulation of adenyl cyclase activity. Chalones would maintain high levels of cAMP which, in turn, would inhibit the nucleoside kinase activity necessary for DNA synthesis.

In keeping with their role in the regulation of growth of tissues, chalones exert an inhibitory effect upon the proliferation of cells in embryonic tissues, thus limiting the expansion of tissue. Extracts of adult tissues do affect the growth of their ancestral lines in the embryo (Bishoff, 1964; Philpott, 1971). Chopra and Simnett (1971) demonstrated that kidney extracts from adult rats inhibit proliferation of cells of the larval kidney (pronephros) of *Xenopus laevis*. Moreover, an antiserum prepared against such an extract is able to stimulate the proliferation of cells in the same system, thereby demonstrating the existence of a chalone in the embryonic tissue. The action of this chalone can be neutralized by addition of the specific antiserum (Chopra and Simnett, 1971).

Neutralization of the chalone activity by an antiserum raised against mouse T.E. in rabbits was studied. The neutralization curve of the chalone activity has a parabolic shape, very similar to the normal curves of immunoprecipitation. The extremes of the curves (excess of antigens and antibodies) correspond to the soluble complexes. Our results imply that, when T.E. is neutralized with an excess of antiserum (soluble complexes), the chalone activity is not impaired. In the zone of equivalence, a marked inhibition of chalone activity was observed. This result suggests that the antibodies that neutralize the chalone activity are not directed against the active center of the chalone molecule. Furthermore, these results are in agreement with the observation that the biological activity of the spermatogonial chalone shows no species specificity. Therefore, it is conceivable that its active site does not possess strong immunogenic properties (Castellon *et al.*, 1986).

Kinetics of the seminiferous epithelium and chalone effect

Because of the apparent relative lack of immunogenic properties of the spermatogonial chalone, it was possible to estimate the biological, active half-life (*in vivo*) of the mouse G_1-specific spermatogonial chalone. The experiments were done by intraperitoneal injection of the chalone and the apparent half-life was 16 hours.

Iversen (1981), in a review on chalones, suggested that the inhibitory effects of the chalones on spermatogonial proliferation make them good candidates for use as male-specific antifertility agents.

Long-term administration of T.E. to mice *in vivo* did not, however, elicit a value of I.F. greater than 0.47, even though the treatment extended over four cycles of the seminiferous epithelium (approximately 32 days), i.e. a full spermatogonic period in these species.

In the same series of experiments, it was shown by radioautographic analysis that the rate of evolution of the different series of spermatogenic cells in the mouse was not affected by prolonged administration of chalone *in vivo* (Bustos-Obregón, 1986). These observations imply that the effect of the chalone is non-cytotoxic and that the germ cell fraction that is allowed to enter G_1 can proceed normally through spermatogenesis.

In conclusion, spermatogonial chalones probably do not have a future as male contraceptives, but because of their physiological effects on the proliferative regulation of germ cells they enhance our understanding of the mechanisms of normal and pathological multiplication of spermatogonia.

Acknowledgements

Thanks are due to Mr E. Castellon for scientific criticism and to Mrs M.L. Chacon for typing the manuscript. Parts of the work reported here were supported by Fondecyt and by D.T.I. (University of Chile).

References

Attallah, A.M. (1976). Regulation of cell growth *in vitro* and *in vivo*: point/counter point. In: Houch, J.C., ed. **Chalones**, Amsterdam, North Holland, p.176.

Bishoff, W.H. (1964). Inhibition of mitosis by homologous tissue extracts. **Journal of Cell Biology** 23:10A.

Bustos-Obregón, E. (1984). Tissue chalones, with special reference to the spermatogonial chalones. In: McKerns, K.W., Aakvaaz, A.& Hansson, V., eds. **Regulation of Target Cell Responsiveness**, New York, Plenum, pp.403–432.

Bustos-Obregón, E. (1986) Spermatogonial proliferation: role of the chalones. In: Paulson, J.D., Negro-Vilar, A., Lucena, E. & Martini, L., eds. **Andrology Male Fertility and Sterility**, New York, Academic Press, pp.293 311.

Castellon, E., Arenas, P., Balbontin, J. & Bustos-Obregón, E. (1986). Propiedades inmunogenicas de la chalona espermatogonial G_1. **Tenth Meeting of ALIRH**, Vina del Mar, R20.

Chopra, D.P. & Simmett, I.D. (1971). Stimulation of cell division in larval kidney (*Xenopus laevis*) by kidney antiserum. **Experimental Cell Research** 64:396–402.

Clermont, Y. & Mauger, A. (1974). Existence of a spermatogonial chalone in the rat testis. **Cell and Tissue Kinetics** 7:165–172.

Clermont, Y. & Mauger, A. (1976). Effect of a spermatogonial chalone on the growing rat testis. **Cell and Tissue Kinetics** 9:99–104.

Finkler, N. & Acker, P. (1978). Chalones: a mini-review. **The Mount Sinai Journal of Medicine** 45:258–264.

Fremuth, F. (1984). Chalones and specific growth factors in normal and tumor growth. **Acta Universitatis Carolinae Medica Monographia CX**, Univerzita Karlova, Praha, Czechoslovakia, pp.111.

Irons, M. & Clermont, Y. (1979). Spermatogonial chalone (S): effect on the phases of the cell cycle of type A spermatogonia in the rat. **Cell and Tissue Kinetics** 12:425–433.

Iversen, O.H. (1969). Chalones of the skin. Homeostatic regulation. In: Wolstenholme, R. & Knight, J., eds. **CIBA Foundation Symposium**, London, J & A Churchill, pp.29–56.

Iversen, O.H. (1981). The chalones. **Handbook of Experimental Pharmacology** 57:491–550.

Philpott, G.W. (1971). Tissue-specific inhibition of cell proliferation in embryonic stomach epithelium *in vitro*. **Gastroenterology** 61:25.

Teel, R.W. (1972). Inhibition of DNA synthesis in hamster cheek pouch tissue in organ culture by dibutyryl cyclic AMP and a homologous extract. **Biochemical and Biophysical Research Communications** 47:1010–1014.

Thumann, A. & Bustos-Obregón, E. (1978). An *in vitro* system for the study of rat spermatogonial proliferative control. **Andrologia** 10:22–25.

Thumann, A. & Bustos-Obregón, E. (1982). *In vitro* assay of rat spermatogonial chalone in prepubertal seminiferous tubules. **Andrologia** 14:35–42.

Thumann, A., Carboni, R. & Bustos-Obregón, E. (1981). *In vitro* characterization of rat G1 spermatogonial chalone. **Andrologia** 13:583–589.

Cellular function of proto-oncogenes

GEOFFREY M. COOPER

Dana-Farber Cancer Institute and Department of Pathology, Harvard Medical School, Boston, MA 02115, USA.

Keywords

Proto-oncogenes, spermatogenesis, oocyte maturation, c-*mos*, c-*raf*.

Oncogenes and proto-oncogenes

Oncogenes were first identified as specific genes of retroviruses that induce neoplastic transformation of virus-infected cells. Subsequently, cellular oncogenes were identified by three approaches: (1) as homologs of retroviral oncogenes; (2) as genes that induce transformation upon transfection of cultured cells; and (3) as genes that are frequently altered in neoplasms by rearrangement or amplification of DNA. Together, these approaches have identified over 60 cellular genes which, as activated oncogenes, can induce at least some aspects of neoplastic transformation. The oncogenes which have been characterized so far encode proteins that can be divided into five functional groups: growth factors; plasma membrane proteins with tyrosine kinase activity; plasma membrane guanine nucleotide-binding proteins; cytoplasmic proteins associated with serine/threonine kinase activity; and nuclear proteins. It is generally believed that these proteins function as signal-transducing regulatory molecules, the activities of which can lead to the proliferation of cells.

Oncogenes are formed from normal cellular genes as a consequence of mutations or rearrangements of DNA which result either in abnormal gene expression or in the synthesis of structurally (and functionally) altered proteins. The ability of activated oncogenes to induce cell transformation suggests that their progenitors in normal cells (proto-oncogenes) function as regulators of the growth and differentiation of normal cells. The notion that proto-oncogenes play important roles in normal cell physiology is supported by the evolutionary conservation of these genes throughout vertebrates and, in some cases, in insects and yeast. The normal cellular role of some proto-oncogenes has been revealed by DNA sequence analysis. Thus, the *sis*, *erbB*, *fms*, *erbA*, *jun* and *fos* oncogenes are derived from genes encoding platelet-derived growth factor, epidermal growth factor receptor, macrophage colony-stimulating factor receptor, thyroid hormone receptor, and transcription factor AP-1 (both *jun* and *fos*), respectively. However, the normal physiological roles of other proto-oncogenes remain unknown.

While some proto-oncogenes are expressed in many types of proliferating cells, others display more restricted patterns of expression, suggesting that they function in specific developmental pathways. For example, the *src* and *ras* proto-oncogenes are expressed at high levels in terminally differentiated neurons and can induce neuronal differentiation of PC12 pheochromocytoma cells in culture, suggesting the possibility that these genes may normally function in neuronal differentiation. Analysis of the normal cell function of proto-oncogenes may, thus, provide an approach to the identification of genes involved in the regulation of developmental processes, as well as in cell growth.

Expression of proto-oncogenes in spermatogenesis

Analysis of gene expression within defined populations of normal cells may allow us to identify genes involved in specific stages of differentiation. The development of male germ cells in the testis provides a system which is particularly well suited for analysis of gene expression within a cell lineage, since cell types can be isolated that represent a spectrum of developmental stages ranging from mitotically proliferating stem cells to mature spermatozoa (Bellvé, 1979). At birth, the male germ cells are represented by the primitive type A spermatogonia which differentiate into the renewing stem cell population of type A spermatogonia. In the mouse, type A spermatogonia undergo four mitotic divisions and differentiate into intermediate and type B spermatogonia. The type B spermatogonia divide once and then enter the prophase of meiosis as preleptotene spermatocytes. Spermatocyte development continues through the leptotene, zygotene and pachytene stages of meiotic prophase, which is followed by two rapid cell divisions that result in the formation of round spermatids, the earliest haploid postmeiotic cells. Differentiation from the round spermatid to the mature spermatozoa then occurs over a 2-week period.

Stage-specific transcription of a number of genes during spermatogenesis has been described principally in pachytene spermatocytes and postmeiotic round spermatids (Hecht, 1986). Earlier studies have also described specific patterns of transcription of four proto-oncogenes in the development of germ cells. The c-*abl* tyrosine kinase proto-oncogene is transcribed as a 4.7-kb RNA in postmeiotic spermatids, whereas transcripts of higher molecular weight are found in a variety of somatic cell types (Ponzetto and Wolgemuth, 1985). The *pim*-1 proto-oncogene, a member of the serine/threonine kinase family, is also transcribed in postmeiotic spermatids as an RNA of 2.4-kb in contrast to the 2.8-kb *pim*-1 transcripts detected in somatic tissues (Sorrentino *et al.*, 1988). The c-*mos* proto-oncogene, another serine/threonine kinase, is expressed most abundantly in male and female germ cells, as a 1.7-kb RNA in round spermatids and as a 1.4-kb RNA in oocytes (Goldman *et al.*, 1987; Mutter and Wolgemuth, 1987; Propst *et al.*, 1987). Transcription of the *int*-1 proto-oncogene has been exclusively detected in postmeiotic male germ cells and in the neural tube of the developing mouse embryo (Wilkinson *et al.*, 1987;

Shackleford and Varmus, 1987). Since these findings suggest the possible function of several proto-oncogenes in the latter stages of spermatogenesis, we undertook a comprehensive analysis of the expression of a series of proto-oncogenes representative of different functional classes in each of the spermatogenic cell types that can be isolated in sufficient quantities for biochemical studies.

We initially examined expression of c-*raf*, since this is the major serine/threonine kinase proto-oncogene in addition to c-*mos*. Transcription of the c-*raf* proto-oncogene was detected in both type A and B spermatogonia and throughout meiotic prophase, with some increase in levels of the transcript in adult pachytene spermatocytes. The c-*raf* transcript was also detected in round spermatids but was no longer present in residual bodies. Thus, c-*raf*, in contrast to c-*mos*, is expressed throughout almost the entire spermatogenic cell lineage (Wolfes *et al*., 1989).

The *ras* gene family consists of three members (*ras*H, *ras*K and *ras*N) that encode plasma membrane guanine nucleotide-binding proteins. The c-*ras*H transcript was detected in mitotically proliferating spermatogonia, in spermatocytes throughout the prophase of meiosis, and postmeiotically in both round spermatids and residual bodies. Thus, c-*ras*H appears to be transcribed throughout spermatogenesis and the RNA is present through the terminal differentiation of postmeiotic spermatids to mature spermatozoa (Wolfes *et al*., 1989). c-*ras*K RNA was also detected in spermatogonia and in spermatocytes at meiotic prophase. However, levels of c-*ras*K RNA were significantly reduced in round spermatids and this RNA was undetectable in residual bodies, indicating that the transcription and/or stability of c-*ras*K RNA is reduced in postmeiotic cells (Wolfes *et al*., 1989). A 5.0-kb transcript of c-*ras*N was present in all cell types studied, including residual bodies. However, three additional transcripts of 1.4, 1.9 and 3.5 kb were specifically detected at meiotic prophase and during postmeiotic stages of germ cell development (Wolfes *et al*., 1989). Although the significance of the different sizes of transcripts of c-*ras*N is unclear, these results indicate that all three c-*ras* proto-oncogenes, like c-*raf*, are expressed throughout most of spermatogenesis.

In contrast to the continuous expression of c-*ras* and c-*raf* proto-oncogenes, three nuclear proto-oncogenes, c-*myc*, c-*fos* and c-*jun*, were found to be specifically expressed at high levels in type B spermatogonia (Wolfes *et al*., 1989). In addition, high levels of c-*myc* and c-*jun* RNAs were detected in preleptotene spermatocytes, which represent the first stage of meiotic prophase. The level of expression of these proto-oncogenes was at least tenfold lower in other types of spermatogenic cell.

The c-*jun* and c-*fos* proto-oncogenes have recently been identified as components of transcription factor AP-1 (Curran and Franza, 1988). The product of the c-*myc* gene has also been found to function as a transcriptional activator in yeast (Lech *et al*., 1988). Transcription of these nuclear proto-oncogenes is rapidly increased by stimuli that induce either proliferation or differentiation, suggesting that they may act as regulators of transcription to modulate changes in gene expression. The high level of specific transcription of these proto-oncogenes in type B spermatogonia suggests, therefore, their potential involvement in mediation of changes in gene expression at this stage of the differentiation of germ cells. Since the type B spermatogonia represent the last mitotic division of stem cells prior to entry into the prophase of meiosis, it is possible that the nuclear proto-oncogenes are involved in altering programs of gene expression at this developmental transition.

The c-*mos* proto-oncogene in oocyte maturation

The c-*mos* proto-oncogene is also specifically transcribed in mouse oocytes and c-*mos* transcripts accumulate at high levels (estimated to be of the order of 100 000 copies per cell) in fully grown oocytes arrested at the diplotene stage of meiotic prophase (Goldman *et al.*, 1987; Mutter and Wolgemuth, 1987). Since most normal types of cell studied have been negative for transcription of c-*mos*, these results suggest a specific role for the c-*mos* proto-oncogene in male and female germ cells. In particular, the accumulation of c-*mos* RNA in oocytes suggests potential roles for this proto-oncogene as a maternal message.

To begin to define the function of the c-*mos* RNA that accumulates in mouse oocytes, we investigated its stability and polyadenylation during oocyte maturation, fertilization and early cleavage (Goldman *et al.*, 1988). Our results indicate that c-*mos* RNA is retained in mature ovulated eggs and zygotes but is degraded at the two-cell embryo stage, consistent with the fate of the bulk of maternal RNA in the mouse. In addition, c-*mos* RNA was found to be post-transcriptionally polyadenylated in concert with oocyte maturation. These results suggest that c-*mos* functions as a maternal mRNA which is probably translated during oocyte maturation or fertilization and which may, therefore, play a role in these or other early developmental processes.

The predicted product of the c-*mos* proto-oncogene is a protein of approximately 37 kDa which is a member of the serine/threonine protein kinase family. A number of proteins are specifically modified by phosphorylation in ovulated and fertilized eggs and phosphorylation of proteins is thought to play a regulatory role in meiosis and early cleavages. It is tempting, therefore, to consider the hypothesis that c-*mos* encodes a regulatory kinase that functions in these early developmental events.

In order to investigate the possible role of c-*mos* during oocyte maturation, we injected murine oocytes with c-*mos* antisense oligonucleotides to degrade maternal c-*mos* RNA (O'Keefe *et al.*, 1989). Such injections of antisense material induced two specific abnormalities: (1) decondensation of metaphase chromosomes and reformation of a nucleus within the body of the egg, 2–3 hours after extrusion of the first polar body; and (2) subsequent cleavage to two cells. Thus, the loss of c-*mos* function in the maturing mouse oocyte prevents meiosis II and leads to decondensation of chromosomes, formation of the nuclear membrane, and oocyte cleavage after completion of the first meiotic division. Therefore, it appears that the c-*mos* proto-oncogene functions as a maternal message required for normal meiotic maturation. Since the phenotypes produced by loss of c-*mos* are similar to those produced by loss of maturation promoting factor (MPF) (Clarke *et al.*, 1988), we are currently investigating the possibility that c-*mos* is involved in the regulation of MPF activity.

References

Bellvé, A.R. (1979). The molecular biology of mammalian spermatogenesis. In: Finn, C.A., ed. **Oxford Reviews of Reproductive Biology**, London, Oxford Press, pp.159–261.

Clarke, H.J., Rossant, J. & Masui, Y. (1988). Suppression of chromosome condensation during meiotic maturation induces parthenogenetic development of mouse oocytes. **Development** 104:97–103.

Curran, T. & Franza, B.R. (1988). Fos and Jun: the AP-1 connection. **Cell** 55:395–397.

Goldman, D.S., Kiessling, A.A. & Cooper, G.M. (1988). Post-transcriptional processing suggests that c-*mos* functions as a maternal message in mouse eggs. **Oncogene** 3:159–162.

Goldman, D.S., Kiessling, A.A., Millette, C.F. & Cooper, G.M. (1987). Expression of c-*mos* RNA in germ cells of male and female mice. **Proceedings of the National Academy of Sciences, USA** 84:4509–4513.

Hecht, N.B. (1986). Regulation of gene expression during mammalian spermatogenesis. In: Rossant, J. & Pederson, R., eds. **Experimental Approaches of Mammalian Embryonic Development**, New York, Cambridge University Press, pp.151–193.

Lech, K., Anderson, K. & Brent, R. (1988). DNA-bound Fos proteins activate transcription in yeast. **Cell** 52:179–184.

Mutter, G.L. & Wolgemuth, D.J. (1987). Distinct developmental patterns of c-*mos* proto-oncogene expression in female and male mouse germ cells. **Proceedings of the National Academy of Sciences, USA** 84:5301–5305.

O'Keefe, S., Wolfes, H., Kiessling, A.A. & Cooper, G.M. (1989). Microinjection of anti-sense c-*mos* oligonucleotides prevents meiosis II in the maturing mouse egg. **Proceedings of the National Academy of Sciences, USA** 86:7038–7042.

Ponzetto, C. & Wolgemuth, D.J. (1985). Haploid expression of a unique c-*abl* transcript in the mouse male germ line. **Molecular Cellular Biology** 5:1791–1794.

Propst, F., Rosenberg, M.P., Iyer, A., Kaul, K. & VandeWoude, G.F. (1987). c-*mos* proto-oncogene RNA transcripts in mouse tissues: structural features, developmental regulation, and localization in specific cell types. **Molecular and Cellular Biology** 7:1629–1637.

Shackleford, G.M. & Varmus, H.E. (1987). Expression of the proto-oncogene *int*-1 is restricted to postmeiotic male germ cells and the neural tube of mid-gestational embryos. **Cell** 50:89–95.

Sorrentino, V., McKinney, M.D., Giorgi, M., Geremia, R. & Fleissner, E. (1988). Expression of cellular proto-oncogenes in the mouse male germ line: a distinctive

2.4-kilobase *pim*-1 transcript is expressed in haploid postmeiotic cells. **Proceedings of the National Academy of Sciences, USA** 85:2191–2195.

Wilkinson, D.G., Bailes, J.A. & McMahon, A.P. (1987). Expression of the proto-oncogene *int*-1 is restricted to specific neural cells in the developing mouse embryo. **Cell** 50:79–88.

Wolfes, H., Kogawa, K., Millette, C.F. & Cooper, G.M. (1989). Proto-oncogene expression in spermatogenesis: specific expression of nuclear proto-oncogenes prior to entry into meiotic prophase. **Science** 245:740–743.

Characteristics of the expression of the c-*abl* and c-*mos* proto-oncogenes in mouse germ cells

A. G. WADEWITZ[1] AND D.J. WOLGEMUTH[1,2]

[1]*Center for Reproductive Sciences and* [2]*Department of Genetics and Development, College of Physicians and Surgeons, Columbia University, New York, NY 10032, USA.*

Keywords

c-*abl*, c-*mos*, germ cell differentiation, oocyte, protein kinase (tyrosine specific), early spermatids, haploid spermatogenic cells.

Introduction

A molecular biological approach to the elucidation of the genetic control of development involves the identification of genes that are expressed in a tissue-specific or cell type-specific manner. Specificity of expression of a gene is regarded as a strong indication that the gene plays a role in determining the phenotype or function of the cells in which it is expressed. Our previous observations of the specific expression in haploid spermatogenic cells of high levels of uniquely sized c-*abl* and c-*mos* transcripts suggested, thus, that these genes may be important for spermiogenic differentiation or subsequent function of male gametes. The presence of high levels of a uniquely sized c-*mos* transcript in mouse oocytes further suggested a possible role for this proto-oncogene in oocyte maturation or early embryogenesis.

The fact that c-*abl* and c-*mos* are proto-oncogenes is of interest at several levels, especially given the potential role of proto-oncogenes in the regulation of the growth and differentiation of cells in a wide variety of systems. A role for these proto-oncogenes in growth control has been directly implicated by the observations that c-*erb*B corresponds to a region of the gene that encodes the epidermal growth factor (Downward *et al.*, 1984) and that c-*sis* codes for one of the two polypeptide chains of platelet-derived growth factor (Doolittle *et al.*, 1983; Waterfield *et al.*, 1983). c-*fms* has been shown to correspond to the receptor for macrophage colony-stimulating factor (Sherr *et al.*, 1985).

Several proto-oncogenes have been examined for their expression during mammalian development (reviewed by Adamson, 1987). Although distinct patterns of expression have been described in various developing germ layers, tissues, organs, etc., the data are insufficient for us to hypothesize about their specific roles in development. It is clear, however, that virtually all proto-oncogenes examined are expressed during cellular differentiation as well as during proliferation. A striking example of this potential diversity of function is exhibited by c-*src*, for which roles in proliferation, commitment, and expression of a differentiated (neuronal) phenotype have been postulated (Adamson, 1987).

Several proto-oncogenes have been associated with protein kinase activity (Bishop, 1983). Protein phosphorylation is believed to play a major role in the mechanisms by which cells receive and interpret extracellular signals, as well as being critical for normal cellular metabolism. The potential protein kinase activity of the products of c-*abl* and c-*mos* and their pattern of expression in germ cells suggest that these genes could be important in such functions as the metabolic activities of spermatogenic cells and/or in the initiation of meiotic and mitotic events in the oocyte and postfertilization embryo.

This chapter provides a brief summary of our current knowledge of the properties of the products of the c-*abl* and c-*mos* genes and the pattern of their expression in the male and female germ lines, together with some additional observations on the protein product of c-*abl*. In summarizing the observations on the c-*abl* and c-*mos* from our laboratory and from those of other investigators, we offer some suggestions as to the potential function of these genes in mammalian gametogenesis and embryogenesis.

Materials and methods

Analysis of c-abl *protein*

Testes were dissected from Swiss Webster mice, either sexually mature (more than 6 weeks old), or prepuberal (day 12–13 of postnatal development). Suspensions of testicular cells were obtained by mechanical disruption of the seminiferous tubules between the frosted surfaces of two microscope slides. Enzymatic treatment with collagenase or trypsin (Wolgemuth *et al.*, 1985) was avoided to minimize potential proteolysis of c-*abl* proteins.

Immunoprecipitates of the c-*abl* protein were obtained by use of previously described *abl*-specific antisera (Konopka *et al.*, 1984; Ponzetto *et al.*, 1989). The procedures used for extraction of cells, immunoprecipitation, and autophosphorylation *in vitro* were performed essentially as described by Konopka and Witte (1985) and modified by Ponzetto *et al.* (1989). In control immunoprecipitations, non-immune or pre-immune sera were used. In some experiments the Triton X-100 used in the kinase lysis buffer was replaced by CHAPS (3-[(3-cholamido-propyl)-dimethylammonio]-1-propanesulfonate).

SDS polyacrylamide gel electrophoresis (SDS-PAGE) was performed as described previously (Ponzetto *et al.*, 1989). Two-dimensional gel electrophoresis was performed according to the method of O'Farrell (1975). Isoelectric focusing gels contained 1.6% pH 5–7 and 0.4% pH 3.5–10 ampholines and were run for a total of 7000 volt-hours. The second dimension was run on 8% SDS-PAGE. Isoelectric points were estimated from results of co-electrophoresis of standards of known molecular weights and pI values.

Gels were treated with 1 mol/l KOH for 1.5 hours at 55°C to select for phosphotyrosine-containing proteins (Yonemoto *et al.*, 1987). Phosphoamino acids were analyzed by the procedure of Cooper *et al.* (1983). Proteins phosphorylated in the kinase assay *in vitro* were electroeluted from gel slices in 5 mmol/l Tris, pH 8.45, 38 mmol/l glycine, 0.01% SDS with 10 μg bovine serum albumin as carrier. The eluted proteins were dried under vacuum, resuspended in 0.1 ml 5.7 N HCl and hydrolyzed at 110°C for 1 hour. The hydrolyzed samples were dried under vacuum and mixed with unlabeled phosphoamino acid markers. Two-dimensional thin-layer electrophoresis on cellulose plates was first carried out in pH 1.9 buffer (50:156:1794, 88% formic acid:glacial acetic acid:H_2O) at 500 V for 1 hour. This step was followed by electrophoresis in pH 3.5 buffer (10:100:1890, pyridine:glacial acetic acid:H_2O) at 500 V for 25 minutes. Phosphoamino acid markers were located by staining of the cellulose with ninhydrin.

Results and discussion

*Expression of the c-***abl** *gene*

c-*abl* is the cellular homolog of the transforming region of the Abelson murine leukemia virus. It is present as a single-copy gene in the mouse (Wang *et al.*, 1984) and human (Heisterkamp *et al.*, 1983) genomes. The gene is expressed at low levels in all tissues and cell lines examined (e.g. Wang and Baltimore, 1983), and it is transcribed as mRNAs of approximately 6 kb and 8 kb. An interesting exception to this pattern is observed in the adult mouse testis, where high levels of a 4.7-kb transcript are found (Muller *et al.*, 1982). We have shown that the pattern of expression of this novel transcript is developmentally regulated and restricted to postmeiotic germ cells (Ponzetto and Wolgemuth, 1985). The haploid-specific expression of c-*abl* has been confirmed by several laboratories (Propst *et al.*, 1987; Shackelford and Varmus, 1987; Goldman *et al.*, 1987).

c-*abl* is a complex gene, spanning >100 kb and yielding at least five distinct mRNAs, as determined by molecular cloning and Northern blot hybridization analysis. We and others have shown that the testicular transcript differs from the somatic transcripts at the 3' end, lacking about 1 kb of the 3' untranslated sequences found in the somatic transcripts (Duggal *et al.*, 1987; Oppi *et al.*, 1987; Meijer *et al.*, 1987). cDNA cloning has provided evidence for the existence of four different classes of c-*abl* mRNAs (types I to IV), based on sequences at their 5' ends (Ben-Neriah *et al.*, 1986; Meijer *et al.*, 1987; Oppi *et al.*, 1987). The different 5' ends are formed by the splicing of alternative 5' exons onto a common second exon. Types II and IV contain additional 5' untranslated regions which account for the larger transcripts observed. Type I mRNAs appear to represent the shorter somatic transcripts. The 4.7-kb testicular transcript has been reported to contain the same 5' sequences as the type I mRNA (Oppi *et al.*, 1987; Meijer *et al.*, 1987). The predicted amino acid sequence obtained from cloning studies (Oppi *et al.*, 1987; Meijer *et al.*, 1987), from analysis of *in-vitro* translation (Meijer *et al.*, 1987), as well as from our studies on testicular c-*abl* proteins (Ponzetto *et al.*, 1989), indicate that the 4.7-kb testicular c-*abl* mRNA would produce a c-*abl* protein indistinguishable from the c-*abl* protein produced from the somatic, type I c-*abl* mRNA on one-dimensional electrophoresis.

The predicted amino acid sequences corresponding to the various c-*abl* mRNAs would yield proteins that differ by only 26 to 45 amino acids at the amino termini. There are no specific features of the predicted amino terminal sequences that suggest any potential known function. For example, none of the amino termini contains obvious transmembrane domains or leader sequences. However, the different amino termini can be divided into two general classes, called A and B in our discussion. The class A proteins are represented by the type I, II, and III cDNAs and are proteins with amino termini characteristic of location in the cytosol as opposed to the membrane. The type I sequence is hydrophilic, suggesting that such proteins would be present in the soluble pool in cell-fractionation experiments (Ben-Neriah *et al.*, 1986; Witte, 1986). Type II proteins are more hydrophobic and could be membrane associated or involved in protein–protein interactions (Witte, 1986). The class B proteins (type IV transcripts), however, would contain an N-terminal glycine, in the sequence met-gly-gln. This sequence serves as an acceptor site for myristylation of gag-*abl* (Schultz and Oroszolan, 1984) and *src* (Buss and Sefton, 1985) proteins. Such a hydrophobic modification may be important for localization to the plasma membrane (Sefton, 1986). It is not known whether both class A and class B proteins are present in testicular cells nor is it known whether any of the testicular c-*abl* proteins contain such modifications.

*Studies on testicular c-*abl *proteins*

Recent experiments in our laboratory, using immunoprecipitation and a kinase assay *in vitro* to detect the presence of c-*abl* proteins, revealed the presence of c-*abl* proteins (P150) in mouse testicular tissue and in spermatogenic cells (Fig. 1, lanes 1 and 2). In addition, a protein exhibiting a relative molecular weight of approximately 74 kD (P74) was labeled. This P74 phosphoprotein was not observed in control lines of cells (Ponzetto *et al.*, 1989).

We found that the recovery of P74 protein was variable and depended most critically on whether one or two cycles of immunoprecipitation were used. If the products of the assay of phosphorylation *in vitro* were analyzed by SDS-PAGE after the first immunoprecipitation, P74 was found to be present at levels higher than those of P150. A second immunoprecipitation with an *abl*-specific antibody, after the first immune complex was dissociated at 95°C with SDS and mercaptoethanol, resulted in the recovery once again of P150 but in the almost complete loss of P74 (Fig. 1, lanes 3 and 4). This result suggested that the P74 protein was probably co-precipitated by the *abl*-specific

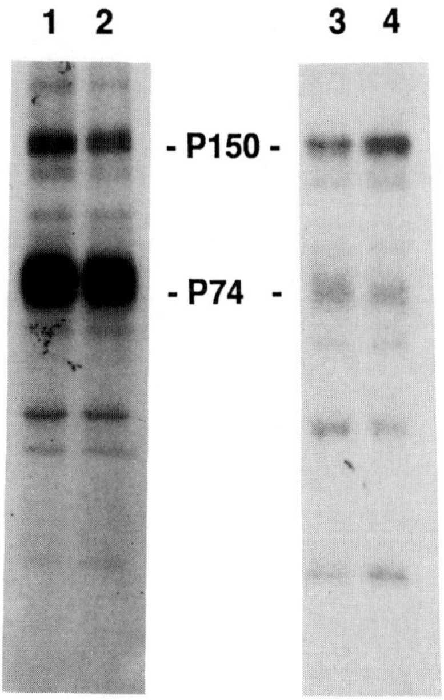

Fig. 1 In-vitro phosphorylation of c-*abl* proteins. Mouse testis cells were lysed in kinase lysis buffer that contained Triton X-100 and immunoprecipitated with the *abl*-specific antibody apEX-4, as described by Ponzetto *et al.* (1989). The immunoprecipitate was subjected to phosphorylation *in vitro* and the products were fractionated by SDS-PAGE on 8% gels (lanes 1 and 2). Alternatively, the labelled immunoprecipitated products were diluted, after denaturation with SDS and mercaptoethanol, and re-precipitated with the same *abl*-specific antibody (lanes 3 and 4). Control immunoprecipitates obtained with pre-immune rabbit serum were negative for P150 and P74 and are not shown.

antibodies by virtue of its close association with P150 in the cellular lysate, and that P74 was not precipitated as a result of recognition by the *abl*-specific antibodies. After denaturation, P74 was apparently no longer associated with P150.

Since the expression of testicular transcripts of c-*abl* has been shown to be developmentally regulated, we examined whether P150 and P74 are found in immunoprecipitates of testes from animals at different developmental stages. The assay of kinase activity *in vitro* was conducted on immunoprecipitates, with *abl*-specific antisera, of extracts from cells from mature and immature mice. The results revealed that P150 is present in lysates from testicular cells from both immature and mature testes, whereas the P74 protein is present at detectable levels only in extracts of mature testes (Ponzetto *et al.*, 1989).

We next examined whether P150 and P74 were present in spermatogenic

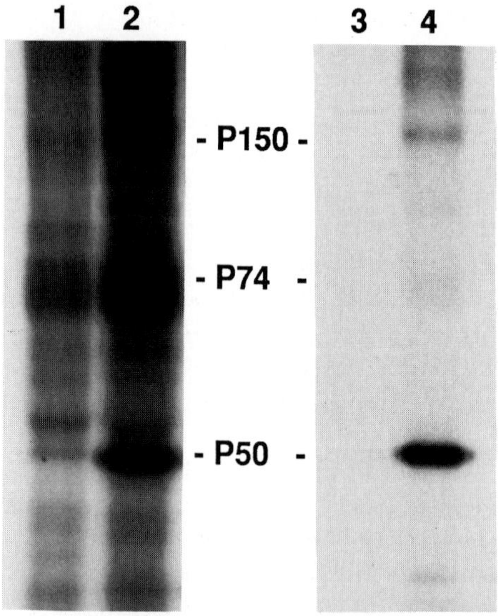

Fig. 2 Effect of substitution of CHAPS for Triton X-100 during immunoprecipitation. The phosphorylation assay was done essentially as described in the text except that the zwitterionic detergent CHAPS was substituted for the Triton X-100 that is normally used. Lanes 1 and 3: lysate of adult mouse testis immunoprecipitated with pre-immune rabbit serum; lanes 2 and 4: lysate of adult mouse testis immunoprecipitated with apEX-4. Lanes 1 and 2: single immunoprecipitation; lanes 3 and 4: double immunoprecipitation. The substitution of CHAPS results in the co-precipitation of a 50-kD phosphoprotein previously found at much lower levels.

cells. Enriched populations of haploid spermatids and of elongating spermatids and residual bodies were obtained and used in the kinase assay. P150 was found to be present in all spermatogenic cells, whereas P74 was observed only in postmeiotic cells (Ponzetto *et al.*, 1989).

Some of our immunoprecipitations were performed in the presence of CHAPS detergent, since it has been reported to be capable of solubilizing functional opiate receptors from brain membranes (Simonds *et al.*, 1980). The phosphorylation was performed as described previously except that CHAPS was substituted for the normally used Triton X-100. After a single immunoprecipitation with *abl*-specific antisera, prominent phosphoproteins included P150, P74 and a 50-kD species not seen in the control in which pre-immune serum was used (Fig. 2, lane 2). However, after a second immunoprecipitation, only the P150 and the 50-kD phosphoprotein (P50) were obtained (Fig. 2, lane 4). The presence of P50 in the second immunoprecipitate, after the original immunoprecipitate was completely denatured with SDS and mercaptoethanol, suggests an extremely strong association between P50 and P150, unlike the association of P74 and P150 which form a complex that does not reform after denaturation. The characteristics of the formation of the complex are unknown and the additional proteins may represent factors that modulate the activity of the kinases and/or they may be substrates.

Two-dimensional electrophoresis was used to characterize the proteins phosphorylated in the kinase assay. As seen in Figure 3a, P74 can be resolved as a complex of phosphoproteins that range in weight from approximately 68 kD to 77 kD and in isoelectric point from approximately 5.2 to 5.8. P50 forms a discrete doublet with an isoelectric point of about 5.2. P150 does not focus under these conditions.

Since the *abl* kinase is tyrosine specific, the autophosphorylated kinase, as well as possible substrates, should contain phosphotyrosine. To determine whether the phosphoproteins actually contained phosphotyrosine, the two-dimensional gels were treated with 1 mol/l KOH for 1.5 hours at 55°C. This treatment selectively hydrolyzes phosphoserine and phosphothreonine, but not phosphotyrosine, from phosphoproteins. Figure 3b shows that only some of the P74 complex contains phosphotyrosine. The P50 doublet appears unchanged, suggesting that it contains significant levels of phosphotyrosine.

To analyze directly the phosphotyrosine content of the products of the kinase assay, the respective proteins were separated on one-dimensional gels, electroeluted from gel slices, hydrolyzed and separated by two-dimensional thin-layer electrophoresis. Figure 4a shows that P150 contains predominantly phosphoserine with approximately equimolar amounts of phosphotyrosine and phosphothreonine. P50 and P74 also contain mostly phosphoserine, but significant amounts of phosphotyrosine were also detected. These results support the hypothesis that P74 and P50 may be substrates of P150. The abundance of phosphoserine is indicative of the presence of an undefined associated serine/threonine protein kinase in the autophosphorylation assay. Either of the co-precipitating phosphoproteins could be responsible for the associated serine/threonine protein kinase activity, but we have no direct evidence to support this possibility.

Recently, Pendergast *et al.* (1987) showed that treatment of NIH-3T3 cells with activators of protein kinase C (PKC) results in a four- to eight-fold increase in levels of the product of c-*abl*. Similarly, purified PKC phosphorylated all c-*abl* proteins at the same two serine residues as those phosphorylated *in vivo*. This result suggested the intriguing possibility that P74, which is similar in size to protein kinase C, may be co-precipitating PKC. This possibility is currently under investigation.

It will be of interest to correlate the presence of specific classes of c-*abl* proteins with the precise morphogenetic changes that occur during spermatogenesis. In particular, it will be critical to determine if c-*abl* proteins are present

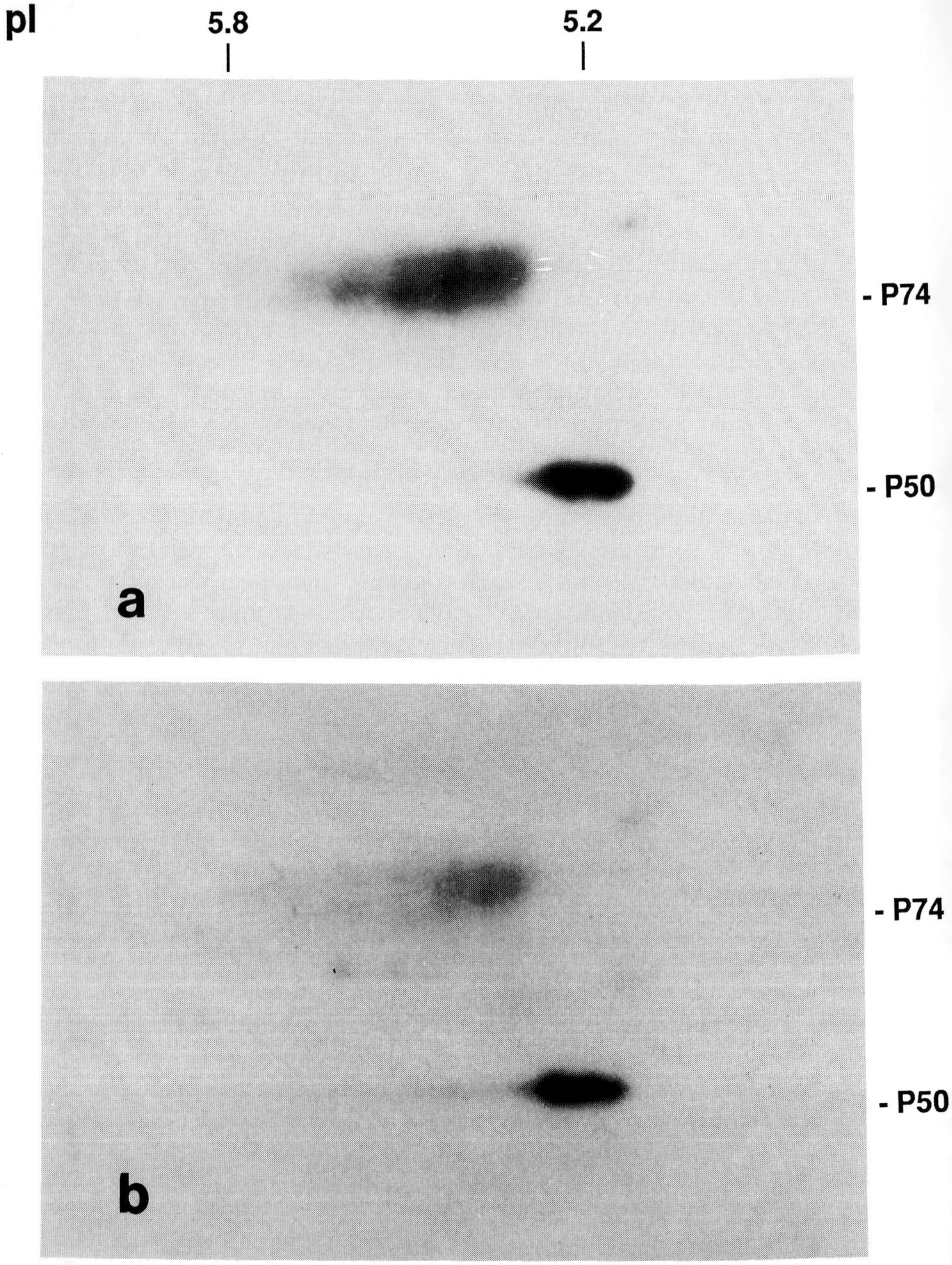

Fig. 3 Two-dimensional analysis of the P74 and P50 phosphoproteins. Mouse testis cells were lysed in CHAPS-substituted kinase lysis buffer, immunoprecipitated with apEX-4 and autophosphorylated as described in the text. Electrophoresis on two-dimensional gels of the products of the autophosphorylation assay *in vitro* was performed according to the procedure of O'Farrell (1975). After initial autoradiography (panel a), the same dried gel was treated with 1 mol/l KOH for 1.5 hours at 55°C to remove selectively both phosphoserine and phosphothreonine and then it was re-exposed to film (panel b).

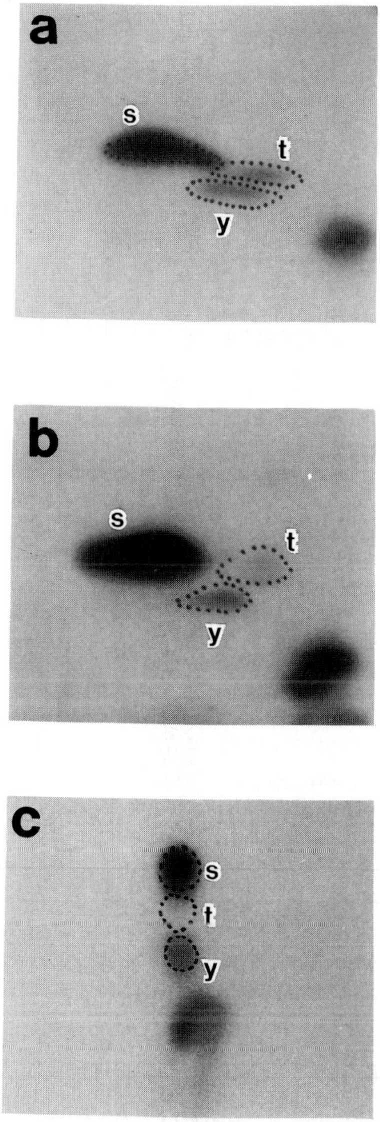

Fig. 4 Phosphoamino acid analysis of P150^{c-abl}, P74 and P50. Acid-hydrolyzed proteins which were phosphorylated in the kinase assay *in vitro* were analyzed by two-dimensional thin-layer electrophoresis as described in Materials and methods. Phosphoamino acid standards were localized by staining with ninhydrin (stipled outlines). Panel (a), P150^{c-abl}; panel (b), P74; and panel (c), P50. (s, phosphoserine; t, phosphothreonine; y, phosphotyrosine.)

in the mature sperm. It has been shown that mammalian testicular cells contain tyrosine kinase activity (Swarup *et al.*, 1983), and that tyrosine phosphorylating activity is observed after fertilization of sea-urchin eggs (Ribot *et al.*, 1984; Kinsey, 1984). Although there are stage-specific changes in protein phosphorylation during mammalian embryogenesis (Lopo and Calarco, 1982; Schultz *et al.*, 1983), it is not known which of the proteins are phosphorylated on tyrosine residues, if any. Tyrosine phosphorylation is typically rare within normal cells, and proteins phosphorylated at tyrosine residues represent $<0.03\%$ of the total cellular population of phosphoproteins (Adamson, 1987). There is no information at present regarding a potential role for c-abl in tyrosine phosphorylation within the testis or in the early embryos.

c-mos

c-*mos* is the normal cellular homolog of transforming sequences of the Moloney murine sarcoma virus. This virus arose by a spontaneous recombination of cellular sequences into the parental strain, Moloney murine leukemia virus, during passage in Balb/c mice (Moloney, 1966; Aaronson and Rowe, 1970). c-*mos* is present as a single gene in the mouse genome (Jones *et al.*, 1980) and has the somewhat unusual structural property of containing no introns. The murine c-*mos* gene contains a single open reading frame which differs in only 25 out of 1157 base pairs (bp) from the corresponding v-*mos* sequence (Van Beveren *et al.*, 1981a). There is also a high level of conservation of c-*mos* sequences among species, for example a 77% sequence similarity exists between coding sequences of murine and human c-*mos* genes (Watson *et al.*, 1982). The high degree of conservation of c-*mos* sequences suggests that the product of the c-*mos* gene may have a similarly conserved function (Van Beveren *et al.*, 1981b; Watson *et al.*, 1982). However, initial efforts to determine the site of expression of c-*mos* in normal mouse tissues failed to detect c-*mos* transcripts (e.g. Gattoni *et al.*, 1982). Expression of c-*mos* has only recently been documented by use of more sensitive methods of detection and examination of previously overlooked tissues (Propst and Vande Woude, 1985).

Transcripts of the c-*mos* gene are detected at their highest levels in the gonads of the adult mouse, and at very low levels in the adult epididymis, in day-19 embryos (Propst and Vande Woude, 1985) and in certain somatic tissues (Propst *et al.*, 1987; Mutter and Wolgemuth, 1987). The pattern of expression of c-*mos* during gametogenesis and embryogenesis is intriguing. In the testis, expression of c-*mos* is most abundant in the postmeiotic, early spermatids (Propst *et al.*, 1987; Goldman *et al.*, 1987; Mutter and Wolgemuth, 1987). In the ovary, c-*mos* transcripts have been shown to accumulate in the cytoplasm of the growing oocytes (Mutter and Wolgemuth, 1987), reaching high levels in fully grown oocytes (Mutter and Wolgemuth, 1987; Goldman *et al.*, 1987). The high levels of c-*mos* mRNAs in the fully grown oocyte suggest the possibility that c-*mos* may be important in subsequent stages of oocyte differentiation or in early embryogenesis.

We have begun to examine a possible function of the c-*mos* gene products at these stages by determining the fate of the oocyte c-*mos* mRNAs during meiotic maturation and in early embryogenesis (Mutter *et al.*, 1988). We have demonstrated that levels of *mos* transcripts drop dramatically by the two-cell stage of embryogenesis. Transcripts of c-*mos* remain undetectable at least through the blastocyst stage. Closer examination of the stages of meiotic maturation revealed that levels of c-*mos* transcripts decreased as oocytes entered the metaphase II stage of meiosis. The drop in levels of c-*mos* mRNA was documented both by in-situ hybridization and by Northern blot hybridization analysis.

The Northern blot hybridization analysis also revealed a slight increase (about 250 nucleotides) in the size of the c-*mos* transcripts in the meiotically mature ova. The difference in size between the transcripts is reminiscent of changes in lengths of poly(A) tails in other systems (Rosenthal *et al.*, 1983; Rosenthal and Ruderman, 1987). The fact that the shift in size occurs when the cells are transcriptionally inactive further suggests that post-transcriptional modification is responsible for this difference. An interesting analogous observation was recently reported by Huarte *et al.* (1988). The gene for tissue plasminogen activator (t-PA) is also expressed abundantly in growing mouse oocytes. In ova, mRNAS for t-PA are longer and the difference in size has been shown to result from an increase in the length of the poly(A) tail. Using antibodies raised against t-PA (Huarte *et al.*, 1985), Huarte *et al.* (1988) were able to demonstrate that the shift in size of the message and the changes in levels of t-PA mRNA were temporally correlated to the appearance of the protein.

Studies on c-*mos* protein have been limited since the presence of c-*mos* transcripts in normal cells has only recently been demonstrated and because existing antibodies against the protein have extensive cross-reactivity with other cellular proteins (Papkoff *et al.*, 1981, 1983). Recently, Herzog *et al.* (1988) demonstrated the presence of proteins of about 42 kD in size in purified populations of spermatids.

Although nothing is known about c-*mos* proteins in oocytes or early embryos, it is interesting to speculate on possible roles for the c-*mos* protein during these stages, given the pattern of transcription of c-*mos* mRNA and the postulated function of c-*mos* as a protein (serine) kinase (Maxwell and Arlinghaus, 1985; Singh *et al.*, 1986). The proteins essential for germinal vesicle breakdown and condensation of chromosomes are present when meiotic maturation begins (Golbus and Stein, 1976; Schultz and Wasserman, 1977a), but stages beyond metaphase I require proteins synthesized after the germinal vesicle has broken down (Schultz and Wasserman, 1977a, 1977b). Phosphoprotein metabolism undergoes drastic changes during meiosis. Resumption of meiosis coincides with a drop in cellular levels of cAMP and in both the phosphorylation and dephosphorylation of several different proteins (Schultz *et al.*, 1983; Bornslaeger *et al.*, 1986a, 1986b). Whether or not c-*mos* protein, as a possible serine kinase, could play a role in these changes is unknown.

Summary

The specificity of expression of c-*abl* and c-*mos* in the germ cell lineage suggests that these genes may play unique roles in the differentiation of the gametes or early in embryonic development. It is now important to characterize the expression of these genes at the RNA level and, especially at the protein level, to identify the possible enzymatic activities of the proteins, and finally to determine if these proteins are associated with other cellular proteins.

Acknowledgements

This work was supported by grants P50 HD05077 and T32 HD07093 from NIH. We thank Dr Carola Ponzetto of the University of Turin for contributions to the data presented in Figure 1 and Dr Owen Witte of the University of California at Los Angeles for supplying *abl*-specific antibodies.

References

Aaronson, S.A. & Rome, W.P. (1970). Nonproducer clones of Murine Sarcoma Virus-transformed BALB/3T3 cells. **Virology** 42:9–19.

Adamson, E.D. (1987). Oncogenes in development. **Development** 99:449–471.

Ben-Neriah, Y.A., Bernards, A., Paskind, M., Daley, G.Q. & Baltimore, D. (1986). Alternative 5' exons in c-*abl* mRNA. **Cell** 44:577–586.

Bishop, J.M. (1983). Cellular oncogenes and retroviruses. **Annual Review of Biochemistry** 52:301–354.

Bornslaeger, E.A., Mattei, P. & Schultz, R.M. (1986a). Involvement of cAMP-dependent protein kinase and protein phosphorylation in regulation of mouse oocyte maturation. **Developmental Biology** 11:453–462.

Bornslaeger, E.A., Poueymirou, W.T., Mattai, P. & Schultz, R.M. (1986b) Effects of protein kinase C activators on germinal vesicle breakdown and polar body emission of mouse oocytes. **Experimental Cell Research** 165:507–517.

Buss, J.E. & Sefton, B.M. (1985). Myristic acid, a rare fatty acid, is the lipid attached to the transforming protein of Rous Sarcoma Virus and its cellular homolog. **Journal of Virology** 53:7–12.

Cooper, J.A., Sefton, B.M. & Hunter, T. (1983). Detection and quantification of phosphotyrosine in proteins. **Methods in Enzymology** 99:387–407.

Doolittle, R.F., Hunkapiller, M.W., Hood, L.E., Devare, S.G., Robbins, K.C., Aaronson, S.A. & Antoniades, H.N. (1983). Simian Sarcoma Virus *onc* gene, v-*sis*, is derived from the gene (or genes) encoding a platelet-derived growth factor. **Science** 221:275–276.

Downward, J., Yarden, Y., Mayes, E., Scrace, G., Totty, N., Stockwell, P., Ullrich, A., Schlessinger, J. & Waterfield, M.D. (1984). Close similarity of epidermal growth factor receptor and v-*erb*-B oncogene protein sequences. **Nature** 307:521–527.

Duggal, R.N., Zakeri, Z.F., Ponzetto, C. & Wolgemuth, D.J. (1987). Differential expression of the c-*abl* proto-oncogene and the homeobox-containing gene Hox 1.4 during mouse spermatogenesis. In: Orgebin-Crist, M.-C. & Danzo, B.J., eds. **Cell Biology of the Testis and Epididymis, Annals of the New York Academy of Sciences** 153:112–127.

Gattoni, S., Kirschmeier, P., Weinstein, I.B., Scobedo, J.E. & Dina, D. (1982). Cellular Moloney Murine Sarcoma (c-*mos*) sequences are hypermethylated and transcriptionally silent in normal and transformed rodent cells. **Molecular and Cellular Biology** 2:42–51.

Golbus, M.S. & Stein, M.P. (1976). Qualitative patterns of protein synthesis in the mouse oocyte. **Journal of Experimental Zoology** 198:337–342.

Goldman, D.S., Kiessling, A.A., Millette, C.F. & Cooper, G.M. (1987). Expression of c-*mos* RNA in germ cells of male and female mice. **Proceedings of the National Academy of Sciences, USA** 84:4509–4513.

Herzog, N.K., Singh, B., Elder, J., Lipkin, I., Trauger, R.T., Millette, C.F., Goldman, D.S., Wolfes, H., Cooper, G.M. & Arlinghaus, R.B. (1988). Identification of the protein product of the c-*mos* proto-oncogene in mouse testes. **Oncogene** 3:225–229.

Heisterkamp, N., Groffen, J. & Stephenson, J.R. (1983). The human v-*abl* cellular homologue. **Journal of Molecular and Applied Genetics** 2:57–68.

Huarte, J., Berlin, D. & Vassalli, J.D. (1985). Plasminogen activator in mouse and rat oocytes: induction during meiotic maturation. **Cell** 43:551–558.

Huarte, J., Berlin, D., Vassalli, A., Strickland, S. & Vassalli, J.D. (1988). Meiotic maturation of mouse oocytes triggers the translation and polyadenylation of dormant tissue-type plasminogen activator mRNA. **Genes and Development** 1:1201–1211.

Jones, M., Von Straaten, F., Galleshaw, J.A. & Verma, I. (1980). Identification and molecular cloning of Moloney Mouse Sarcoma Virus-specific sequences from uninfected mouse cells. **Proceedings of the National Academy of Sciences, USA** 77:2651–2655.

Kinsey, W.H. (1984). Regulation of tyrosine-specific kinase activity at fertilization. **Developmental Biology** 105:137–143.

Konopka, J.B., Davis, R.L., Watanabe, S.M., Ponticelli, A.M., Shiff-Maker, L., Ronsenberg, N. & Witte, O.N. (1984). Only site-directed antibodies reactive with the highly conserved *src*-homologous region of the v-*abl* protein neutralize kinase activity. **Journal of Virology** 51:223–232.

Konopka, J. & Witte, O.N. (1985). Detection of c-*abl* tyrosine kinase activity *in vitro* permits direct comparison of normal and altered *abl* gene products. **Molecular and Cellular Biology** 5:3116–3123.

Lopo, A.C. & Calarco, P.G. (1982). Stage-specific changes in protein phosphorylation during preimplantation development in the mouse. **Gamete Research** 5:283–290.

Maxwell, S.A. & Arlinghaus, R.B. (1985). A cAMP-independent serine/threonine kinase activity is associated with the *mos* sequences of ts 110 Moloney Murine Sarcoma Virus-encoded $p85^{gag-mos}$. **Journal of General Virology** 66:2135–2146.

Meijer, P., Hermans, A., Von Lindern, M., Van Agthoven, T., De Klein, A., Mackenbach, P., Grootegoed, A., Talarico, D., Della Valle, G. & Grosveld, G. (1987). Molecular characterization of the testis-specific c-*abl* mRNA in mouse. **European Molecular Biology Organization Journal** 6:4041–4048.

Moloney, J.B.B. (1966). A virus-induced rhabdomyosarcoma of mice. **National Cancer Institute Monographs** 22:139–142.

Muller, R., Slamon, D.J., Tremblay, J.M., Cline, M.J. & Verma, I.M. (1982). Differential expression of cellular oncogenes during pre- and postnatal development of the mouse. **Nature** 299:640–644.

Mutter, G.L., Grills, G.S. & Wolgemuth, D.J. (1988). Evidence for the involvement of the proto-oncogene c-*mos* in mammalian meiotic maturation and possibly very early embryogenesis. **European Molecular Biology Organization Journal** 7:283–689.

Mutter, G.L. & Wolgemuth, D.J. (1987). Distinct developmental patterns of c-*mos* proto-oncogene expression in female and male mouse germ cells. **Proceedings of the National Academy of Sciences, USA** 84:5301–5305.

O'Farrell, P.H. (1975). High-resolution two-dimensional electrophoresis of proteins. **Journal of Biological Chemistry**, 250:4007–4021.

Oppi, C.S., Shore, K. & Reddy, P. (1987). Nucleotide sequence of testis-derived c-*abl* cDNAs: implications for testis-specific transcription and *abl* oncogene activation. **Proceedings of the National Academy of Sciences, USA** 84:8200–8204.

Papkoff, J., Mei, H., Hunter, T. & Verma, I. (1981). Analysis of transforming gene products from Moloney Murine Sarcoma Virus. **Cell** 27:109–119.

Papkoff, J., Nigg, E.A. & Hunter, T. (1983). The transforming protein of Moloney Murine Sarcoma Virus is a soluble protein. **Cell** 33:161–172.

Pendergast, A.M., Traugh, J.A. & Witte, O.N. (1987). Normal cellular and transformation-associated *abl* proteins share common sites for protein kinase C phosphorylation. **Molecular and Cellular Biology** 7:4280–4289.

Ponzetto, C., Wadewitz, A.G., Pendergast, A.M., Witte, O.N. & Wolgemuth, D.J. (1989). $P150^{c-abl}$ is detected in mouse male germ cells by an *in vitro* kinase assay and is associated with stage-specific phosphoproteins in haploid cells. **Oncogene** 4:685–690.

Ponzetto, C. & Wolgemuth, D.J. (1985). Haploid expression of a unique c-*abl* transcript in the mouse male germ line. **Molecular and Cellular Biology** 5:1791–1794.

Propst, F., Rosenberg, M.P., Iyer, A., Kaul, K. & Vande Woude, G. (1987). c-*mos* proto-oncogene RNA transcripts in murine tissues: structural features, developmental regulation, and localization in specific cell types. **Molecular and Cellular Biology** 7:1629–1637.

Propst, F. & Vande Woude, G.F. (1985). Expression of c-*mos* proto-oncogene transcripts in mouse tissues. **Nature** 315:516–518.

Ribot, H.D., Eisenman, E.A. & Kinsey, W.H. (1984). Fertilization results in increased tyrosine phosphorylation of egg proteins. **Journal of Biological Chemistry** 259:5333–5338.

Rosenthal, E.T., Ransey, T.R. & Ruderman, J.V. (1983). Sequence-specific adenylations and deadenylations accompany changes in the translation of maternal messenger RNA after fertilization of *Spisula* oocytes. **Journal of Molecular Biology** 166:309–327.

Rosenthal, E.T. & Ruderman, J.V. (1987). Widespread changes in the translation and adenylation of maternal messenger RNAs following fertilization of *Spisula* oocytes. **Developmental Biology** 121:237–246.

Schultz, A. & Oroszolan, S. (1984). Myristylation of *gag-onc* fusion proteins in mammalian transforming retroviruses. **Virology** 133:431–437.

Schultz, R.M., Montgomery, R.R. & Belanoff, J.R. (1983). Regulation of mouse oocyte meiotic maturation: implications of a decrease in oocyte cAMP and protein dephosphorylation in commitment to resume meiosis. **Developmental Biology** 97:264–273.

Schultz, R.M. & Wasserman, P.M. (1977a). Biochemical studies of mammalian oogenesis: protein synthesis during oocyte growth and meiotic maturation in the mouse. **Journal of Cell Science** 24:167–194.

Schultz, R.M. & Wasserman, P.M. (1977b). Specific changes in the pattern of protein synthesis during meiotic maturation of mammalian oocytes *in vitro*. **Proceedings of the National Academy of Sciences, USA** 74:538–541.

Sefton, B.M. (1986). The viral tyrosine protein kinases. **Current Topics in Microbiology and Immunology** 123:39–72.

Shackelford, G.M. & Varmus, H.E. (1987). Expression of the proto-oncogene *int*-1 is restricted to postmeiotic male germ cells and the neural tube of mid-gestational embryos. **Cell** 50:89–95.

Sherr, C.J., Rettienmeier, G.W., Sala, R., Roussel, M.F., Look, A.T. & Stanley, E.R. (1985). The c-*fms* proto-oncogene product is related to the receptor for the mononuclear phagocyte growth factor, CSF-1. **Cell** 41:665–675.

Simonds, W.F., Koski, G., Streaty, R.A., Hjelmeland, L.M. & Kleen, W.A. (1980). Solubilization of active opiate receptors. **Proceedings of the National Academy of Sciences, USA** 77:4623–4627.

Singh, B., Hannink, M., Donoghue, D.J. & Arlinghaus, R.B. (1986). $P37^{mos}$-associated serine/threonine protein kinase activity correlates with the cellular transformation function of v-*mos*. **Journal of Virology** 60:1148–1152.

Swarup, G., Dasgupta, J.D. & Garbers, D.L. (1983). Tyrosine protein kinase activity of rat spleen and other tissues. **Journal of Biological Chemistry** 258:10341–10347.

Van Beveren, C., Van Straaten, F., Galleshaw, J.A. & Verma, I. (1981a). Nucleotide sequence of the genome of a Murine Sarcoma Virus. **Cell** 27:97–108.

Van Beveren, C., Galleshaw, J.A., Jonas, V., Berns, A.J.M., Doolittle, R.F., Donoghue, D.J. & Verma, I.M. (1981b). Nucleotide sequence and formation of the transforming gene of a mouse sarcoma virus. **Nature** 289:258–262.

Wang, J. & Baltimore, D. (1983). Cellular RNA homologous to the Abelson Murine Leukemia Virus transforming gene: expression and relationship to the viral sequence. **Molecular and Cellular Biology** 3:773–779.

Wang, J.Y., Ledley, F., Goff, S., Lee, R., Groner, Y. & Baltimore, D. (1984). The mouse c-*abl* locus: molecular cloning and characterization. **Cell**, 36:349–356.

Waterfield, M.D., Scrace, G.T., Whittle, N., Stroobant, P., Johnson, A., Wasteson, A., Westermark, B., Heldin, C.H., Huang, J.S. & Deuel, T.F. (1983). Platelet-derived growth factor is structurally related to the putative transforming protein $p28^{sis}$ of Simian Sarcoma Virus. **Nature** 304:35–39.

Watson, R., Oskarrson, M. & Vande Woude, G. (1982). Human DNA sequences homologous to the transforming gene (*mos*) of Moloney Murine Sarcoma Virus. **Proceedings of the National Academy of Sciences, USA** 79:4078–4082.

Witte, O.N. (1986). Functions of the *abl* oncogene. **Cancer Survey** 5:183–197.

Wolgemuth, D.J., Gizang-Ginsberg, E., Engelmeyer, E., Gavin, B.J. & Ponzetto, C. (1985). Separation of mouse testis cells on a Celsep apparatus and their usefulness as a source of high-molecular-weight DNA or RNA. **Gamete Research** 12:1–10.

Yonemoto, W., Filson, A.J., Queral-Lustig, A.E., Wang, J.Y.J. & Brugge, J.S. (1987). Detection of phosphotyrosine-containing proteins in polyoma virus middle tumor antigen-transformed cells after treatment with a phosphotyrosine phosphatase inhibitor. **Journal of Molecular and Cellular Biology** 7:905–913.

II Mechanisms of hormone action

Mechanisms of action of estrogens and antiestrogens

J. GORSKI, H. AHRENS, D. MEIER, F. MURDOCH AND M. SEYFRED

College of Agricultural and Life Sciences, Departments of Biochemistry and Animal Sciences, University of Wisconsin, Madison, WI 53706, USA.

Keywords

Estrogen receptors, receptor localization, antiestrogens, mechanism of estrogen action.

Introduction

Estrogenic hormones coordinate an array of physiological functions that are involved in female vertebrate reproduction. As coordinating regulators, estrogens must affect different tissues, at different times, in manifestly different ways. For example, within the pituitary gland, lactotrophs are stimulated by estrogens to increase the production of prolactin via the increased expression of the prolactin gene (Shull and Gorski, 1986). In addition, the turnover of prolactin mRNA appears to be slower under the influence of estrogen, and the lactotrophs increase their rate of replication as a result of stimulation by estrogen. Within neighboring gonadotrophs in the pituitary, production of the gonadotropins FSH and LH is decreased by estrogens (Miller *et al.*, 1977). At the same time, in other tissues, estrogen causes a similarly complex array of increases and decreases in gene expression that leads to modifications in cell function.

In contrast to the complexity of cellular response to estrogens, the estrogen receptor appears to be the product of a single gene and is probably just a single species of protein (Green *et al.*, 1986). This latter point is still a matter of some controversy and more definitive data are needed. However, we will assume that a single receptor species is involved in all estrogenic hormonal responses. If we make this assumption, it is apparent that the formation of the receptor–estrogen complex must result in a conformational change that is capable of initiating the diverse responses that occur across the various target tissues (Hansen and Gorski, 1985). It is also apparent that the complexity of response must occur at a step subsequent to the formation of the estrogenic ligand–receptor complex. Although by no means definitely proven, it is a popular, currently held assumption that a common genomic response element or nucleotide sequence found in hormone-sensitive genes, which binds to the estrogen receptor, provides the integrating factor in hormonal response (Klein-Hitpass *et al.*, 1986).

In reality, our understanding of the mechanisms of estrogen action is, at

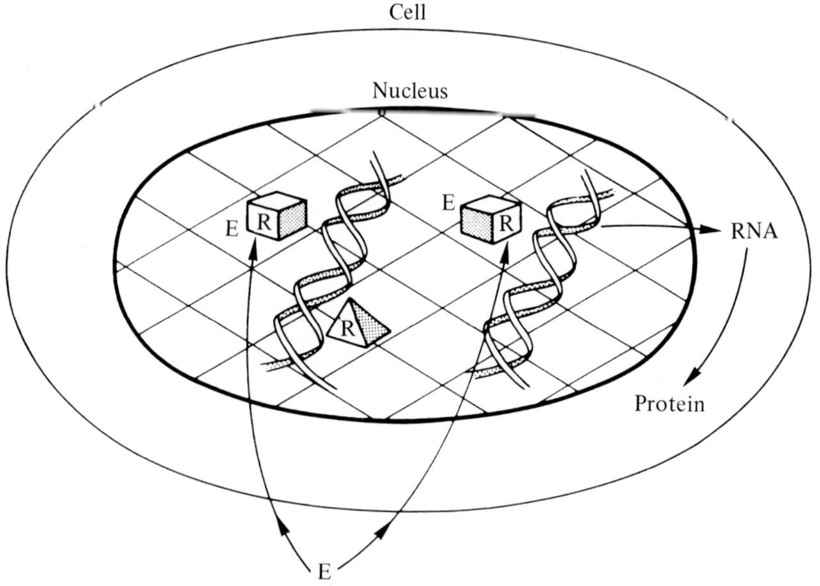

Fig. 1 Current model of estrogen receptor action at the cellular level. (E, estrogen; R, receptor.)

best, superficial. We have only limited information about most of the steps involved, beginning with the localization of the receptor in the target cells. We shall discuss certain of these points in order to clarify what is known and not known about steroid hormone mechanisms.

Localization of estrogen receptors

The unoccupied estrogen receptor is a nuclear protein (Fig. 1) as judged by density enucleation studies and recent immunocytochemical localization (Welshons *et al.*, 1984; King and Greene, 1984). It should be noted that older immunocytochemical studies indicated that all estrogen receptors were in the cytoplasm. More recent studies, using newer techniques, have indicated that both unoccupied and occupied receptors are located exclusively in the nuclear compartment. Similarly, the results of cell enucleation studies indicate that estrogen receptors are not present in the cytoplasm, but are present in the subcellular fraction that contains nuclei. The occupation of the estrogen receptor by steroid causes a change in the affinity of the receptor for nuclear components, such that the receptor can only be extracted by buffers of high ionic strength. In contrast, the unoccupied receptor can readily be extracted by buffers of low ionic strength. However, results of immunocytochemical studies of the glucocorticoid receptor have been less definitive, and both nuclear and cytoplasmic receptors have been reported (Gustafsson *et al.*, 1987).

Subnuclear localization

It is important to note that 20 000 or more estrogen receptors are found tightly bound to the nucleus of a typical target cell after the administration of estrogen. Whether or not all of these receptors are functional is not clear, but dose–response experiments indicate a direct proportionality between receptor occupancy and cell response (Katzenellenbogen and Gorski, 1975).

The estrogen receptors appear to be widely distributed within the nucleus and no specific localization has been observed by immunocytochemical methods (King and Greene, 1984). Furthermore, there does not appear to be any change in the localization of receptors after estrogen binding. A variety of biochemical investigations has also revealed a wide array of nuclear constituents that bind to the estrogen receptor. These constituents include histones, RNA, chromatin proteins, nuclear matrix, and DNA (Gorski and Gannon, 1976). In most of these studies the receptors are present in relatively crude preparations, so it is difficult to determine whether it is the receptor alone or other components of the preparation that are interacting with the nuclear constituent. The most popular subject for such studies has been certain specific DNA sequences that have been deduced to be hormone-response elements in target genes (Yamamoto, 1985). The estrogen response element (ERE) is a DNA sequence located in the regulatory regions of genes that are known to respond to treatment with estrogen. These sequences, when placed upstream from a variety of genes, cause those genes to respond to estrogen. This response can take place in any cell that contains estrogen receptors. Such a response was demonstrated in yeast cells, in which estrogen receptors were present as a result of transfection *in vitro* with expression vectors containing gene for the estrogen receptor. However, the hormone-sensitive transcription complex, presumably including the estrogen receptor, the ERE, and ancillary factors, has yet to be defined. Furthermore, such complexes would account for only a fraction of the 20 000 receptors that are tightly bound to the nucleus after the administration of estrogen.

An estrogenic response was observed in yeast cells that were transfected with both estrogen receptor genes and response elements. Studies in this system strongly support the concept that the receptor contains a domain that directly recognizes the specific sequences of the ERE in the face of a large amount of non-specific DNA sequences. It is also highly probable that other chromatin proteins or transcription factors are involved in this recognition complex. However, it seems unlikely that there is a specific binding protein for every regulated gene in the genome. It is more likely that a specific array or complex of proteins present in a certain cell may associate with a regulatory sequence of a gene to present a unique complex or code, specific for the expression of that gene (Struhl, 1987). Thus, the response element itself may vary, as has been observed for the response elements in all the steroid hormone-responsive genes. The array of proteins might vary from cell to cell, and this variation could account for the diversity of response, as well as for the range in the magnitude of response, which is seen with the different genes that are regulated by a single steroid hormone.

The role of the hormone in the response to estrogen may be more complex than originally imagined. Recent data reported by Chambon's group suggest that the binding of hormone to the receptor initiates at least two important modifications in receptor function (Webster *et al.*, 1988). Estrogen binding to the steroid-binding domain of the receptor appears to initiate interactions of that same domain with transcription factors and/or the RNA polymerase II molecule. In addition, estrogen binding positively affects the activity of the adjacent DNA-binding domain of the receptor. These conclusions are based on the observation that chimeric proteins, which contain the steroid-binding domain of the receptor, linked to the DNA-binding domains of other transcription factors, such as the yeast Gal 4 protein, act as hormone-sensitive Gal 4 transcription factors. Similarly, Yamamoto and associates observed that the steroid-binding domain appears to function independently of the DNA-binding domain (Godowski *et al.*, 1988). They showed that the domains can be shuffled so that the relationship of one domain to another is different, yet enhancement of the transcriptional activity of the reporter gene by the rearranged receptor remains hormone sensitive.

Although steroid receptors are widely thought to function as DNA binding proteins, evidence that estrogen binding influences interaction of the receptor with chromatin is minimal. Again, recent work by Chambon has provided very persuasive evidence that the estrogen binding affects the interaction of the nuclear-binding domain of the receptor with the DNA–chromatin complex that is associated with the response element (Webster *et al.*, 1988). In these experiments, a chimeric gene product containing an estrogen-binding domain linked to the yeast Gal 4 DNA-binding domain was shown to compete with normal Gal 4 protein for binding to a Gal 4 response element. This competition occurred with antiestrogen as well as with estrogen, even though the antiestrogen, unlike estrogen, cannot induce the expression of the Gal 4 responsive gene. These results are of particular significance because they appear to mimic the observations *in vivo* that antiestrogens cause the same high-affinity association of the receptor with the nucleus as do the estrogens, but they do not induce most estrogenic responses. The model presented in Figure 2 illustrates how the estrogen receptor might interact with two regions of the chromatin of a target gene and how this interaction could, in turn, be influenced by the binding of an appropriate ligand.

Antiestrogens

Antiestrogens are competitive inhibitors of the estrogen receptor, and they bind with high affinity to the ligand-binding domain of the receptor (Jordan *et al.*, 1986). This interaction causes changes in the receptor's affinity for the

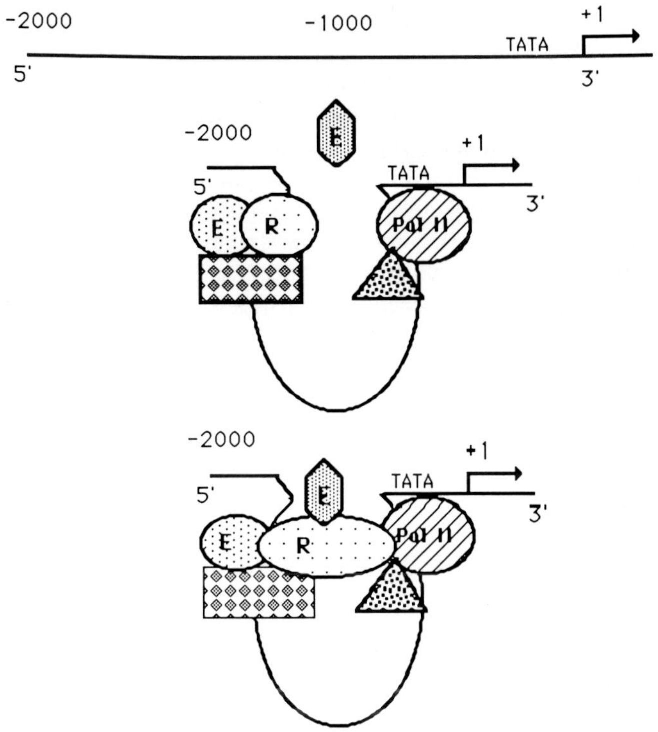

Fig. 2 Model of the interaction of the estrogen receptor with the chromatin of a target gene. An estrogen response element (ERE) is located approximately 1500–2000 base pairs upstream from the site of initiation of transcription. The polymerase II (Pol II) molecule is associated with the promoter region of the gene immediately upstream from the site of initiation of transcription. An estrogen molecule (E) binds to the steroid-binding domain of the receptor (ER) and causes a conformational change in the receptor that changes the receptor's interaction with both the upstream response element and the polymerase II–transcription factor complex.

nucleus, which are similar to the changes induced by estrogens. Thus, the receptor–antiestrogen complex, just like the estrogen–receptor complex, can only be extracted by buffers of high ionic strength. However, antiestrogens do not have the effects on gene expression or induce other cellular responses that are comparable to those of estrogens. Chambon's recent work with a chimeric estrogen receptor protein suggests that the binding of antiestrogen may cause a change in the receptor's DNA-binding domain, which leads to a higher affinity of the receptor for the nucleus. However, in contrast to the binding of an estrogen, the binding of an antiestrogen does not induce the appropriate changes in the receptor domains that modulate transcription. We believe that the steroid-binding domain itself is most likely to be the site on the receptor that is responsible for these transcriptional effects. This conclusion is based, in part, on observations that estrogen causes a drastic change in the conformation of the steroid-binding domain, which is notably different from the conformation induced by the antiestrogens (Hansen and Gorski, 1986). In addition, a variety of transfection studies with truncated or chimeric receptor genes suggests that the steroid-binding domain contains much of the functional transcription-regulating activity of the receptor.

If the above hypotheses are correct, then antiestrogens may possibly have a dual function. In addition to their role as competitive inhibitors, the antiestrogen–receptor complex may interfere with the regulation of a gene's constitutive expression or the regulation of such a gene by other regulators. For example, the prolactin gene is regulated by estrogen, glucocorticoids, epidermal growth factor, calcium ions, as well as other factors (Shull and Gorski, 1986). The presence of an antiestrogen–receptor complex on the chromatin of the prolactin gene might interfere with the ability of other regulatory factors to interact with the regulatory elements of the gene.

The complex agonistic and antagonistic properties of certain antiestrogens may also be explained by the different structural features of a particular antiestrogen–receptor complex when placed in specific but different chromatin environments.

Summary

Our understanding of how steroid hormones act at the cellular and molecular level has increased dramatically in the last few years. There are controversies as well as gaps in our knowledge that require further exploration. However, the models presented here illustrate some recent progress and indicate problems that future workers are likely to address.

Acknowledgements

This work was supported in part by the College of Agricultural and Life Sciences, University of Wisconsin, Madison; by NIH grants HD08192 and CA18110; and by a grant from the National Foundation for Cancer Research awarded to JG, and by NIH Postdoctoral Fellowships awarded to DM (HD06972), FM (HD07136), and MS (HD06973).

References

Godowski, P.J., Picard, D. & Yamamoto, K.R. (1988). Signal transduction and transcriptional regulation by glucocorticoid receptor-LexA fusion proteins. **Science** 241:812–816.

Gorski, J. & Gannon, F. (1976). Current models of steroid hormone action: a critique. **Annual Review of Physiology** 38:425–450.

Green, S., Walter, P., Kumar, V., Bornert, J.-M., Argos, P. & Chambon, P. (1986). Human oestrogen receptor cDNA: sequence, expression and homology to V-*erb-A*. **Nature** 320:134–139.

Gustafsson, J.-A., Carlstedt-Duke, J., Poellinger, L., Okret, S., Wikstrom, A.-C., Bronnegard, M., Gillner, M., Dong, Y., Fuxe, K., Cintra, A., Harfstrand, A. & Agnati, L. (1987). Biochemistry, molecular biology, and physiology of the glucocorticoid receptor. **Endocrine Reviews** 8:185–234.

Hansen, J.C. & Gorski, J. (1985). Conformational and electrostatic properties of unoccupied and liganded estrogen receptors determined by aqueous two-phase partitioning. **Biochemistry** 24:6078–6085.

Hansen, J.C. & Gorski, J. (1986). Conformational transitions of the estrogen receptor monomer. **Journal of Biological Chemistry** 61:13990–13996.

Jordan, V.C., Koch, R. & Lieberman, M.E. (1986). Structure–activity relationships of nonestroidal estrogens and antiestrogens. In: Jordan, V.C., ed. **Estrogen/Antiestrogen Action and Breast Cancer Therapy**, University of Wisconsin Press, Madison, WI, pp.19–41.

Katzenellenbogen, B.S. & Gorski, J. (1975). Estrogen actions on syntheses of macromolecules in target cells. In: Litwack, ed. **Biochemical Actions of Hormones**, Vol. III, New York, Academic Press, pp.187–243.

King, W.J. & Greene, G.L. (1984). Monoclonal antibodies localize oestrogen receptor in the nuclei of target cells. **Nature** 307:745–747.

Klein-Hitpass, L., Schorpp, M., Wagner, U. & Ryffel, G.U. (1986). An estrogen-responsive element derived from the 5' flanking region of the *Xenopus* vitellogen A2 gene functions in transfected human cells. **Cell** 46:1053–1061.

Miller, W.L., Knight, M.M., Grimek, H.J. & Gorski, J. (1977). Estrogen regulation of FSH in cell cultures of sheep pituitaries. **Endocrinology** 100:1306–1316.

Shull, J.D. & Gorski, J. (1986). The hormonal regulation of prolactin gene expression: an examination of mechanisms controlling prolactin synthesis and the possible relationship of estrogen to these mechanisms. In: Aurbach, G.D. & McCormick, D.B., eds. **Vitamins and Hormones: Advances in Research and Applications**, Vol. 43, New York, Academic Press, pp.197–249.

Struhl, K. (1987). Promotors, activator proteins, and the mechanism of transcriptional initiation in yeast. **Cell** 49:295–297.

Webster, N.J.G., Green, S., Jin, J.R. & Chambon, P. (1988). The hormone-binding domains of the estrogen and glucocorticoid receptors contain an inducible transcription activation function. **Cell** 54:199–207.

Welshons, W., Lieberman, M.E. & Gorski, J. (1984). Nuclear localization of unoccupied estrogen receptors: cytochalasin enucleation of GH3 cells. **Nature** 307:747–749.

Yamamoto, K.R. (1985). Steroid receptor-regulated transcription of specific genes and gene networks. **Annual Review of Genetics** 19:209–252.

Are receptor-associated nuclear proteins associated with the earliest effects of steroid hormones?

E.E. BAULIEU, N. BINART, F. CADEPOND, M.G. CATELLI, B. CHAMBRAUD, J. GARNIER,[1] J.M. GASC, G. GROYER-SCHWEIZER, M.E. OBLIN, C. RADANYI, G. REDEUILH, J.M. RENOIR AND M. SABBAH

Laboratorie Hormones, INSERM U33 and Faculté de Médecine, 94270 Bicêtre, France; [1]INRA, 78350 Jouy en Josas, France.

Keywords

Heat-shock protein 90, receptors, ligand-binding domain, DNA-binding domain, RU 486.

Introduction

The functional importance of the interaction of heat-shock protein 90 (hsp90) with receptors for steroid hormones in the action of these hormones has been suggested. This hypothesis, although not yet proven, is supported by new data obtained in our laboratory and in the laboratories of others, whereas no conflicting experimental results have been presented. Our recent studies have dealt with the cloning of hsp90, the translation of normal and mutated receptors, the effects of the antihormone RU 486, and immunohistochemistry.

This chapter deals with very early steps in the action of steroid hormones (and antihormone), immediately after the binding of the hormone (or antihormone) to the receptor (R). We review data related to our current working hypothesis about the role of hsp90 in receptor function.

We are concerned with the receptors for estrogen (E), progestin (P), glucocorticosteroid (G), mineralocorticosteroid (M), and androgen (A). All these receptors belong to the *erb*-A superfamily (Evans, 1988) and, thus, they have the same overall structural organization (Fig. 1). We suggest that they may mediate the activity of their corresponding hormones through a common mechanism.

Five years ago we presented the first data demonstrating the interaction between four steroid receptors (chick ER, PR, GR, and AR; Baulieu *et al.*, 1983) with a non-steroid binding protein of 90 kDa. We chose to study the 'non-transformed' 8S-form of steroid hormone receptors (8S-Rs), of calculated molecular weight of about 300 kDa (see Sherman *et al.*, 1983, for review), because we felt that it would be relatively easy to separate large, 'non-transformed' steroid-binding complexes from other soluble proteins. The first evidence for the 8S form of steroid receptors was provided for ER by Toft *et al.*

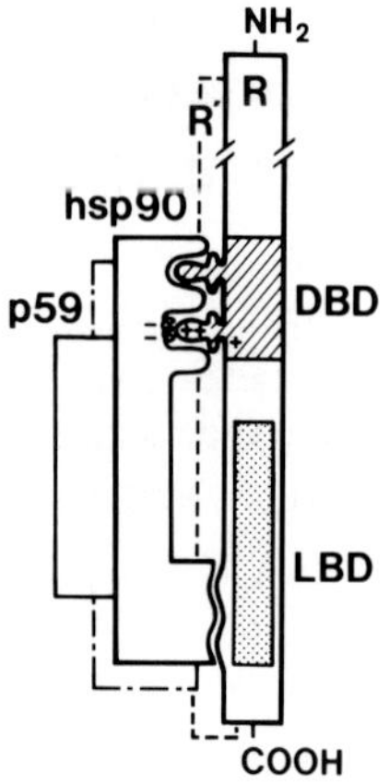

Fig. 1 Diagrammatic representation of a steroid hormone receptor. The receptor itself includes a DNA-binding domain (DBD) and a ligand-binding domain (LBD). In the case of ER, a second ER subunit (R') (Redeuilh *et al.*, 1987) is represented by a dotted frame. The difference in sizes of steroid hormone receptors is shown by the interrupted line in the N-terminal domain. Interaction with the heat-shock protein of about 90 kDa (hsp90) occurs at two sites, with LBD and DBD (the possibly ionic interaction between the positively charged amino acid of DBD with the negatively charged amino acids of the hsp90 A region is shown by + and −). The postulated dimeric state of hsp90 is indicated (-·-). The interacton between hsp90 and p59 (a nuclear protein of about 59 kDa) is also represented.

(1967) and then generalized to other steroid receptors (Baulieu *et al.*, 1971). 8S-Rs are recovered in the cytosol of target cells which have not been exposed to hormone and have, thus, been envisioned as biologically inactive forms. These receptors, with a sedimentation coefficient in the 7S–10S range, have been described as oligomers (Baulieu *et al.*, 1971; Sherman *et al.*, 1983) or called 'aggregates' (Schrader *et al.*, 1975). Until 1983, no experimental data were available to describe the subunit composition of 8S-Rs. The purification of the 8S-PR from chick oviduct (Wolfson *et al.*, 1980; Renoir *et al.*, 1984) allowed a monoclonal antibody to be produced (Radanyi *et al.*, 1983) and the subsequent demonstration of a 90-kDa subunit common to the 8S-Rs for the five steroid hormones (Baulieu *et al.*, 1983; Joab *et al.*, 1984; Groyer *et al.*, 1985; Rafestin-Oblin *et al.*, 1989). The work of Toft and colleagues led to a similar conclusion with respect to the chick PR (Dougherty *et al.*, 1984). Soon thereafter, important observations were made. (1) The 90-kDa protein and the 8S-Rs do not bind DNA, in contrast to the 'transformed' receptor form with sedimentation coefficient of about 4S (4S-R, or 5S-R for the dimeric form of the ER), which binds both to non-specific DNA and to hormone-response element (HRE) DNA (Beato, 1987). (2) The 90-kDa protein is a heat-shock protein of about 90 kDa (hsp90), as demonstrated by biochemical, immunological and cloning techniques (Catelli *et al.*, 1985a, 1985b; Schuh *et al.*, 1985; Sanchez *et al.*, 1985). Our working hypothesis, recently reviewed in detail (Baulieu, 1987; Baulieu and Catelli, 1988), is that hsp90 is responsible for the absence of binding to DNA by the 8S-Rs and is released when the steroid hormone binds to the receptor, thus unmasking the DNA-binding site of the 4S-R. In this chapter, we present some new data from our laboratory which confirm and extend our original description of the hetero-oligomeric form of steroid receptors and we discuss some controversial issues concerning the function of the 8S-Rs.

Steroid receptors and hsp90 are nuclear proteins. Do they associate physiologically to form '8S-receptors'?

It was known for some time that hormone–receptor complexes (H–Rs) are nuclear rather than cytoplasmic (Edelman *et al.*, 1963; Jungblut *et al.*, 1967), as 'logically' expected for gene transactivators that bind to DNA (Yamamoto and Alberts, 1976), and this localization was confirmed by combined immunohistochemical and autoradiographic techniques (Gasc *et al.*, 1983). We then demonstrated that the chick oviduct PR is essentially located in target-cell nuclei, even in the absence of hormone (Gasc *et al.*, 1983, 1989), as was also found for the mammalian PR (Perrot-Applanat *et al.*, 1985) and ER (King and Greene, 1984; Welshons *et al.*, 1984). In the case of GR, a number of observations (reviewed in Gustafsson *et al.*, 1987; Picard and Yamamoto, 1987) have indicated that it is mostly, if not totally, cyctoplasmic prior to exposure of target cells to hormone. Furthermore, it has been suggested that the receptor is translocated to the nucleus upon exposure to hormone. We have found (Fig. 2; Gasc *et al.*, 1989) that GR is nuclear but, in the absence of the hormone, it is not as firmly bound to the nucleus as ER and PR, a difference that could explain why GR is sometimes observed in the cytoplasm; nuclear GR may leak out of the nucleus during the fixation step which precedes immunocytochemistry. Thus, increased staining of the nucleus after exposure to glucocorticosteroid may be due to stronger nuclear attachment of the hormone–GR complexes, rather than to translocation of the GR from the cytoplasm to the nucleus. We have observed that the cytoplasmic GR-like antigen, as detected by immunohistochemistry, does not seem to participate in a translocation process when cells are exposed to hormone (the antibody may detect a variant of the GR in the cytoplasm, such as, for example, GR-β which does not bind the steroid) (Hollenberg *et al.*, 1985).

If, in the absence of hormone, the receptors are nuclear and present in the 8S-R form (Wolfson, 1984), some hsp90 should be detectable in the nucleus. Hsp90 is a cytoplasmic protein. However, it has been observed in nuclei of heat-stressed chick fibroblasts (Collier and Schlesinger, 1986). Immunohisto-

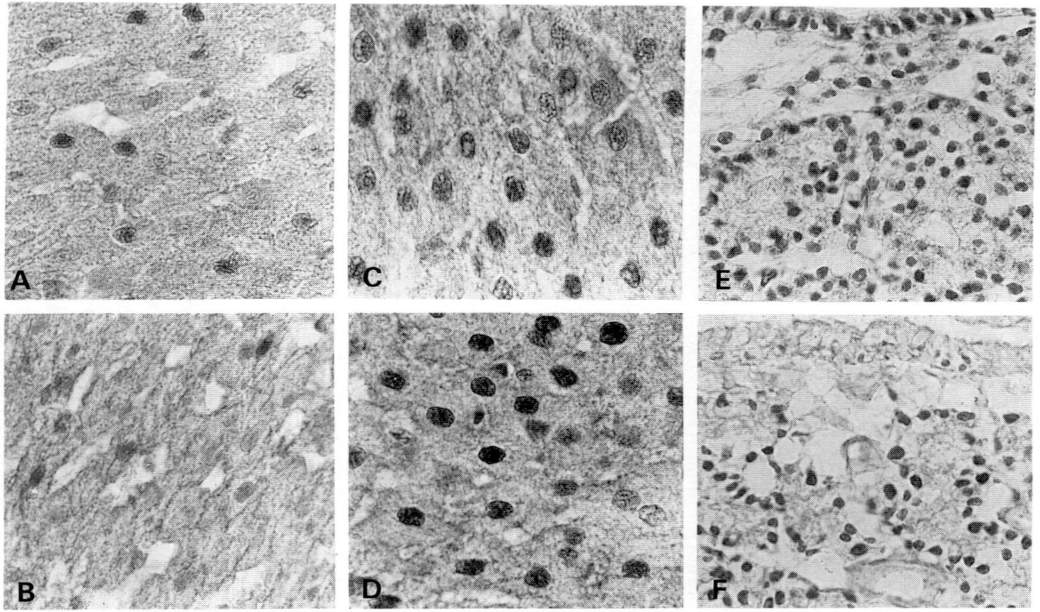

Fig. 2 The glucocorticosteroid receptor: a nuclear protein. Comparison of the retention, in the nucleus, of hormone-free and hormone-occupied receptors. In frozen sections of the liver from a control and an adrenalectomized (Adx) rat (A), the immunostaining of the GR is completely lost if the section is pre-incubated in a buffered solution (PBS-sucrose) for 2.5 minutes before fixation (B). The same pre-incubation treatment has no effect on immunostaining of GR if the Adx rat has received dexamethasone (compare C, without, and D, with pre-incubation). The difference between B and D illustrates the low affinity of the binding of the hormone-free compared to the hormone-occupied nuclear GR. After treatment with dexamethasone, a higher affinity of the GR for nuclear structures allows better retention of receptors, i.e. an apparent increase, often interpreted as a result of nuclear translocation. Under the same conditions, in the chick oviduct, there is no substantial decrease in immunostaining of PR after pre-incubation in PBS-sucrose (compare E, without pre-incubation and F, with pre-incubation), although the immature chicken had not received progesterone. No increase in nuclear immunostaining of PR is observed after treatment with progesterone. Bar = 10 μm (Gasc *et al.*, 1989).

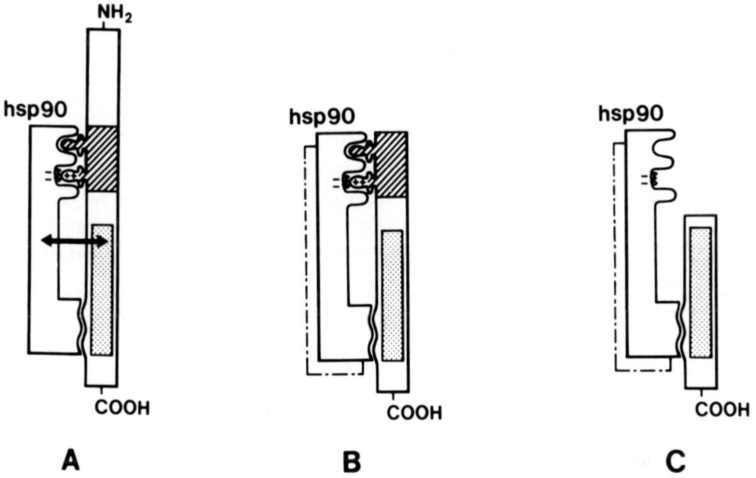

Fig. 3 Diagrammatic representation of steroid receptors. (A) '7S–PR' form (with one hsp90 molecule), obtained after purification, followed by cross-linking treatment with dimethyl pimelimidate (Aranyi *et al.*, 1988). (B) GR nt_i mutant, lacking the N-terminal region (Gehring and Arndt, 1985). (C) Trypsinized receptor, isolated after proteolysis of 8S–GR (cited in Denis *et al.*, 1988).

logically, we detected the presence of hsp90 in the nucleus of all the cells we have examined in the chick (Gasc *et al.*, 1983; Gasc *et al.*, in preparation). Hsp90 is abundant (from 0.5% to 2% of soluble protein, depending on the tissue) and the presence of a small quantity in the nucleus would suffice to ensure interaction with steroid Rs (concentrations of receptors are 100- to 1000-fold lower than that of hsp90). However, the mere presence of immunoreactive Rs and hsp90 in nuclei, while necessary for our hypothesis, does not prove the occurrence of 8S-Rs that contain hsp90.

Even if they are intrinsic nuclear proteins, 8S-Rs are found in the low-salt cytosol after homogenization of target cells which have not been exposed to hormone; they can also be demonstrated in the cytosol, at 0–4°C, under isotonic conditions (e.g. in 0.15 mol/l KCl) (Joab *et al.*, 1984). The complexes are stabilized by oxyanions – molybdate ions (Dahmer *et al.*, 1984); tungstate ions (Nishigori and Toft, 1980) – or cross-linking agents (Aranyi *et al.*, 1988; Fig. 3A; Rexin *et al.*, 1988). It was found that the binding of hormone agonists, increased temperature, and/or increased ionic strength favor the 8S to 4S transformation (see reviews in Milgrom, 1981; Eriksson and Gustafsson, 1983); the hormone-dependent transformation of Rs from 8S to 4S forms occurs more rapidly as the temperature increases (Mougdil *et al.*, 1985; Denis *et al.*, 1988). *In vitro* it is possible to transform the 8S-Rs into 4S-Rs subunits,

$$\underset{8S}{(R,\ hsp)} \overset{\pm H}{\longleftrightarrow} \underset{H\text{-}8S}{(H\text{-}R,\ hsp)} \longleftrightarrow \underset{H\text{-}8S^{+}}{(H\text{-}R^{+},\ hsp)} \overset{hsp}{\longleftrightarrow} \underset{H\text{-}4S^{+}}{H\text{-}R^{+}} \longrightarrow \underset{H\text{-}4S^{*}}{H\text{-}R^{*}}$$

Fig. 4 Series of reactions leading from the inactive, hetero-oligomeric 8S receptor to active hormone–receptor complexes. The stoichiometry of R and hsp90 in the 8S-R is not indicated (see text). The plus sign indicates that there is some activation of the receptor within the 8S complex (Redeuilh *et al.*, 1987). The asterisk indicates that the receptor is now in a form that is either biologically active or inactive, but in both cases unable to reassociate with hsp90.

even in the absence of hormone, by increasing the ionic strength (e.g. with 0.3–0.4 mol/l KCl) at low temperature (Yang *et al.*, 1982). *In vitro*, transformed receptors, whether devoid of ligand or bound to hormone or antihormone, can bind identically to hormone-response elements (Willmann and Beato, 1986; Bailly *et al.*, 1986). However, no direct demonstration that hormone-free 4S-R has biological activity has yet been provided. Indirect evidence strongly suggests that, in target cells, the hormone–4S-R complexes are biologically active (see review in Yamamoto, 1985; Corthesy *et al.*, 1988).

A number of studies favor the possibility that the 8S-R represents the physiological structure of receptors in target cells in the absence of hormone (Mendel *et al.*, 1986, 1987), in particular, studies in which the stabilizing effects of RU 486 are exploited (Lefebvre *et al.*, 1988), protein labelling (Mendel and Orti, 1988; Howard and Distelhorst, 1988), and cross-linking of proteins in intact cells (Rexin *et al.*, 1988). We believe that the hormone-induced dissociation of hsp90–receptor complexes is reversible (Fig. 4), as has been shown with ER (Rochefort and Baulieu, 1971; Sabbah *et al.*, 1987; Redeuilh, unpublished data). It may be more difficult to demonstrate this reversibility with the GR, which is highly unstable after the release of hsp90 (Leach *et al.*, 1979). It is not known whether, after release of 4S-R from the 8S structure, there is further reversible or irreversible transformation related to the activity and/or inactivation of the receptor (Fig. 4; *R). Futhermore, we interpret the constitutive activity of receptors devoid of the ligand-binding domain (see Fig. 1; Hollenberg *et al.*, 1987; Kumar *et al.*, 1987) as an indication of hsp90–receptor interaction in cells (as discussed in the next section).

Interactions of hsp90 with ligand-binding (LBD) and DNA-binding (DBD) domains of steroid receptors

In all tested organs and species, cytosol 8S-Rs include at least one molecule of hsp90. The remarkable evolutionary conservation of hsp90s is demonstrated by comparison of nucleotide sequences obtained from different species (Binart *et al.*, 1989). The results of experiments in which heterospecific receptors (human GR, human ER, and chick PR) were introduced into receptor-negative/poor cells (monkey, hamster and yeast, and human, respectively; Pratt *et al.*, 1988; Greene *et al.*, 1986; Gronemeyer *et al.*, 1987; Chambon, personal communication) suggest that transfected receptors bind endogenous and, therefore, heterologous hsp90s. This result provides the premise for the suggestion that receptors for steroid hormones function via a common mechanism in all species.

In order to define which domain(s) of steroid receptors is (are) involved in the formation of complexes with hsp90, we performed transfection experiments using plasmids that encode wild-type and mutated GR and ER (Hollenberg *et al.*, 1987; Kumar *et al.*, 1987). After transfection of GR-specific cDNAs that lack LBDs (mutants 532* and 532-597 in Hollenberg *et al.*, 1987), no 8S-GR was found, and the receptor was in a 4S form (Pratt *et al.*, 1988). The same result was obtained with the HE15 and HE21 plasmids (Kumar *et al.*, 1987), which carry the gene for an estrogen receptor devoid of a steroid-binding region (Chambraud, unpublished data). Thus, we propose that there is binding of hsp90 to the LBD of normal GR and ER (see Fig. 1).

In the course of transfection experiments, some differences in hsp90–DBD interactions were observed when the GR and ER were compared. After transfection of cDNA that lacked DBD (Pratt *et al.*, 1988), the GR expressed in COS cells is in the 8S form – the initially reported instability is probably related to the increased susceptibility of mutated GR to proteolysis (Cadepond and Groyer-Schweizer, unpublished data). Similarly, under the same conditions as those in which the GR–DBD appears to play a very minor role in the stability of 8S-R, we have observed that ER without DBD (HE4 in Kumar *et al.*, 1987) also is found in 8S form (Chambraud, unpublished data). Transfection experiments with mutated receptors only give indirect evidence for the regions involved and provide correlation with transcriptional activity. The receptor may normally need a specific conformation for binding to hsp90. We also have observed that certain deletions in the DBD of GR can modify the steroid-binding properties of the LBD (Cadepond and Groyer-Schweizer, unpublished data). It has been confirmed biochemically that GR–LBD can bind hsp90, since complexes containing LBD–hsp90 have been obtained after selective proteolysis of the 8S-GR (cited in Denis *et al.*, 1988; Fig. 3C). Results of transfection experiments with GR and ER (to be published), as well as the demonstration of the 8S-form of the nt_i mutant of GR, which is devoid of the N-terminal end of GR, indicate that the N-terminal portion of receptors probably does not play an important role in formation of the 8S form (Gehring and Arndt, 1985; Fig. 3B).

Other data may be discussed in the context of interactions between receptors and hsp90. Cloning and determination of the nucleotide sequence revealed a region A of 70 amino acids in chick and other hsp90s (Fig. 5) which

	K	K	K	K	K
	N	N	N	N	N
	L	L	L	L	L
285	E	E	E	E	E
284	E	E	E	E	E
	E	Q	Q	D	I
282	D	D	D	E	E
	I	I	I	T	Q
	Y	Y	Y	Y	V
	L	K	K	K	E
278	E	E	E	E	E
	K	K	K	K	K
	I	I	I	I	V
	K	K	K	-	K
	K	K	K	-	K
	-	T	T	T	T
	K	K	K	K	K
	K	K	K	K	P
	K	K	K	K	K
	K	K	K	K	K
	-	-	-	A	-
	D	D	D	D	-
	G	K	K	K	-
	D	G	G	D	-
	K	S	S	K	-
	K	D	D	K	-
264	E	D	D	D	E
	E	E	E	A	E
	E	E	E	D	E
	E	-	-	E	E
260	D	D	D	D	D
	S	S	S	E	-
	G	G	G	G	-
	V	V	V	V	V
	D	D	D	D	E
255	E	E	E	E	E
	I	I	I	I	L
	E	K	K	K	K
→ 252	P	P	P	P	P
	K	K	K	-	K
	D	E	E	E	K
	E	E	E	D	D
	T	X	D	T	D
	-	E	D	E	E
	K	K	K	M	D
	-	D	D	-	K
	-	X	E	-	K
246	E	E	E	E	E
	E	E	E	-	E
	K	K	K	K	D
	E	E	E	K	K
	E	G	G	E	-
	K	K	K	D	K
	E	E	E	G	E
	E	E	E	E	E
	E	E	E	K	D
	K	-	-	K	K
	-	-	-	-	K
	E	-	-	E	E
	E	-	-	D	E
	-	-	-	D	-
	A	A	A	A	-
233	E	E	E	E	E
	D	D	D	D	P
	D	D	D	D	I
	S	S	S	S	P
	V	I	I	V	V
	E	E	E	E	E
	K	K	K	K	K
	D	E	E	E	E
	R	R	R	R	V
	E	X	E	E	E
	K	K	K	K	K
	E	E	E	E	T
	V	L	L	V	V
	221	205	217	210	209
	CHICK	MOUSE	HUMAN	DROSO	YEAST

Fig. 5 Conservation of negative charges in the A region of five hsp90s (numbers refer to the first amino acid of the region; in the mouse sequence, X indicates an undetermined amino acid). Conserved, negatively charged amino acids are represented by bold-faced letters (underlined numbers in the chick hsp90) (Binart *et al.*, submitted).

is highly charged, with a predominance of negatively charged residues (Binart *et al.*, 1989). Predictions of possible structures suggest two α helices separated by a proline turn. Carboxyl groups of nine of the negatively charged amino acids, fully conserved throughout all species examined, can be aligned with the phosphate groups of a segment of a B-DNA double helix, as indicated by computer-assisted, three-dimensional modeling (Binart *et al.*, 1989; Levin and Garnier, 1988; Fig. 6). We propose that the A region interacts with the DBD of steroid receptors, particularly at the level of the positively charged amino acids present in the second Zn-finger and the C-terminal region of the DBD. Experimental results are compatible with this hypothesis. An antibody raised against the A region of hsp90, which recognizes free hsp90, does not bind to hsp90 when it is included in 8S-PR (Catelli *et al.*, 1988). Similarly, an antibody against a sequence of amino acids that corresponds to the second finger of the chick PR, while able to bind to 4S-PR, does not bind to the 8S-PR (Smith *et al.*, 1988). It is difficult to assess the part played by ionic bonds in the formation and stability of 8S-Rs, and there are probably differences between receptors – molybdate-stabilized 8S-ER dissociates more easily in a milieu of high ionic strength than does chick 8S-PR (Redeuilh *et al.*, 1981). However, bonds other than ionic ones are probably involved and may obscure the electrostatic characteristics of interactions between DBD and hsp90.

Hsp90 in 8S-receptors: functional aspects

From the previous discussion, it appears that the role of hsp90 in receptor physiology could be to cap, and thus mask, the DBD of the receptor in its DNA-non-binding 8S form. In the absence of hormone, hsp90 would be a negative regulator of DNA-binding receptors, since, in preventing binding of receptors to HREs, it would presumably preclude biological activity. We suggest that the attachment of hsp90 to the LBD is critical for the favorable positioning of hsp90, in order to direct the interaction of the A region of hsp90 with the DBD of the receptor. The remarkable correlation between the constitutive activity of truncated LBD-negative receptors (Hollenberg *et al.*, 1987; Kumar *et al.*, 1987; Godowski *et al.*, 1987; Adler *et al.*, 1988) with the absence of formation of the 8S-complex in transfection experiments (Pratt *et al.*, 1988; Chambraud, in preparation) is an important argument in favor of our hypothesis. Binding of the hsp90 to LBD could also explain: (1) why chimeras of LBD and DNA-binding (Gal4 or LexA) or transcription regulatory (E1A) elements (not all of the Zn-finger type; Webster *et al.*, 1988; Picard *et al.*, 1988; Godowski *et al.*, 1988) are inactive in the absence of hormone (the ionic interaction with hsp90 being, probably, relatively non-specific); and (2) how they are activated by the proper steroid ligand (activation would involve release of hsp90).

Pharmacological results obtained with RU 486, an antiglucocorticosteroid and antiprogesterone steroid (see reviews in Baulieu and Segal, 1984) are compatible with our model. When cytosol GR or PR binds RU 486 instead of

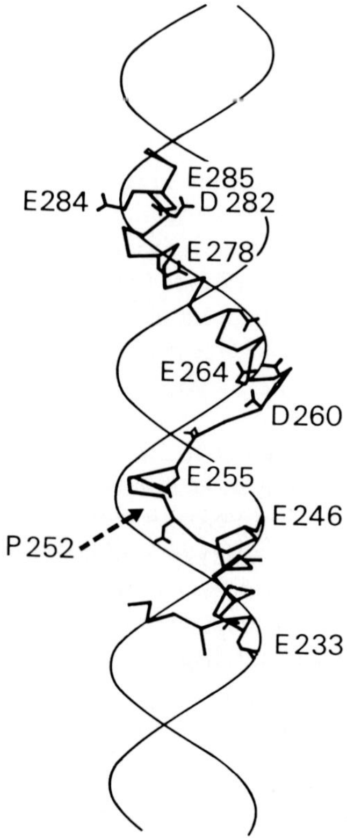

Fig. 6 Sketch of the segment 228–290 of zone A of chick hsp90. The model of the segment was generated with the graphic system PS 390 of Evans and Sutherland and the MANOSK program. Segment 228–232, predicted with a low probability as helical, was modeled as a coil. Phi and psi angles of the loop region were manually adjusted in order to obtain the fitting of a maximum of negatively charged residues to the phosphate backbone (continuous double-helical line) of a B-DNA structure. During the fitting, the two α helices (amino acids 233–247 and 261–287) were considered as rigid bodies. Only the α-carbon of the polypeptide backbone and the negatively charged side-chains are represented (chi angles of -50, 180, 180 and -50, 156 for Glu and Asp residues, respectively). The numbered residues are the nine most conserved negative amino acids between the five species; they are aligned with the DNA phosphate groups (Binart *et al.*, 1988).

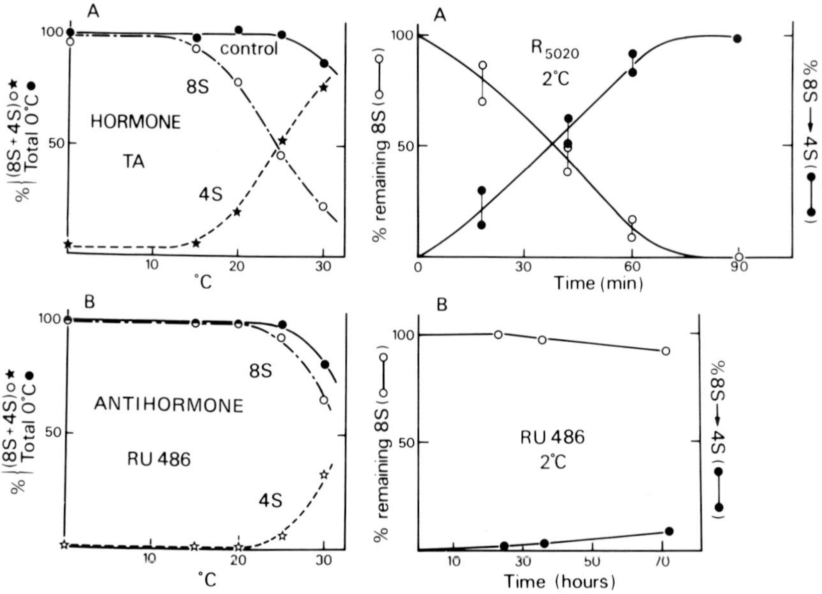

Fig. 7 Effect of binding of RU 486 on transformations of 8S–GR (left) and 8S–PR (right) transformation to their 4S forms (B), compared to the effects of agonists (A). (TA, triamcinolone acetonide; R_{5020}, progestin (Groyer *et al.*, 1987; Renoir *et al.*, 1989a).)

the corresponding agonist, the 8S to 4S transition is significantly impeded (Fig. 7), even if the 8S to 4S transformation is stimulated by increasing the temperature or the concentration of KCl (Groyer *et al.*, 1987; Renoir *et al.*, 1989a). The difference between the kinetics of transformation of agonist- and antagonist-bound 8S-Rs may explain an aspect of the antagonistic activity of RU 486 at the receptor level. DNA of the glucocorticoid responsive element (GRE) in the TAT promoter is not protected from chemical methylation in HTC cells exposed to RU 486 (Becker *et al.*, 1986) or cultured in the absence of glucocorticosteroid, in contrast to the protection apparently provided by agonist–receptor complexes. The lack of protection may be due to the DBD-capping activity of hsp90 (Fig. 8A). It has recently been suggested that, in intact cells, RU 486-GR (Webster *et al.*, 1988) or RU 486-PR (Bailly *et al.*, 1989) complexes, while being biologically inactive, can bind to the corresponding HRE. In Figure 8B, we indicate that such a possibility does not exclude the hsp90-mediated mechanism of receptor function: binding of hsp90 to receptor may be conserved (or even reinforced), even if the antagonist-induced transconformation of LBD would lead to a weakening of hsp90–DBD interaction; the complex of the hsp90–RU 486-receptor would not, however, be able to induce transcription (because of interference with the function of

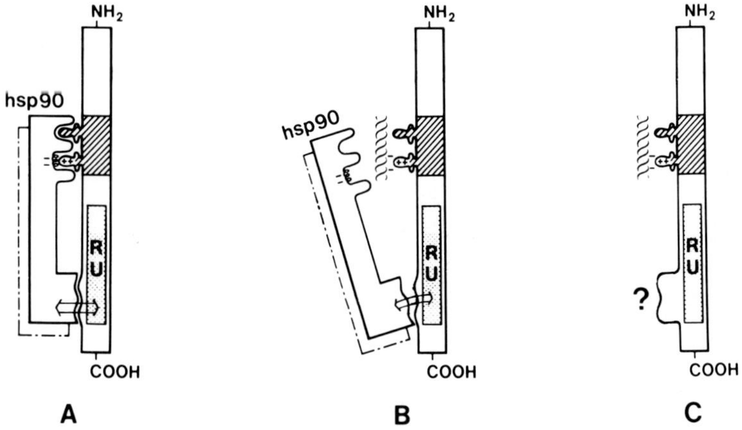

Fig. 8 Mechanism of action of an antisteroid hormone mechanism at the receptor level: three possible models. (A) Stabilization of receptor–hsp90 interactions (Groyer *et al.*, 1987). (B) Hsp90–LBD binding is maintained, but the DBD of the receptor is available for binding to DNA of the hormone-response element (Webster *et al.*, 1988; Bailly *et al.*, 1988). (C) Release of hsp90, availability of the DBD for binding to DNA, and transconformation of the receptor, precluding any effect on transcription. (RU, antisteroid hormone RU 486.)

transcription factors). We are aware that the stabilization of 8S-PR or 8S-GR by binding of RU 486 may not be the only mechanism of antihormone action, and that other antihormones may act by a different mechanism; for example, binding of antihormone to LBD may induce a transconformation of the receptor (Fig. 8C) which would impede efficient interaction of the receptor with other components of the gene transcription machinery, in contrast to the effect of an agonist.

In summary, capping of DBD, whether by ionic bonding or other interactions, and/or steric hindrance can be considered as a putative mechanism by which hsp90 could affect binding of receptor to HRE and, consequently, the function of the receptor. Binding of hsp90 to LBD would permit the proper positioning of hsp90, preventing binding by the receptor to DNA. Hormone agonists would trigger the response, through binding to LBD, and the subsequent release of hsp90. Differences between agonistic and antagonistic functions may also be interpreted at this level.

Stoichiometry of the complex of receptor and associated proteins

Hsp90 is found as a dimer, whether isolated from the large pool of cytoplasmic hsp90 or released from purified 8S-R (Radanyi *et al.*, 1989). We do not know whether or not hsp90 is a dimer within the 8S–PR or 8S–GR complexes since, experimentally, only one molecule of hsp90-specific monoclonal antibody BF_4 can be bound to hsp90, regardless of whether the latter is free or included in 8S-Rs. Thus, we cannot exclude the possibility that the 8S-R contains a single molecule of hsp90, which, upon release from 8S-R, may combine with another hsp90 molecule to produce a dimer. Originally, we proposed that the 8S–PR (Renoir *et al.*, 1984) and 8S–GR (Idziorek, unpublished data) contain one molecule of receptor and two molecules of hsp90, and this proposal has been confirmed for the GR (Mendel and Orti, 1988; Denis *et al.*, 1987). Our evidence for both 8S–GR and 8S–PR is based on the densitometric scanning of stained electrophoretic gels and on the specific activity of purified 8S-R for chick PR, with one binding site per 250 kDa, explainable by molecular weights of 100 kDa for the steroid-binding protein and 180 kDa for the non-steroid-binding components (two molecules of hsp90). The issue is different with the 8-9S–ER (Sabbah *et al.*, 1987; Redeuilh *et al.*, 1987), since we demonstrated that it includes two molecules of ER in the hsp90-containing 8-9S form. That the original inactive forms of PR and GR also include two molecules of receptor and two of hsp90 is not excluded, since one molecule of receptor may be lost during the purification process, and the GR (Wrange *et al.*, 1988), like the ER (Kumar and Chambon, 1988; Sabbah *et al.*, 1989), may possibly be active in a dimeric form.

Another open question arises from the discovery that, in rabbit cytosol, a monoclonal antibody against a p59 protein interacts with 8S–PR and other 8S-Rs in the rabbit uterine cytosol (Tai *et al.*, 1986). This observation has been extended (Renoir *et al.*, unpublished data) to several other mammalian (human, calf) cytosol receptors (the monoclonal antibody does not react with chick and rat proteins). We have not previously detected p59 after SDS-polyacrylamide gel electrophoresis of purified 8S-R because, in the course of purification, there is an obligatory washing of the hormone-affinity column (Renoir *et al.*, 1986), which can remove p59 (unpublished data). Indeed, recent studies by immunoaffinity chromatography with an antibody against p59 have provided us with 8S-hetero-oligomeric receptors (rabbit PR and calf ER), which contain the p59 antigen in addition to hsp90 and the receptor itself (Renoir *et al.*, 1989b). It has been found also that, unlike the 4S-receptors, hsp90 binds p59 in accordance with the model represented in Figure 1. It has also been found that p59 is present in many types of cell, always in the nucleus (Gasc, unpublished data).

Two different forms of nuclear receptor

We suggest that there are two different forms of nuclear steroid receptors. In the absence of hormone, there is a nuclear, non-transformed form of steroid receptor, which always includes hsp90 (probably in a dimeric form), the steroid–DNA-binding unit(s), and possibly p59 (in cells where it is expressed)

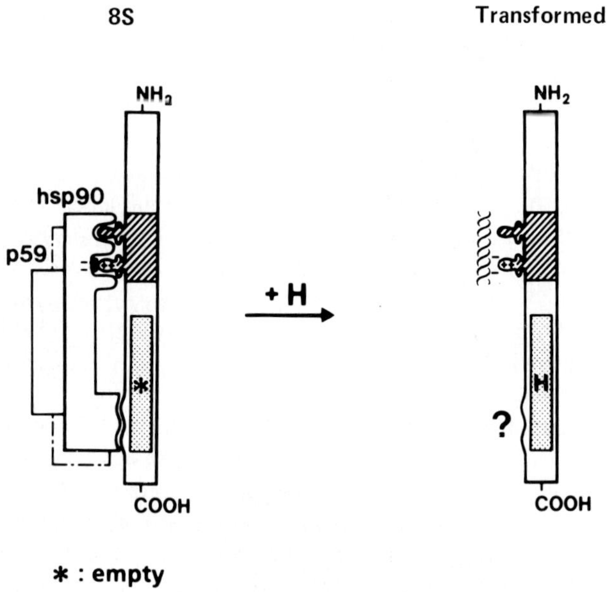

Fig. 9 Transformation/activation of a steroid hormone receptor. The diagram represents the non-active 8S-receptor, as in Figure 1, and the release of the active hormone–4S-receptor complex upon binding of the hormone (H). Whether there is further transconformation of the '4S-R' is not known. (* = empty.)

(see Fig. 1). This nuclear 8S form is inactive, but it is present in target cells prior to exposure to hormone; p59 may contribute to its nuclear location; it may be stabilized by binding of RU 486 in the case of the GR and PR. It differs from the nuclear, DNA-binding, transformed 4S form of the receptor (Fig. 9), which, after dissociation of the non-transformed receptor subsequent to binding of the agonist, is 'activated' and is, indeed, active at the transcriptional level.

Two functions may be ascribed to the binding of hsp90 to steroid receptors. First, in the absence of ligand, hsp90 may contribute to the stabilization of the receptor protein: a number of experiments indicate a greater resistance of receptors to chemicals or increased temperature in their 8S form, as opposed to their 4S form (Leach *et al.*, 1979; Buchou *et al.*, 1983; Aranyi *et al.*, 1988). This protective effect may also explain the longer half-life of the receptor in the absence than in the presence of hormone (Milgrom *et al.*, 1973; Read *et al.*, 1988). Secondly, binding of hsp90 would provide repression of receptor activity in the absence of hormone. The conformational change provoked by steroid binding would trigger the response to the hormone by bringing about the release of hsp90 and, thus, the receptor would be able to bind the HRE, an interaction that probably leads to appropriate changes in the chromatin (Archer *et al.*, 1989) and, eventually, a transcriptional response.

Further studies are currently underway in order to verify our hypothesis and to explore the possible physiological, pharmacological and pathological consequences of our model. The hsp90 hypothesis may explain how the DBD of steroid receptors is hidden and does not function in the absence of hormone and, conversely, how it becomes available for binding to DNA in a hormone-dependent manner. Hsp90 would function at the level of the DBD of receptor proteins. Correct positioning of hsp90, in order to cap the DBD, would be directed by binding of hsp90 to the LBD. The LBD, which binds the steroid, would provide, presumably through a conformational change, the response to the hormone with the release of hsp90. Hsp90 may, thus, provide an extramolecular mechanism involved in the control of the function of composite proteins such as steroid receptors. The remarkable functional tolerance of the structure of steroid receptors to topological changes (Evans, 1988) is an important argument in favor of the hsp90 mechanism. Whether this abundant heat-shock protein plays a similar role with other acidophilic proteins (including other transcription regulators) is unknown – however, interactions with a number of tyrosine protein kinases of viral oncogene origin, the eIF-2α kinase and F-actin have been described (reviewed in Pratt, 1987). It is proposed that, in the receptor molecule, LBD plays a signaling and transducing role, while DBD plays a functional (executive) role and hsp90 is an extrinsic repressor, released after binding of the hormone.

Acknowledgements

We are grateful to P. Leclerc and C. Legris for their help in preparing the manuscript and to J.C. Lambert for the illustrations. We thank M.C. Lebeau, H. Richard-Foy and P. Robel for their critical review of the text. We also thank M. Beato, P. Chambon, R. Evans, L. Faber, J. Greene, J.A. Gustafsson, C. Nolan and D. Toft for the gift of various biological materials.

References

Adler, S., Waterman, M.L., He, X. & Rosenfeld, M. (1988). **Cell** 52:685–695.

Aranyi, P., Radanyi, C., Renoir, J.M., Devin, J. & Baulieu, E.E. (1988). **Biochemistry** 27:1330–1336.

Archer, T.K., Cordingley, M.G., Marsaud, V., Richard-Foy, H. & Hager, G.L. (1989). In: Carlsedt-Duke, J., Eriksson, H. & Gustafsson, J.A., eds., **The Steroid/Thyroid Hormone Receptor Family and Gene Regulation**, Basel, Birkhäuser Verlag, pp.221–238.

Bailly, A., Guiochon-Mantel, A., Misrahi, M., Loosfelt, H., Atger, M., Savouret, J.F., Perrot-Applanat, M., Vu Hai, M.T., Rauch, M., Lorenzo, F., Logeat, F. & Milgrom, E. (1989). In: Carlstedt-Duke, J., Eriksson, H. & Gustafsson, J.A., eds., **The Steroid/Thyroid Hormone Receptor Family and Gene Regulation**, Basel, Birkhäuser Verlag, pp.271–279.

Bailly, A., Lepage, C., Rauch, M. & Milgrom, E. (1986). **Embo Journal** 5:3235–3241.
Baulieu, E.E. (1987). **Journal of Cell Biochemistry** 35:161–174.
Baulieu, E.E., Alberga, A., Jung, I., Lebeau, M.C., Mercier-Bodard, C., Milgrom, E., Raynaud, J.P., Raynaud-Jammet, C., Rochefort, H., Truong, H. & Robel, P. (1971). **Recent Progress in Hormone Research** 27:351–419.
Baulieu, E.E., Binart, N., Buchou, T., Catelli, M.G., Garcia, T., Gasc, J.M., Groyer, A., Joab, I., Montcharmont, B., Radanyi, C., Renoir, J.M., Tuohimaa, P. & Mester, J. (1983). In: Eriksson, H. & Gustafsson, J.A., eds. **Steroid Hormone Receptors: Structure and Function**, Amsterdam, Elsevier, pp.45–72.
Baulieu, E.E. & Catelli, M.G. (1988). In: Pardue, M.L., Feramisco, J.R. & Lindquist, S., eds. **Stress-Induced Proteins**, New York, Alan R. Liss, pp.203–219.
Baulieu, E.E. & Segal, S.J., eds. (1984). **The Antiprogestin Steroid RU486 and Human Fertility Control**, New York, Plenum Press.
Beato, M. (1987). **Biochemica et Biophysica Acta** 910:95–102.
Becker, P.B., Gloss, B., Schmid, W., Strähle, U. & Schitz, G. (1986). **Nature** 324:686–688.
Binart, N., Chambraud, B., Dumas, B., Rowlands, D.A., Bigogne, C., Levin, J.M., Garnier, J., Baulieu, E.E. & Catelli, M.G. (1989). **Biochemical and Biophysical Research Communications** 159:140–147.
Buchou, T., Mester, J., Renoir, J.M. & Baulieu, E.E. (1983). **Biochemical and Biophysical Research Communications** 114:479–487.
Catelli, M.G., Binart, N., Feramisco, J.R. & Helfman, D. (1985a). **Nucleic Acids Research** 13:6035–6047.
Catelli, M.G., Binart, N., Jung-Testas, I., Renoir, J.M., Baulieu, E.E., Feramisco, J.R. & Welch, W.J. (1985b). **Embo Journal** 4:3131–3135.
Catelli, M.G., Radanyi, C., Renoir, J.M., Binart, N. & Baulieu, E.E. (1988). **UCLA Symposium on Stress-Induced Proteins** April 10–16, Keystone, Abstract no. 304, p.276.
Collier, N.C. & Schlesinger, M.J. (1986). **Journal of Cell Biology** 103:1495–1507.
Corthesy, B., Hipskind, R., Theulaz, I. & Wahli, W. (1988). **Science** 239:1137–1139.
Dahmer, M.K., Housley, P.R. & Pratt, W.B. (1984). **Annual Review of Physiology** 46:67–81.
Denis, M., Wikström, A.C. & Gustafsson, J.A. (1987). **Journal of Biological Chemistry** 262:11803–11806.
Denis, M., Poellinger, L., Wikström, A.C. & Gustafsson, J.A. (1988). **Nature** 333:686–688.
Dougherty, J.J., Puri, R.K. & Toft, D.O. (1984). **Journal of Biological Chemistry** 259:8004–8009.
Edelman, I.S., Bogoroch, R. & Porter, G.A. (1963). **Proceedings of the National Academy of Sciences, USA** 50:1169–1177.
Eriksson, H. & Gustafsson, J.A., eds. (1983). **Steroid Hormone Receptors: Structure and Function** Amsterdam, Elsevier.
Evans, R.M. (1988). **Science** 240:889–895.
Gasc, J.M., Ennis, B.W., Baulieu, E.E. & Stumpf, W.E. (1983). **Comptes Rendus de l'Academie des Sciences de Paris** 297:477–482.
Gasc, J.M., Delahaye, F. & Baulieu, E.E. (1989). **Experimental Cell Research** 181:492–504.
Gehring, U. & Arndt, H. (1985). **FEBS Letters** 179:138–142.
Godowski, P.J., Picard, D. & Yamamoto, K.R. (1988). **Science** 241:812–816.

Godowski, P.J., Rusconi, S., Miesfield, R. & Yamamoto, K.R. (1987). **Nature** 325:365–368.

Greene, G.L., Gilna, P., Waterfield, N., Becker, A., Hort, Y. & Shine, J. (1986). **Science** 231:1150–1154.

Gronemeyer, H., Turcotte, B., Quirin-Stricker, C., Bocquel, M.T., Meyer, M.E., Krozowski, Z., Jeltsch, J.M., Lerouge, T., Garnier, J. & Chambon, P. (1987). **Embo Journal** 6:3985–3994.

Groyer, A., Le Bouc, Y., Joab, I., Radanyi, C., Renoir, J.M., Robel, P. & Baulieu, E.E. (1985). **European Journal of Biochemistry** 149:445–451.

Groyer, A., Schweizer-Groyer, G., Cadepond, F., Mariller, M. & Baulieu, E.E. (1987). **Nature** 8:624–626.

Gustafsson, J.A., Carlstedt-Duke, J., Poellinger, L., Okret, S., Wikstrom, A.C., Bronnegard, M., Gillner, M., Dong, Y., Fuxe, K., Cintra, A., Harfstrand, A. & Agnati, L. (1987). **Endocrine Reviews** 8:185–234.

Hollenberg, S.M., Giguere, V., Segui, P. & Evans, R.M. (1987). **Cell** 49:39–46.

Hollenberg, S.M., Weingerger, C., Ong, E.S., Cerelli, G., Oro, A., Lebo, R., Thompson, E.B., Rosenfeld, M.G. & Evans, R.M. (1985). **Nature** 318:635–641.

Howard, K.J. & Distelhorst, C.W. (1988). **Journal of Biological Chemistry** 263:3474–3481.

Joab, I., Radany, C., Renoir, J.M., Buchou, T., Catelli, M.G., Binart, N., Mester, J. & Baulieu, E.E. (1984). **Nature** 308:850–853.

Jungblut, P.W., Hätzel, I., De Sombre, E.R. & Jensen, E.V. (1967). In: Karlson, P., ed. **Wirkungs-mechanismen der Hormone**, Berlin, Springer Verlag, pp.58–86.

King, W.J. & Greene, G.L. (1984). **Nature** 307:745–747.

Kumar, V. & Chambon, P. (1988). **Cell** 55:145–156.

Leach, K.L., Dahmer, M.K., Hammond, N., Sando, J.J. & Pratt, W.B. (1979). **Journal of Biological Chemistry** 254:11884–11890.

Lefebvre, P., Formstecher, P., Richard, C. & Dautrevaux, M. (1988). **Biochemical and Biophysical Research Communications** 150:1221–1229.

Levin, J.M. & Garnier, J. (1988). **Biochemica et Biophysica Acta** 955:263–295.

Mendel, D.B., Bodwell, J.E., Gametchu, B., Harrisson, R.W. & Munck, A. (1986). **Journal of Biological Chemistry** 261:3758–3763.

Mendel, D.B. & Orti, E. (1988). **Journal of Biological Chemistry** 263:6695–6701.

Milgrom, E.E. (1981). In: Litwack, G., ed. **Biochemical Action of Hormones** Vol. VIII, New York, Academic Press, pp.466–491.

Milgrom, E., Luu Thi, M., Atger, M. & Baulieu, E.E. (1973). **Journal of Biological Chemistry** 248:6366–6374.

Mougdil, V.K., Eessalu, T.E., Buchou, T., Renoir, J.M., Mester, J. & Baulieu, E.E. (1985). **Endocrinology** 116:1267–1274.

Nishigori, H. & Toft, D. (1980). **Biochemistry** 19:77–83.

Perrot-Applanat, M., Logeat, F., Groyer-Picard, M.T. & Milgrom, E. (1985). **Endocrinology** 116:1473–1484.

Picard, D., Salser, S.J. & Yamamoto, K.R. (1988). **Cell** 54:1073–1080.

Picard, D. & Yamamoto, K.R. (1987). **EMBO Journal** 6:3333–3340.

Pratt, W.B. (1987). **Journal of Cell Biochemistry** 35:51–68.

Pratt, W.B., Jolly, D.J., Pratt, D.V., Hollenberg, S.M., Giguere, V., Cadepond, F.M., Schweizer-Groyer, G., Catelli, M.G., Evans, R.M. & Baulieu, E.E. (1988). **Journal of Biological Chemistry** 263:267–273.

Radanyi, C., Joab, I., Renoir, J.M., Richard-Foy, H. & Baulieu, E.E. (1983).

Proceedings of the National Academy of Sciences, USA 80:2854–2858.
Rafestin-Oblin, M.E., Couette, B., Radanyi, C., Lombes, M. & Baulieu, E.E. (1989). **Journal of Biological Chemistry** 264:9304–9309.
Read, L.D., Snider, C.E., Miller, J.S., Greene, J.L. & Katzenellenbogen, B.S. (1988). **Molecular Endocrinology** 2.263–271.
Redeuilh, G., Moncharmont, B., Secco, C. & Baulieu, E.E. (1987). **Journal of Biological Chemistry** 262:6969–6975.
Redeuilh, G., Secco, C., Baulieu, E.E. & Richard-Foy, H. (1981). **Journal of Biological Chemistry** 256:11496–11502.
Renoir, J.M., Buchou, T. & Baulieu, E.E. (1986). **Biochemistry** 25:6405–6413.
Renoir, J.M., Buchou, T., Mester, J., Radanyi, C. & Baulieu, E.E. (1984). **Biochemistry** 23:6016–6023.
Renoir, J.M., Radanyi, C. & Baulieu, E.E. (1989a). **Steroids** 53:1–20.
Renoir, J.M., Jung-Testas, I., Radanyi, C., Soltani, M., Awa, Y., Faber, L.E. & Baulieu, E.E. (1989b). **71st Meeting of the Endocrine Society**, Seattle, Washington, June 21–24, 1989, Abstract no. 992, p.270.
Rexin, M., Busch, W. & Gehring, U. (1988). **Biochemistry** 27:5593–5601.
Rochefort, H. & Baulieu, E.E. (1971). **Biochimie** 53:893–907.
Sabbah, M., Redeuilh, G. & Baulieu, E.E. (1989). **Journal of Biological Chemistry** 264:2397–2400.
Sabbah, M., Redeuilh, G., Secco, C. & Baulieu, E.E. (1987). **Journal of Biological Chemistry** 262:8631–8635.
Sanchez, E.R., Toft, D.O., Schlessinger, M.J. & Pratt, W.B. (1985). **Journal of Biological Chemistry** 260:12398–12401.
Schrader, W.T., Heuer, S.S. & O'Malley, B.W. (1975). **Biology of Reproduction** 12:134–142.
Schuh, S., Yonemoto, W., Brugge, J., Bauer, V.J., Riehl, R.M., Sullivan, W.P. & Toft, D.O. (1985). **Journal of Biological Chemistry** 260:14292–14296.
Sherman, M.R., Tuazon, F.B., Stevens, Y.W. & Niu, E.M. (1983). In: Eriksson, H. & Gustafsson, J.A., eds. **Steroid Hormone Receptors: Structure and Function**, Amsterdam, Elsevier, pp.3–24.
Smith, D.F., Lubahn, D.B., McCormick, D.J., Wilson, E.M. & Toft, D.O. (1988). **Endocrinology** 122:2816–2825.
Tai, P.K.K., Maeda, Y., Nakao, K., Wakim, N.G., Dugring, J.L. & Faber, L. (1986). **Biochemistry** 25:5269–5275.
Toft, D., Shyamala, G. & Gorski, J. (1967). **Proceedings of the National Academy of Sciences, USA** 57:1740.
Webster, N.J.G., Green, S., Jin, J.R. & Chambon, P. (1988). **Cell** 54:199–207.
Welshons, W.V., Lieberman, M.E. & Gorski, J. (1984). **Nature** 307:747–749.
Willmann, T. & Beato, M. (1986). **Nature** 324:688–690.
Wolfson, A. (1984). **Journal of Steroid Biochemistry** 21:519–521.
Wolfson, A., Mester, J., Yang, C.R. & Baulieu, E.E. (1980). **Biochemical and Biophysical Research Communications** 95:1577–1584.
Wrange, O., Eriksson, P. & Perlmann, T. (1988). **Symposium on the Steroid/Thyroid Hormone Receptor Family and Gene Regulation** November 4–5, Stockholm, Abstract no. 30, p.99.
Yamamoto, K.R. & Alberts, B.M. (1976). **Annual Review of Biochemistry** 45:721–746.
Yang, C.R., Mester, J., Wolfson, A., Renoir, J.M. & Baulieu, E.E. (1982). **Biochemical Journal** 208:399–406.

Hormonal control of gene expression in the ovary

J.S. RICHARDS

Department of Cell Biology, Baylor College of Medicine, Houston, Texas 77030, USA.

Keywords

P450 genes, cAMP, prostaglandin endoperoxide synthase, aromatase, estradiol, follicle, corpus luteum, theca cells, granulosa cells, differentiation.

Introduction

The biological challenge to be met by the mammalian ovary is to maintain the continuous development of small follicles and, at the same time, to allow other follicles to ovulate and become corpora lutea. The dynamics of this system are orchestrated by many interwoven processes which allow less than 1% of the total number of follicles contained within the ovary to ovulate. The key to the development of a follicle that succeeds in ovulating lies in the ability of that follicle to gain new functional capabilities. These new capabilities include the synthesis and action of estradiol in preovulatory follicles, which are combined with enhanced production of cAMP in response to gonadotropins and the induction of specific proteins in response to cAMP (Richards, 1980; Hsueh *et al.*, 1984; Richards *et al.*, 1987b; Richards and Hedin, 1988). Some of the proteins known to be regulated by cAMP during the development of preovulatory follicles, ovulation and luteinization are summarized in Figure 1. These proteins have been categorized according to the cell type (theca, granulosa and lutea) in which they appear and the functional domains (response system, steroidogenesis, ovulation, and peptide synthesis) that they control. Note, in particular, that cAMP regulates the synthesis of many proteins in theca cells and granulosa cells of preovulatory follicles but has little known effect on these same, or other, proteins in luteal tissue.

From these observations we propose that the transition from the follicular to the luteal stage of differentiation marks an abrupt shift from gonadotropic hormone-dependent and cAMP-dependent regulation of follicular cell function to cAMP-independent regulation of the corpus luteum (Fig. 2). This transition is induced by the luteinizing hormone (LH) surge and elevated levels of intracellular cAMP and only occurs in preovulatory follicles. The molecular mechanisms underlying these changes in cell function remain to be clearly defined. A schematic representation of the molecular events that occur in theca cells and granulosa cells of preovulatory follicles is shown in Figure 3. This model provides a conceptual framework to which we can refer as we discuss the tissue- and hormone-specific regulation of several genes during follicular

	Theca cells	Granulosa cells	Luteal cells
Response system	LH receptor Adenylyl cyclase RIIβ ($RII_{51/52}$)	LH receptor Adenylyl cyclase RIIβ ($RII_{51/52}$)	LH receptor Adenylyl cyclase
Steroido-genesis	$P450_{scc}$ $P450_{17\alpha}$	$P450_{scc}$ $P450_{arom}$	
Ovulation		Plasminogen activators Prostaglandin synthase	
Peptides	TGF_{β}	Inhibin IGF-1	

Fig. 1 Proteins regulated by cAMP in the rat ovary.

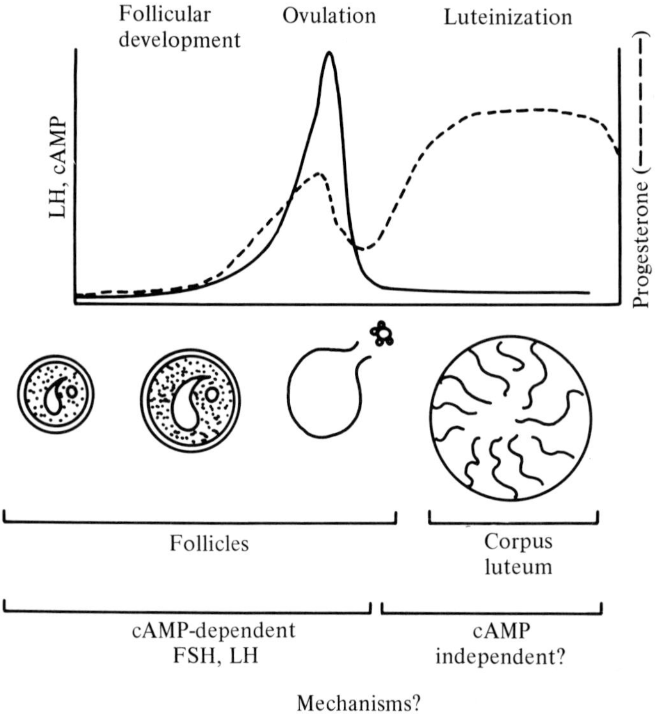

Fig. 2 Schematic diagram of follicular development, ovulation and luteinization: shift from cAMP-dependent to cAMP-independent mechanisms.

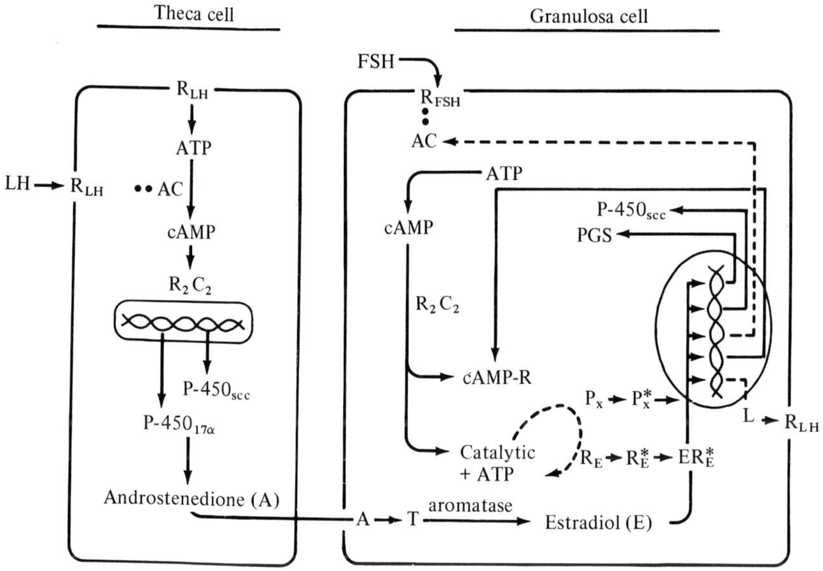

Fig. 3 Schematic representation of the molecular events that coordinate the actions of estradiol, FSH and LH in theca and granulosa cells of preovulatory follicles. LH acts on theca cells via cAMP to regulate levels of mRNA for both $P450_{scc}$ and $P450_{17\alpha}$, leading to increased biosynthesis of androstenedione. The mechanisms by which cAMP acts in theca cells remain to be determined but appear to involve an increase in the levels of RIIβ, $P450_{scc}$, and $P450_{17\alpha}$. In granulosa cells, androstenedione is converted to estradiol by the aromatase P450 enzyme system. Estradiol, in turn, binds to estradiol receptors (R_E) in granulosa cells and may thereby regulate gene expression. However, despite the presence of estradiol and estradiol receptors, little or no effect of estradiol is observed unless FSH acts via the FSH receptor to increase intracellular concentrations of cAMP. In a manner not yet understood, cAMP appears to enhance the actions of estradiol. The action of estradiol may be enhanced by cAMP-dependent phosphorylation of the estradiol receptor (R_E*), since recent cloning of the estradiol receptor has revealed putative sites for cAMP-dependent phosphorylation. Alternatively, increased levels of cAMP may lead to the phosphorylation of other trans-acting regulatory proteins (P_x – P_x*) which, in conjunction with the estradiol receptor, increase the rate of transcription of the LH receptor, adenylyl cyclase components, RII_β, PGS, $P450_{scc}$, and $P450_{arom}$. It is also possible that one or more of the trans-acting regulatory proteins which are phosphorylated by cAMP-dependent protein kinase is induced by estradiol or by the sequential actions of estradiol and cAMP. Such a mechanism would explain the developmental changes that occur in granulosa cells in response to the same signal, cAMP.

development and luteinization. The genes to be analyzed include: RII_β, the regulatory subunit of cAMP-dependent protein kinase type II, aromatase cytochrome P450 ($P450_{arom}$), cholesterol side-chain cleavage cytochrome P450 ($P450_{scc}$), 17α-hydroxylase cytochrome P450 ($P450_{17\alpha}$) and prostaglandin endoperoxide synthase (PGS).

Results and discussion

Cyclic AMP-dependent protein kinases

As already mentioned, the development of preovulatory follicles is associated with enhanced responsiveness to gonadotropins, which is mediated, in part, by induction of receptors for luteinizing hormone (Richards, 1980; Richards and Bogovich, 1982; Richards *et al.*, 1987) and by enhanced activation of adenylyl cyclase (Jonassen *et al.*, 1982). The latter process may involve an increase in the stimulatory, alpha subunit of adenylyl cyclase $G_{\alpha s}$ (Richards and Hedin, 1988). Granulosa and theca cells of preovulatory follicles are also associated with a marked increase in the content of RII_β (RII_{51}; mol. wt = 51 000), the regulatory subunit of cAMP-dependent protein kinase type II (Richards and Rolfes, 1980). This RII_β subunit has been shown to be structurally and immunologically similar to the RII subunit found in rat and bovine brain (Jahnsen *et al.*, 1985, 1986a, 1986b) but is distinct from RII_α (RII_{54}; mol. wt = 54 000), the R subunit characteristic of rat and bovine heart (Jahnsen *et al.*, 1986a, 1986b).

Recent studies have shown that the increase in subunit content of RII_β is associated with an increase in RII_β mRNA in theca and granulosa cells of preovulatory follicles (Hedin *et al.*, 1987a). The increase in levels of RII_β subunits and mRNA in granulosa cells has been shown *in vivo* and *in vitro* to be dependent on the synergistic actions of estradiol and follicle-stimulating hormone (FSH)/cAMP (Richards and Rolfes, 1980; Ratoosh and Richards, 1985; Ratoosh *et al.*, 1987) and is mediated, in part, by increased transcription of the RII_β gene (Hedin *et al.*, 1987a).

As a consequence of the LH surge and in association with follicular cell luteinization, levels of RII_β subunit (Richards and Kirchick, 1984) and mRNA (Hedin *et al.*, 1987a) decline rapidly and remain low in functional corpora lutea of pregnancy (Hedin *et al.*, 1987a) and in luteinized cells in culture (our unpublished data). Thus, the transition of the follicle from a cAMP-dependent structure to a cAMP-independent tissue is associated with a specific decrease in the level of the cAMP binding, regulatory subunit of protein kinase.

These observations reveal an underlying paradox. The regulatory subunit acts in the holoenzyme to inhibit kinase activity of the catalytic (C) subunit. cAMP mediates dissociation of the enzyme and activation of the free C subunit. Therefore, why is the level of the RII_β subunit increased in preovulatory follicles when these cells appear most responsive to gonadotropins and cAMP? Conversely, why is transcription of RII_β mRNA turned off as a consequence of the LH surge and luteinization when cells appear to lose responsiveness to cAMP? It is possible that changes in the R subunit represent a biochemical feedback mechanism designed to ensure that the catalytic subunit remains under strict regulation by the R subunit. Accordingly, an increase in cAMP would lead to increased synthesis of the R subunit. This increased synthesis would prevent inappropriate activation of the catalytic subunit in the absence of cAMP. In the ovarian follicle, this mechanism may represent an important way in which the follicle synchronizes specific cAMP-mediated events – such as ovulation and luteinization – and it may ensure that these events do not occur prematurely but only in response to the LH surge and markedly increased concentrations of intracellular cAMP. Although data obtained in previous studies do not support the notion that the induction of RII_{β} is associated with a marked shift in the cAMP-mediated dose– response activation of protein kinase (Richards *et al.*, 1984), the hypothesis remains attractive. Transfection studies using an RII_{β} expression vector will provide a useful approach for the re-examination of this question in greater detail. Recent transfection studies using mutant forms of RI have demonstrated that overexpression of a dominant mutant phenotype can inhibit cAMP-mediated activation of kinase activity and lead to decreased responsiveness to cAMP (Clegg *et al.*, 1987).

Having described how changes in protein kinase occur in association with the transition of the follicle to the corpus luteum, we will next examine how this transition relates to changes in the expression of genes known to be regulated by cAMP in the follicle (Fig. 3) but not in the corpus luteum.

17α-Hydroxylase cytochrome P450

Recent purification (Nakajin and Hall, 1981), cloning (Zuber *et al.*, 1986a) and subsequent transfection studies (Zuber *et al.*, 1986b) have all elegantly shown that $P450_{17\alpha}$ is a single peptide which can perform two enzymatic functions, that of a 17α-hydroxylase and that of a $C_{17/20}$-lyase, which converts progesterone to androstenedione. Conversion of androstenedione to testosterone by 17-keto steroid reductase occurs in both theca cells and granulosa cells (Bogovich and Richards, 1981). Recent studies have shown that, unlike aromatase and $P450_{17\alpha}$, 17-keto steroid reductase appears to be a constitutive enzyme present in granulosa cells of all types of follicles including those present after hypophysectomy. On a per-follicle basis, there is more 17-keto steroid reductase in granulosa cells than in theca cells (Bogovich and Richards, 1981). This difference may ensure that most of the conversion of androstenedione to testosterone occurs close to the site of conversion of testosterone to estradiol, thereby minimizing circulating levels of active androgens.

The development of conditions for serum-free tissue culture of granulosa cells (Hsueh *et al.*, 1984) and for low-serum cultures of theca cells and granulosa cells (Richards *et al.*, 1986) has allowed clear documentation of the

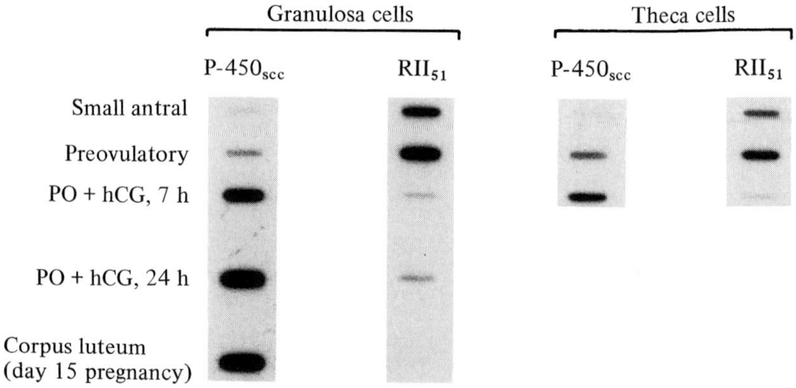

Fig. 4 Changes in levels of mRNA for RII_β and $P450_{scc}$ during follicular development and luteinization. (PO, preovulatory; hCG, human chorionic gonadotropin; RII_{51}, RII_β.)

two-cell theory of steroidogenesis (for review, see Richards, 1980). It has been shown that FSH or cAMP (in the presence of testosterone) can induce aromatase activity exclusively in granulosa cells (Armstrong and Dorrington, 1979; Hsueh *et al.*, 1984; Richards *et al.*, 1986) whereas LH induces 17α-hydroxylase cytochrome P450 ($P450_{17\alpha}$) activity in theca cells (Carson *et al.*, 1981; Erickson *et al.*, 1985; Richards *et al.*, 1986). From a number of different physiological studies (Bogovich and Richards, 1981; Carson *et al.*, 1981; Richards and Bogovich, 1982), it has been shown that slight increases in serum LH and stimulation by LH of the production of androgen are the rate-limiting factors that regulate the initial increase in the biosynthesis of estradiol in small antral follicles of the rat. For example, the rate of biosynthesis of androgen is increased in small antral follicles of immature or pregnant rats injected with low doses of human chorionic gonadotropin (hCG) twice daily for 2 days (Bogovich and Richards, 1981; Richards and Bogovich, 1982). Recent studies have shown that the increase in activity of follicular $P450_{17\alpha}$ is associated with increased levels of the enzyme in theca cells, as measured by immunoblots (Hedin *et al.*, 1987b; Rodgers *et al.*, 1986) using a $P450_{17\alpha}$-antibody (Nakajin and Hall, 1981), and by increased levels of $P450_{17\alpha}$ mRNA (Hedin *et al.*, 1987b), as measured by filter hybridization using a cDNA for $P450_{17\alpha}$ (Zuber *et al.*, 1986a).

As a consequence of the LH surge and the elevated level of cAMP, there is a rapid decrease in $P450_{17\alpha}$ activity (Eckstein and Tsafriri, 1986), the level of $P450_{17\alpha}$ as measured by immunoblots, and $P450_{17\alpha}$ mRNA (Hedin *et al.*, 1987b). Furthermore, high doses of LH/hCG or cAMP induce a rapid loss of $P450_{17\alpha}$ in follicles incubated *in vitro*. This loss can be partially inhibited by the

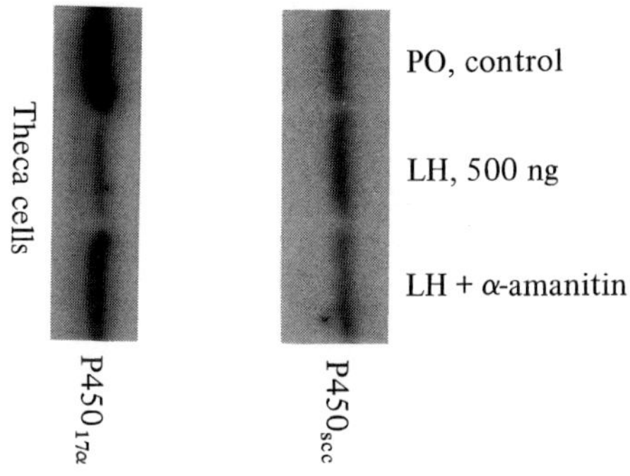

Fig. 5 Changes in levels of 17α-hydroxylase and aromatase in response to LH and α-amanitin. Follicles were incubated with LH (500 ng/ml) alone or in LH plus α-amanitin (25 μg/ml) for 5 hours. Granulosa cells were separated from theca cells and levels of enzymes were analyzed by immunoblotting with specific antibodies.

simultaneous addition of α-amanitin or cycloheximide to the culture medium (Fig. 5).

Taken together, these results indicate that low levels of LH act to increase levels of $P450_{17\alpha}$ in small antral to preovulatory follicles whereas the LH surge or elevated levels of cAMP rapidly inhibit synthesis of $P450_{17\alpha}$ by preovulatory follicles. Because both processes appear to be mediated by transcription of the $P450_{17\alpha}$ gene, two sites (mechanisms?) of regulation by cAMP of the transcription of the $P450_{17\alpha}$ gene must be involved. This biphasic regulation of cytochrome $P450_{17\alpha}$ by LH in theca cells represents a physiological pattern unique to the ovary (as compared to the adrenal and testis) and is not mimicked by other microsomal enzymes (HMG CoA reductase) or mitochondrial enzymes (cytochrome $P450_{scc}$ and adrenodoxin) involved in follicular steroidogenesis (Hedin *et al.*, 1987b; Goldring *et al.*, 1987). However, this biphasic pattern is reminiscent of that observed for the hormonal regulation of RII_β protein and mRNA in theca cells and granulosa cells (described above). The molecular factors mediating the effects of high versus low levels of LH/cAMP in theca cells remain to be resolved.

The LH-mediated loss of $P450_{17\alpha}$ in luteinized theca does not, however, appear to be an irreversible process of differentiation. Preovulatory theca, isolated 7 hours after an ovulatory dose of hCG (at a time when the levels of $P450_{17\alpha}$ protein and mRNA are already reduced) (Hedin *et al.*, 1987b) and placed in tissue culture, not only regain their ability to synthesize androgens but do so for as long as 30 days, even in the absence of LH or agents such as forskolin that increase levels of cAMP (Richards *et al.*, 1986). These same theca also produce large amounts of progesterone for 30 days in culture in the absence of hormones or cAMP. Thus, theca cells, as well as granulosa cells, appear to luteinize – and they appear to maintain their steroidogenic capacity in a constitutive manner.

Although prolactin (PRL) has previously been shown to inhibit the production of androgen by dispersed ovarian cells in serum free cultures (Erickson *et al.*, 1985), it had little or no effect on the biosynthesis of androgen by more purified thecal explants (Hedin *et al.*, 1987b). Therefore, the loss of $P450_{17\alpha}$ and continued low production of androgens by corpora lutea *in situ* may involve the action of PRL on cells other than theca cells.

Aromatase cytochrome P450

In contrast to $P450_{17\alpha}$, aromatase cytochrome P450 (P450) has been localized exclusively to granulosa cells of rat ovarian follicles and its levels are modulated by FSH in the presence of low amounts of androgen (Richards, 1980; Hsueh *et al.*, 1984; Richards *et al.*, 1987a). Antibodies against purified human placental $P450_{arom}$ (Evans *et al.*, 1986), as well as a 62-mer deoxyoligonucleotide probe synthesized from amino acid sequence information derived from peptide cleavage products (Chen *et al.*, 1986), have been used to isolate cDNA clones for the human placental enzyme (Evans *et al.*, 1986, Chen *et al.*, 1988) and the rat ovarian enzyme (Richards *et al.*, 1987a; Hickey *et al.*, 1988).

Using a rat 1.2-kb cDNA clone, we have shown that mRNA for aromatase is induced in granulosa cells of preovulatory follicles; its level is transiently reduced during early stages of luteinization and is then markedly increased in corpora lutea isolated on days 15–21 of gestation (Hickey *et al.*, 1989). These changes in the amount of mRNA are associated with corresponding changes in the amount of the enzyme measured by immunoblot analyses using rabbit IgG raised against human placental aromatase (Fig. 6). Increased levels of enzyme in preovulatory follicles were also associated with a dramatic increase in the ability of follicles to synthesize estradiol from endogenous or exogenous androgen substrates. Unexpectedly, although the amount of aromatase in corpora lutea isolated on days 15–21 of gestation was five- to tenfold greater than that in the preovulatory follicle (Hickey *et al.*, 1989), the rate of synthesis of estradiol by these corpora lutea incubated with a saturating concentration (300 ng/ml) of testosterone was at least 40-fold lower than that in preovulatory follicles (Fig. 7). This difference equates to a 400-fold difference in the rate of biosynthesis of estradiol when the levels of aromatase in the two tissues normalized.

Another unexpected result was the increase in luteal aromatase activity that occurred immediately postpartum, a time when amounts of aromatase enzyme have declined and the corpus luteum is presumed to be undergoing functional luteolysis (Fig. 7). However, because the rise in LH preceding parturition and the postpartum LH surge are known to stimulate the development of preovulatory follicles and induce increases in follicular aromatase levels and activity, we hypothesized that LH might also be

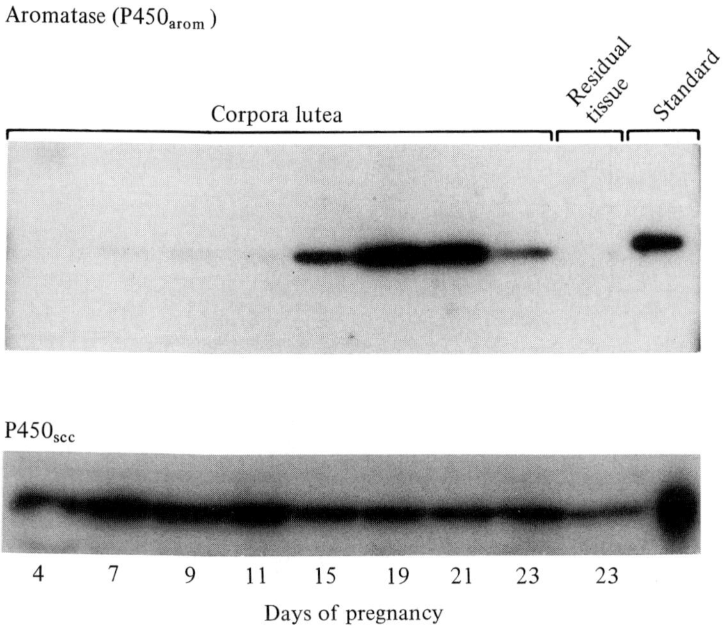

Fig. 6 Changes in levels of aromatase and $P450_{scc}$ enzymes in corpora lutea of pregnant rats.

regulating aromatase activity in the postpartum corpus luteum. To analyze this possibility, LH-specific antibody was administered to pregnant rats from day 19 to day 23. Whereas the antibody completely blocked follicular growth and induction of follicular aromatase activity, it had no effect on aromatase activity in the corpus luteum (Fig. 7; Hickey *et al.*, 1989). The absence of a direct effect of LH/cAMP on aromatase levels and activity in the corpus luteum is underscored by the inability of hCG to increase aromatase levels or activity in corpora lutea of pregnant rats when administered on days 8–10 or days 13–15, despite the ability of hCG to stimulate follicular growth and to induce follicular aromatase activity in these same animals (Bogovich and Richards, 1981).

Taken together, these observations provide additional evidence that a gene known to be regulated by cAMP in the follicle is subsequently regulated by other hormones in the corpus luteum. Most recently, we have shown that the induction of aromatase mRNA and its level in the corpus luteum are dependent on the placental hormones, rat placental lactogen (rPL) and testosterone (Hickey *et al.*, 1989). Despite regulation of the amount of aromatase enzyme by these hormones, rates of biosynthesis of estradiol remained low.

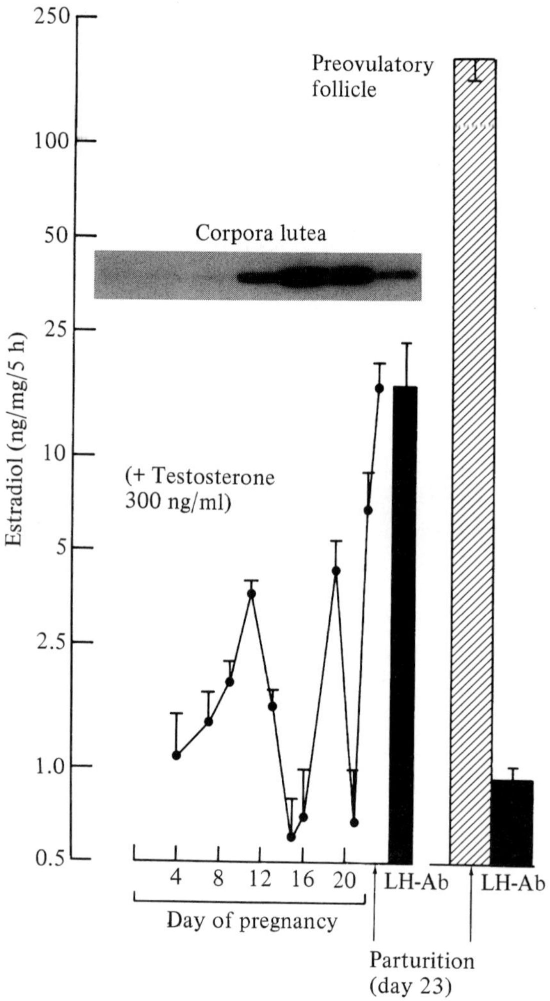

Fig. 7 Changes in rates of biosynthesis of estradiol in corpora lutea and follicles isolated during pregnancy and at parturition. LH-Ab was administered from day 19 to 23 (solid bars). Adapted from Hickey *et al.* (1989).

Cholesterol side-chain cleavage cytochrome P450

The cholesterol side-chain cleavage cytochrome P450 ($P450_{scc}$) enzyme converts cholesterol to pregnenolone in a key, rate-limiting step in the biosynthesis of progesterone in ovarian cells (Waterman and Simpson, 1985). Recently, antibodies raised against purified rat $P450_{scc}$ antigens (Farkash *et al.*, 1986) have been used for immunofluorescence localization of cytochrome $P450_{scc}$ in specific ovarian tissues (Zlotkin *et al.*, 1986), in granulosa cells in culture (Goldring *et al.*, 1986), and within the inner mitochondrial membranes of these cells (Farkash *et al.*, 1986). The immunofluorescence localization studies have demonstrated that levels of cytochrome $P450_{scc}$ are greater in preovulatory follicles than in small follicles but it is present in its highest amount in corpora lutea (Zlotkin *et al.*, 1986). Immunoblot analysis of both rat (Hedin *et al.*, 1987b) and bovine (Rodgers *et al.*, 1986) follicles and corpora lutea has demonstrated further that, whereas the amount of cytochrome $P450_{scc}$ increases markedly during luteinization, the level of the electron donor for this enzyme, adrenodoxin, exhibits only a small change.

A human cDNA probe (Matteson *et al.*, 1984) and an affinity-purified antibody against $P450_{scc}$ from rat were used to isolate a rat cytochrome $P450_{scc}$ cDNA clone for an analysis of the hormonal regulation of cytochrome $P450_{scc}$ mRNA during ovarian follicular development and luteinization (Goldring *et al.*, 1987). Levels of $P450_{scc}$ mRNA are negligible in theca and granulosa cells of small antral follicles and are low but measurable in both cell types in preovulatory follicles (see Fig. 4). Data obtained from hypophysectomized rats *in vivo* and granulosa cells *in vitro* suggest that the initial induction of the mRNA in granulosa cells is dependent on the synergistic actions of estradiol and FSH (Goldring *et al.*, 1987). However, the most dramatic increase in the amount of $P450_{scc}$ mRNA occurs in response to the LH surge and during early luteinization (Fig. 4). Elevated expression of the $P450_{scc}$ gene then appears to be constitutively maintained in corpora lutea throughout gestation (Goldring *et al.*, 1987). A similar pattern is observed for the level of the $P450_{scc}$ enzyme (Fig. 6). The elevated and apparently stable maintenance of concentrations of $P450_{scc}$ mRNA and protein throughout pregnancy and parturition is in marked contrast to the changes in concentrations of progesterone in serum during gestation and at parturition (Goldring *et al.*, 1987), suggesting that once transcription of the $P450_{sc}$ gene is turned on by the LH surge, it is maintained irrespective of marked changes in serum levels of placental hormones.

The constitutive expression of cytochrome $P450_{scc}$ mRNA in corpora lutea during gestation is also supported directly (Voutilainen *et al.*, 1986) and indirectly (Richards *et al.*, 1986) by results of studies *in vitro*. For example, when theca and granulosa cells are isolated separately from rat preovulatory follicles 7 hours after an ovulatory dose of hCG and then incubated separately in culture, they maintain an elevated rate of synthesis of progesterone for 30 days, even in the absence of hormones (FSH, LH, prolactin) and agonists that increase levels of cAMP (Richards *et al.*, 1986). In contrast, theca and granulosa cells isolated from either small antral or preovulatory follicles and cultured under similar conditions fail to synthesize progesterone unless either hormones or forskolin are added to the culture media (Richards *et al.*, 1986; Goldring *et al.*, 1987).

Analysis of RNA prepared from similar cultures shows that forskolin is required to maintain levels of transcription of $P450_{scc}$ mRNA in granulosa cells isolated from preovulatory follicles, whereas levels of $P450_{scc}$ mRNA and

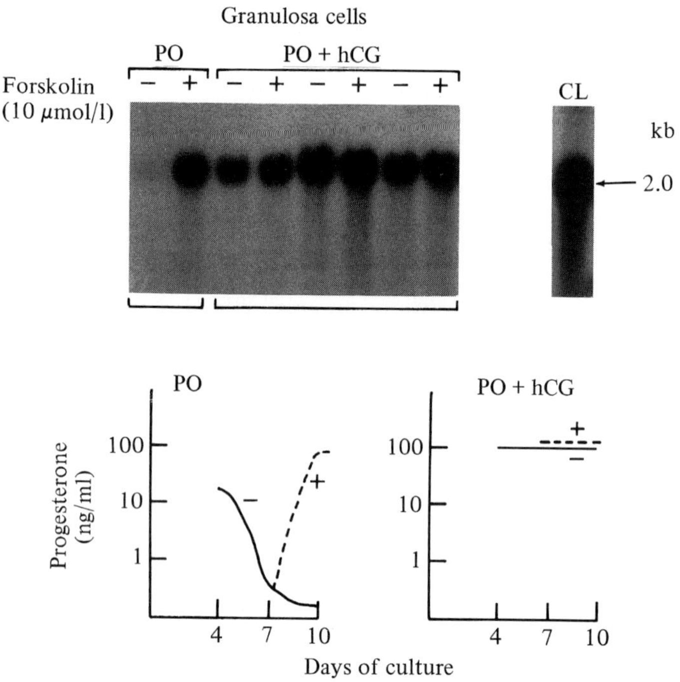

Fig. 8 Levels of mRNA for $P450_{scc}$ in cultured granulosa cells. Granulosa cells of preovulatory (PO) follicles or from PO follicles exposed to an ovulatory dose of hCG for 7 hours *in vivo* were isolated and cultured in DMEM:F12 that contained 1% fetal bovine serum for 10 days. Forskolin (10 μmol/l) was added to the media of half the cultures on day 7. RNA was prepared on day 10. Progesterone was measured in the media by radioimmunoassay.

the biosynthesis of progesterone are constitutively maintained in luteinized granulosa cells isolated from preovulatory follicles exposed for 7 hours *in vivo* to an ovulatory dose of hCG (Fig. 8; Oonk *et al.*, 1989). Addition of forskolin to the luteinized cultures had no effect on either the level of $P450_{scc}$ mRNA or the rate of synthesis of progesterone (Fig. 8). These observations extend and complement the pioneering studies of Channing (1968) and more recent studies by Voutilainen *et al.*, (1986) who have shown that the biosynthesis of progesterone and transcription of cytochrome $P450_{scc}$ mRNA continue in luteinized human granulosa cells for at least 10 days. These changes in the expression of cytochrome $P450_{scc}$ mRNA in ovarian cells contrast with those in adrenal (John *et al.*, 1986) and placental (Chung *et al.*, 1986) tissues in which levels of cytochrome $P450_{scc}$ are regulated by cAMP alone, without any enhancement by estradiol.

The factors and mechanisms involved in the switch from hormone-dependent regulation of cytochrome $P450_{scc}$ mRNA transcription in granulosa and theca cells of preovulatory follicles to a stable, constitutive (cAMP-independent?) mode in corpora lutea appear to be unique to ovarian tissue. The whole series of events raises the possibility that the luteotropic effects of estradiol and PRL in the rat, and of LH in the primate, may act *in vivo* to inhibit luteolytic events that do not occur in tissue culture. The results of studies both *in vivo* and *in vitro* suggest further that the marked changes that occur in concentrations of progesterone in serum during pregnancy in the rat are controlled at additional sites in the steroidogenic pathway, for example, including conversion to 20α-dihydroprogesterone (20α-DHP) (Goldring and Orly, 1985), and by other mechanisms governed, for example, by somatomedin C (Adashi *et al.*, 1985), estradiol (Gibori *et al.*, 1988), lipoproteins (Schuler *et al.*, 1981) and their receptors (Gibori *et al.*, 1984), and by cholesterol transport (Tanaka *et al.*, 1984). These latter processes have also been implicated in the maintenance of steroidogenesis in a Leydig cell tumor cell line (R2C) in which $P450_{scc}$ is constitutively expressed and not markedly altered by inhibitors of protein synthesis, even when the accumulation of pregnenolone was blocked (Freeman, 1987). The identification of a rapidly turning over regulatory protein has yet to be made.

Prostaglandin endoperoxide synthase

Prostaglandin endoperoxide synthase (PGS; mol. wt = 70 000) catalyzes the rate-limiting step in the conversion of arachidonic acid to prostaglandins E2 and $F_{2\alpha}$, thromboxane A2 and prostacyclin (PGI_2) (Smith, 1986) and, therefore, plays a key role in inflammatory responses. Prostaglandins are also associated with and required for LH-induced ovulation of preovulatory follicles, a process similar to an inflammatory response (for review, see Espey, 1980). Prostaglandins are not required for luteinization (Richards, 1980). Therefore, one might predict that the production of prostaglandins is stimulated rapidly by the LH surge, that it occurs only in follicles that are capable of ovulating, and that its production is transient. To analyze this hypothesis we have measured the production of PGS by follicles at defined stages of development (Richards and Bogovich, 1982) and quantitated LH-induced changes in the level of PGS in follicular cells using a rabbit anti-sheep affinity-purified PGS IgG (Hedin *et al.*, 1987c).

Preovulatory follicles, but not small antral follicles, synthesize PGE and $PGF_{2\alpha}$ when incubated with ovulatory doses of LH or FSH (Richards and Bogovich, 1982). Synthesis of prostaglandins is associated with a dose- and time-dependent induction of the PGS enzyme in preovulatory follicles (Fig. 9). Maximal increases in levels of PGS occur 7 hours after administration of an ovulatory dose of hCG *in vivo* (Hedin *et al.*, 1987c) or in response to large amounts of LH (1 μg/ml), FSH (500 ng/ml) and forskolin (10 μmol/l) *in vitro*

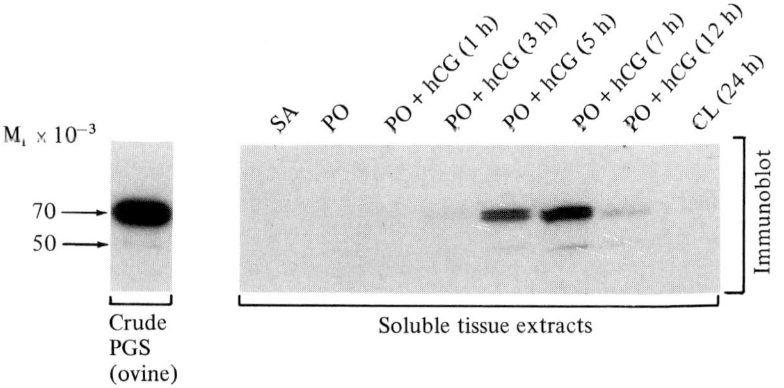

Fig. 9 Time course of induction of prostaglandin endoperoxidase synthase (PGS) in preovulatory follicles by an ovulatory dose of hCG.

(Wong *et al.*, 1989). PGS has been localized exclusively to granulosa cells of follicles prior to ovulation; its levels decline by the time ovulation occurs (12 hours) and are negligible in corpora lutea (Hedin *et al.*, 1987c). Induction of PGS in follicles *in vitro* by either LH or forskolin is inhibited by α-amanitin or cycloheximide, a result suggesting that the appearance of the enzyme in granulosa cells is dependent on a transcriptional event, possibly one that involves activation of the PGS gene itself. Indomethacin, which covalently binds to the enzyme and blocks catalytic activity, does not block induction by LH or forskolin. Furthermore, neither PGE nor $PGF_{2\alpha}$ alters hormonally induced increases in levels of PGS, a result that suggests that the enzyme is not regulated by end-product feedback mechanisms (Wong *et al.*, 1989).

Most recently, cDNAs encoding the sheep PGS enzyme have been cloned (DeWitt and Smith, 1988) and their use should allow us to determine if LH is regulating the increase in levels of PGS at the transcriptional or at the translational level.

Summary

In the foregoing discussion (and as summarized in Fig. 10) we have presented results showing that the levels of mRNA and enzyme for $P450_{17\alpha}$, $P450_{scc}$ and $P450_{arom}$ increase during the development of preovulatory follicles. These changes occur in response to FSH, to low but increasing concentrations of LH (cAMP), and to estradiol. The LH surge and elevated concentrations of cAMP terminate follicular growth and stimulate distinct changes in the expression of each gene. $P450_{17\alpha}$ is repressed, $P450_{scc}$ is markedly induced and its levels remain elevated in a constitutive manner, the amount of $P450_{arom}$ declines transiently and is subsequently increased by the action of placental-derived

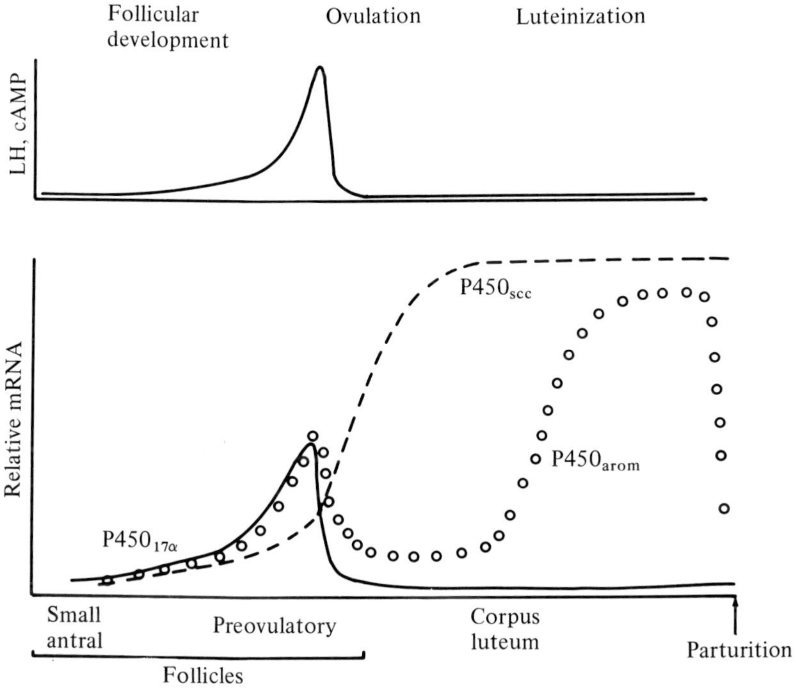

Fig. 10 Schematic diagram of changes in levels of mRNA transcribed from P450 genes during follicular development and luteinization.

hormones, rat placental lactogen (rPL) and testosterone (or estradiol). These results provide evidence to support the hypothesis that the 'transformation' of a preovulatory follicle to a corpus luteum is associated with a shift from cAMP-dependent regulation of cell function (see Fig. 3) to cAMP-independent mechanisms which involve other signal–transduction pathways.

The molecular basis for the diverse mechanisms that regulate levels of PGS and the P450 enzymes during differentiation of ovarian cells remains to be determined. However, the changes depicted in Figure 11 suggest that there are tissue- and hormone-specific domains that regulate the transcription of each gene. Expression of $P450_{17\alpha}$ occurs only in theca cells. Therefore, within the 5' flanking sequence of the $P450_{17\alpha}$ gene there must be cis-acting elements that respond to theca-specific transcription factors. Aromatase and PGS are induced exclusively in granulosa cells, indicating that there must be cis-acting elements in these two genes which respond to granulosa cell-specific transcription factors. The $P450_{scc}$ gene is regulated by factors common to both theca and granulosa cells.

Each of these genes also appears to have one or more cAMP regulatory elements (CRE). One CRE responds to low concentrations of cAMP and acts

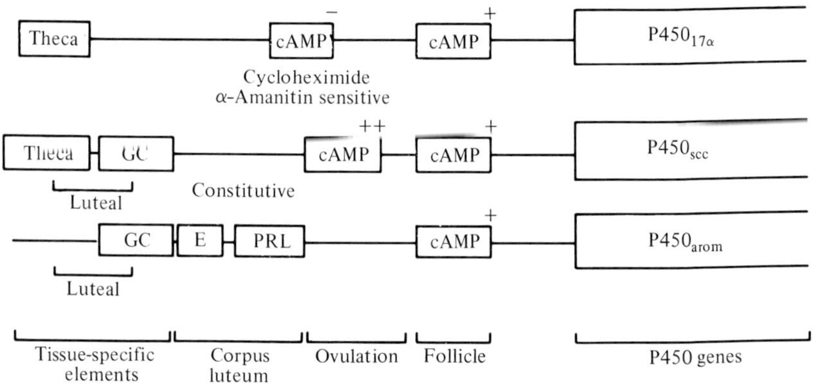

Fig. 11 Diverse mechanisms regulating the expression of P450 genes: identification of putative cis-acting regulatory elements involved in tissue- and hormone-specific regulation of each gene.

to increase the rate of transcription of each gene during follicular development. In contrast, other CRE domains, presumably interacting with distinct cAMP-regulated transcription factors, are altered only as a consequence of elevated intracellular concentrations of cAMP. These putative factors which are modulated (phosphorylated?) by cAMP (see Fig. 3) appear to act either as repressors (in the case of P450$_{17\alpha}$) or as activators (in the case of P450$_{scc}$) of transcription, depending on the tissue in which the particular gene is being expressed. The aromatase gene contains, in addition, regulatory elements responsive to the actions of PRL and estradiol.

Isolation of genomic clones for each of these genes should make it possible to begin characterizing both the cis-acting DNA sequences and the trans-acting factors which bind to these sequences and which ultimately control transcription of each gene in a tissue- and hormone-specific manner.

Acknowledgements

The author wishes to thank the postdoctoral fellows (Katryna Bogovich, Tore Jahnsen, Lars Hedin, Gerard J. Hickey, and Ria B. Oonk) and graduate students (Sheri Ratoosh, Richard Kurten, Jami Lifka, Winona Wong, Dana Gaddy-Kurten and Noga B. Goldring) who have participated in these studies at Baylor College of Medicine and the many generous collaborators from other institutions: Dr Suzanane M. Lohmann and Dr Ulrich Walter, Departments of Physiological Chemistry and Medicine, University of Wurzburg, Wurzburg, West Germany, for the bovine heart RII antibody and assistance in the initial purification of ovarian RII subunits; Dr G. Stanley McKnight, Department of Pharmacology, University of Washington, Seattle, Washington, for his assistance with the solution hybridization and transcriptional assays as well as for the cDNA probes for RI and C_α subunits; Dr Joseph

Orly, Department of Biological Chemistry, The Hebrew University of Jerusalem, Jerusalem, Israel, for the cholesterol side-chain cleavage cytochrome P450 antibody; Dr Walter L. Miller, Department of Pediatrics, University of California, San Francisco, California, for the human cDNA for $P450_{scc}$; Dr Charles B. Kasper, McArdle Laboratory for Cancer Research, University of Wisconsin, Madison, Wisconsin, for the rat genomic library; Dr Raymond J. Rodgers, Dr Evan R. Simpson, and Dr Michael R. Waterman for assistance with the 17α-hydroxylase studies; Dr Shiuan Chen, Beckman City of Hope, Duarte, California, for the human aromatase oligonucleotide; and Dr Peter F. Hall, University of New South Wales, Sydney, Australia, for aromatase-specific antibodies. We thank also Georgietta Brown for typing the manuscript, David Scarff for preparing the art work, and Deborah Delmore for photographic services. This work was supported by grants from NIH-HD, 16229 and 16272, and from the American Cancer Society (to JSR).

References

Adashi, E.Y., Resnick, C.E., D'Ercole, A.J., Svododa, M.E. & Van Wyck, J.J. (1985). Insulin-like growth factors as intraovarian regulators of granulosa cell functions. **Endocrine Reviews** 6:400–420.

Armstrong, D.T. & Dorrington, J.H. (1977). Estrogen biosynthesis in ovaries and testis. **Advances in Sex Hormone Research** 3:217–230.

Bogovich, K. & Richards, J.S. (1981). Obligatory role of luteinizng hormone (LH) in the initiation of preovulatory follicular growth in the pregnant rat: specific effects of human chorionic gonadotropin and follicle-stimulating hormone on LH receptors and steroidogenesis in theca, granulosa and luteal cells. **Endocrinology** 109:860–867.

Carson, R.S., Richards, J.S. & Kahn, L.E. (1981). Functional and morphological differentiation of theca and granulosa cells during pregnancy in the rat: dependence on increased basal luteinizing hormone activity. **Endocrinology** 109:1433–1441.

Channing, C.P. (1969). Steroidogenesis and morphology of human ovarian cell types in tissue culture. **Journal of Endocrinology** 45:297–308.

Chen, S., Besman, M.J., Sparkes, R.S., Zoller, S., Klisak, I., Mohandras, T., Hall, P.F. & Shively, J.E. (1988). Human aromatase: cDNA cloning, Southern blot analysis and assignment of the gene to chromosome 15. **DNA** 7:27–38.

Chen, S., Shively, J.E., Nakajin, S., Shinoda, M. & Hall, P.F. (1986). Amino acid terminal sequence analysis of human placenta aromatase. **Biochemical Biophysical Research Communications** 135:713–719.

Chung, B.C., Matteson, K.J., Voutilainen, R., Mohandas,TK. & Miller, W.L. (1986). Human cholesterol side-chain cleavage enzyme $P450_{scc}$: cDNA cloning, assignment of the gene to chromosome 15 and expression in the placenta. **Proceedings of the National Academy of Science, USA** 83:8962–8966.

Clegg, C.H., Leslay, A.C., Cadd, G.G. & McKnight, G.S. (1987). Inhibition of intracellular cAMP-dependent protein kinase using mutant genes of the regulatory type I subunit. **Journal of Biological Sciences** 262:13111–13119.

DeWitt, D.L. & Smith, W.L. (1988). Primary structure of prostaglandin G/H synthase from sheep vesicular gland determined from the complementary DNA sequence. **Proceedings of the National Academy of Science, USA** 85:1412–1416.

Eckstein, B. & Tsafriri, A. (1986). The steroid C-17,20 lyase complex in isolated Graafian follicles: effects of human chorionic gonadotropin. **Endocrinology** 118:1266–1270.

Erickson, G.F., Magoffin, D.A., Dyer, C. & Hofeditz, C. (1985). The ovarian androgen-producing cells: a review of structure function relationships. **Endocrine Reviews** 6:371–399.

Espey, L.L. (1980). Ovulation as an inflammatory reaction – a hypothesis. **Biology of Reproduction** 22:73–106.

Evans, C.T., Ledesma, D.B., Schulz, T.Z., Simpson, E.R. & Mendelson, C.R. (1986). Isolation and characterization of a complementary DNA specific for human aromatase-system cytochrome P450 mRNA. **Proceedings of the National Academy of Science, USA** 83:6387–6391.

Farkash, Y., Timberg, K. & Orly, J. (1986). Preparation of antiserum to rat cytochrome P450 cholesterol side-chain cleavage and its use for ultrastructural localization of the immunoreactive enzyme by protein A gold technique. **Endocrinology** 118:1353–1356.

Freeman, D.A. (1987). Constitutive steroidogenesis in the R2C Leydig tumor cell line is maintained by the adenosine 3',5'-monophosphate-independent production of a cycloheximide-sensitive factor that enhances mitochrondrial pregnenolone biosynthesis. **Endocrinology** 120:124–132.

Gibori, G., Chan, Y.D., Khan, I., Azhar, S. & Reaven, G.M. (1984). Regulation of luteal cell lipoprotein receptors, sterol contents and steroidogenesis by estradiol in the pregnant rat. **Endocrinology** 114:609–617.

Gibori, G., Khan, I., Warshaw, M.L., McLean, M.P., Puryear, T.K., Nelson, S., Durkee, T.J., Azhar, S., Steinschneider, A. & Rao, M.C. (1988). Placental-derived regulators and the complex control of luteal cell function. **Recent Progress in Hormone Research** 44:376–429.

Goldring, N.B., Durica, J.M., Lifka, J., Hedin, L., Ratoosh, S.L., *et al.* (1987). Cholesterol side-chain cleavage P450 ($P450_{scc}$) mRNA: evidence for hormonal regulation in rat ovarian follicles and constitutive expression in corpora lutea. **Endocrinology** 120:1942–1950.

Goldring, N.B., Farkash, Y., Goldschmidt, D. & Orly, J. (1986). Immunofluorescent probing of the mitochondrial cholesterol side-chain cleavage cytochrome P450 in differentiating granulosa cells in culture. **Endocrinology** 119:2821–2832.

Goldring, N.B. & Orly, J. (1985). Concerted metabolism of steroid hormones produced by cocultured ovarian cell types. **Journal of Biological Chemistry** 260:913–921.

Hedin, L., Kurten, D.G., Kurten, R. & Richards, J.S. (1987c). Prostaglandin synthase in rat ovarian follicles: Content, cellular distribution and induction by hormones. **Endocrinology** 121:722–731.

Hedin, L., McKnight, G.S., Lifka, J., Durica, J.M. & Richards, J.S. (1987a). Tissue distribution and hormonal regulation of mRNA for regulatory and catalytic subunits of cAMP-dependent protein kinases during ovarian follicular development and luteinization in the rat. **Endocrinology** 120:1928–1935.

Hedin, L., Rodgers, R.J., Simpson, E.R. & Richards, J.S. (1987b). Changes in content of cytochrome $P450_{17\alpha}$, cytochrome $P450_{scc}$ and HMG CoA reductase in developing rat ovarian follicles and corpora lutea: correlation to theca cell steriodogenesis. **Biology of Reproduction** 38:211–223.

Hickey, G.J., Chen, S., Besman, M.J., Shively, J.E., Hall, P.F., Gaddy-Kurten, D. & Richards, J.S. (1988). Hormonal regulation, tissue distribution and content of aromatase cytochrome P450 messenger RNA and enzyme in rat ovarian follicles and corpora lutea: relationship to estradiol biosynthesis. **Endocrinology** 122:1426–1436.

Hickey, G.J., Oonk, R.B., Hall, P.F. & Richards, J.S. (1989). Aromatase cytochrome P450 and cholesterol side-chain cleavage P450 in corpora lutea of pregnant rats: diverse regulation by peptide and steroid hormones. **Endocrinology** 125:1673–1682.

Hsueh, A.J.W., Adashi, E.Y., Jones, P.B.C. & Welsh, J.R. Th (1984). Hormonal regulation of the differentiation of cultured ovarian granulosa cells. **Endocrine Reviews** 5:76–127.

Jahnsen, T., Hedin, L., Kidd, V.J., Beattie, W.G., Lohmann, S.M. *et al.* (1986a). Molecular cloning, cDNA structure and regulation of the regulatory subunit of type I cAMP-dependent protein kinase from rat ovarian granulosa cells. **Journal of Biological Chemistry** 261:12352–12361.

Jahnsen, T., Hedin, L., Lohmann, S.M., Walter, U. & Richards, J.S. (1986b). The neural type II regulatory subunit of cAMP-dependent protein kinase is present and regulated by hormones in the rat ovary. **Journal of Biological Chemistry** 261:6637–6639.

Jahnsen, T., Lohmann, S.M., Walter, U., Hedin, L. & Richards, J.S. (1985). Purification and characterization of hormone-regulated isoforms of the regulatory subunit of type II cAMP-dependent protein kinase from rat ovaries. **Journal of Biological Chemistry** 260:15980–15987.

John, M.E., John, M.C., Boggaram, V., Simpson, E.R. & Waterman, M.R. (1986). Transcriptional regulation of steroid hydroxylase genes by corticotropin. **Proceedings of the National Academy of Science, USA** 83:4715–4719.

Matteson, K.J., Chung, B. & Miller, W.L. (1984). Molecular cloning of DNA complementary to bovine adrenal $P450_{scc}$ mRNA. **Biochemical Biophysical Research Communications** 120:264–270.

Nakajin, S. & Hall, P.F. (1981). Microsomal P450 from neonatal pig thesis. Purification and properties of C21 steroid side-chain cleavage (17α-hydroxylase $C_{17/20}$ lyase). **Journal of Biological Chemistry** 256:3871–3876.

Oonk, R.B., Beattie, W.G. & Richards, J.S. (1989). Cyclic AMP-dependent and -independent regulation of cholesterol side chain cleavage cytochrome P450 ($P450_{scc}$) in rat ovarian granulosa cells and corpora lutea: cDNA and deduced amino acid sequence of rat $P450_{scc}$. **Journal of Biological Chemistry** 264:21934–21942.

Ratoosh, S.L., Likfa, J., Hedin, L., Jahnsen, T. & Richards, J.S. (1987). Hormonal regulation of the synthesis and mRNA content of the regulatory subunit of cyclic AMP-dependent protein kinase type II in cultured rat ovarian granulosa cells. **Journal of Biological Chemistry** 262:7306–7313.

Ratoosh, S.L. & Richards, J.S. (1985). Regulation of the content and phosphorylation of RII by adenosine 3'5'-monophosphate, follicle stimulating hormone and estradiol in cultured granulosa cells. **Endocrinology** 117:917–927.

Richards, J.S. (1980). Maturation of ovarian follicles: action and interactions of pituitary and ovarian hormones on follicular cell differentiation. **Physiological Reviews** 60:51–89.

Richards, J.S. & Bogovich, K. (1982). Effects of human chorionic gonadotropin and progesterone on follicular development in the immature rat. **Endocrinology** 111:1429–1438.

Richards, J.S., Haddox, M., Tash, J.S., Walter, U. & Lohmann, S.M. (1984). Adenosine 3'5'-monophosphate-dependent protein kinase and granulosa cell responsiveness to gonadotropins. **Endocrinology** 114:2190–2198.

Richards, J.S. & Hedin, L. (1988). Molecular aspects of hormone action in ovarian follicular development, ovulation and luteinization. **Annual Review of Physiology** 50:441–463.

Richards, J.S., Hedin, L. & Caston, L. (1986). Differentiation of rat ovarian thecal cells: evidence for functional luteinization. **Endocrinology** 118:1660–1668.

Richards, J.S., Hickey, G.J., Chen, S., Shively, J.E., Hall, P.F. *et al.* (1987a). Hormonal regulation of estradiol biosynthesis, aromatase activity and aromatase mRNA in rat follicles and corpora lutea. **Steroids** 50:393–409.

Richards, J.S., Jahnsen, T., Hedin, L., Lifka, J., Ratoosh, S.L. *et al.* (1987b). Ovarian follicular development: from physiology to molecular biology. **Recent Progress in Hormone Research** 43:231–276.

Richards, J.S. & Kirchick, H.J. (1984). Changes in content and phosphorylation of cytosol proteins in luteinizing follicles and corpora lutea. **Biology of Reproduction** 30:737–751.

Richards, J.S. & Rolfes, A.I. (1980). Hormonal regulation of cyclic AMP binding to specific receptor proteins in rat ovarian follicles. **Journal of Biological Chemistry** 255:5481–5489.

Rodgers, R.J., Waterman, M.R. & Simpson, E.R. (1986). Cytochrome $P450_{scc}$, $P450_{17a}$, adrenodoxin and reduced nicotinamide adenine dinucleotide phosphate P450 reductase in bovine follicles and corpora lutea. Changes in specific contents during the ovarian cycle. **Endocrinology** 118:1366–1377.

Schuler, L.A., Langerberg, K.K., Gynee, J.T. & Strauss, III Jr. (1981). High-density lipoprotein utilization by dispersed rat luteal cells. **Biochemica Biophysica Acta** 664:583–601.

Smith, W.L. (1986). Prostaglandin biosynthesis and its compartmentation in vascular smooth-muscle and endothelial cells. **Annual Review of Physiology** 48:251–262.

Tanaka, T., Billheimer, J.T. & Strauss, III Jr. (1984). Luteinized rat ovaries contain a sterol carrier protein. **Endocrinology** 114:533–540.

Voutilainen, R., Tapaneinen, J., Chung, B.C., Matteson, K.J. & Miller, W.L. (1986). Hormonal regulation of $P450_{scc}$ (20,22 desmolase) and $P450_{17a}$ (17α-hydroxylase/17,20 lyase) in cultured human granulosa cells. **Journal of Clinical Endocrinology and Metabolism** 63:202–207.

Waterman, M.R. & Simpson, E.R. (1985). Regulation of the biosynthesis of cytochromes P450 involved in steroid hormone synthesis. **Molecular and Cellular Endocrinology** 39:81–89.

Wong, W., Dewitt, D., Smith, W. & Richards, J.S. (1989). Induction of prostaglandin endoperoxide synthase (PGS) in preovulatory follicles *in vitro*: evidence for rapid transcriptional regulation by LH and cAMP. **Molecular Endocrinology** 3:1714–1723.

Zlotkin, T., Farkash, Y. & Orly, J. (1986). Cell-specific expression of immunoreactive cholesterol side-chain cleavage cytochrome P450 during follicular development in the rat ovary. **Endocrinology** 119:2809–2820.

Zuber, M.X., John, M.E., Okamura, T., Simpson, E.R. & Waterman, M.R. (1986a). Bovine adrenal cytochrome $P450_{17\alpha}$: regulation of gene expression by ACTH and elucidation of primary sequence. **Journal of Biological Chemistry** 261:2475–2482.

Zuber, M.X., Simpson, E.R. & Waterman, M.R. (1986b). Expression of bovine 17α-hydroxylase cytochrome P-450 cDNA in nonsteroidogenic (COS I) cells. **Science** 234:1258–1261.

The hormonal control of human luteal cells

H.-Z. WANG,[1] Y.-F. WU,[2] S.-H. LU, Z.-D. SUN, W.-X. SHEN, W. ZHOU AND Y.-T. GONG

Institute of Planned Parenthood Research; [1] Ren-ji Hospital, Shanghai No. 2 Medical University; [2] Shanghai Lu-wan District Maternity and Child Health Hospital; Shanghai, People's Republic of China.

Keywords

Human luteal cells, estradiol, oxytocin, 3β-hydroxysteroid dehydrogenase, functional differentiation, progesterone.

Introduction

The function of the mammalian corpus luteum is coordinated by many hormonal factors, including gonadotropins – luteinizing hormone (LH)/ human chorionic gonadotropin (hCG) – prostaglandins, steroids and various ovarian peptides (reviewed by Richardson, 1986). The complicated interaction among these factors, *in vivo*, makes it difficult to assess their respective roles, particularly in humans. Preparations of dispersed cells have been used to study the inhibitory effects of estradiol (Stouffer *et al.*, 1977; Karsch *et al.*, 1978; Williams *et al.*, 1979; Richardson and Masson, 1980; Laherty *et al.*, 1985). Estradiol-induced luteolysis, possibly mediated by PGF-2α, does not appear to occur in human luteal cells (Thibier *et al.*, 1980). Estradiol may also inhibit the activity of $\Delta^5$3β-hydroxysteroid dehydrogenase-$\Delta^{5,4}$-isomerase (3β-HSD) (Depp *et al.*, 1973).

The differences between species are another problem to be considered. The results from humans are often distinct from those from animals. The potential involvement of oxytocin in luteal regression in ruminants has been investigated (Sheldrick and Flint, 1980; Tan and Biggs, 1982; Wathes and Swann, 1982; Wathes, 1984). Much of the data about the effect of oxytocin on human luteal cells is controversial, especially from experiments *in vitro* (reviewed by Auletta and Flint, 1988). Further work is therefore required before a conclusion can be drawn.

This chapter includes a discussion of some of our recent work on the hormonal control of the production of progesterone in dispersed, human luteal cells *in vitro*. In particular, we examined: (a) the responsiveness to gonadotropin, (b) the inhibitory effect of estradiol on 3β-HSD, (c) the effect of oxytocin, and (d) the functional differentiation of the two major types of luteal cell.

Materials and methods

Preparation of dispersed human luteal cells

Biopsies of corpora lutea were obtained from women who underwent laparotomy in the midluteal phase of the menstrual cycle (cycle days 19–23), for a variety of non-malignant conditions. All had given consent in accordance with a procedure approved by the ethics committee of the hospital and local public health authorities. None of the women had received hormonal treatment before surgery. The corpora lutea were kept in ice-cold medium and immediately brought to the laboratory. A suspension of cells was prepared from each luteal biopsy according to the method described previously (Wang *et al.*, 1988). Briefly, each sample of tissue was dispersed using collagenase, deoxyribonuclease (Sigma Chemical Co., London) and protease (Boehringer Mannheim, West Germany). After washing by repeated centrifugation and resuspension, the number of luteal cells was counted under the light microscope. The viability of the cells was 75–85% as judged by trypan-blue exclusion (Tennant, 1964).

Separation of small and large luteal cells

Concentrated fractions of large and small luteal cells were prepared by centrifugation on a stepwise gradient of Percoll (Pharmacia Fine Chemical, Uppsala, Sweden), by the method of Ohara *et al.* (1987) with slight modifications. The solutions of Percoll, dissolved in 0.15 mol/l NaCl at concentrations of 10%, 15%, 20% and 40% (v/v), were layered sequentially in the tubes. The suspensions of luteal cells were placed on the surface of the Percoll solutions in the polystyrene tubes (15 mm i.d.x150 mm). The tubes were centrifuged at 400 g for 2x1 minute. The types of cell were roughly designated by cell size, which was measured using an eye-piece micrometer (1 division = 2.5 μm). The cells recovered in 12% Percoll and at the interphase between 10% and 15% Percoll were combined and designated as the large-cell fraction (18–25 μm in diameter). The cells recovered in 20% Percoll and between 20% and 40% Percoll were designated as the small cells (5–15 μm in diameter). The small fraction was 8% ± 2% (S.E.) cross-contaminated with large cells and the large fraction was 21% ± 2% (S.E.) contaminated with small cells.

Incubation of cell suspensions

Human chorionic gonadotropin (5380 i.u./mg; Shanghai Biochemical and Pharmaceutical Laboratories) and oxytocin (a. Sigma Chemical Co., London; b. Shanghai Pharmaceutical Industry Co., China) were diluted to appropriate concentrations in culture medium before incubation. The steroids were dissolved in polyethylene glycol and ethanol (50:50 v/v) and then diluted in the culture medium. After preincubation for 1 hour at 37°C, approximately 0.5–

$1x10^5$ cells (0.3 ml of the cell suspension) were dispensed to each tube and incubated with additions of various hormones in 30 μl for a further 3 hours, with shaking, in a water bath. All experiments were carried out in triplicate. After incubation, the samples of cell suspension were stored at −20°C until radioimmunoassay (RIA) for steroids.

Assays for steroids and 3β-HSD

Progesterone or estradiol produced in each tube (in cells and medium together) was extracted with ether and then assayed using a validated RIA, according to the protocol in the WHO Manual (1986). The activity of 3β-HSD was expressed in terms of the rate of conversion of pregnenolone to progesterone in 30 minutes. The inhibitory effects of 3β-HSD were expressed as the reduction in this conversion rate. The average rate of formation of progesterone was compared with that in the control, which was taken as 100% (Shinada *et al.*, 1978). The progesterone content was assayed as described above. The specific antiserum (Shanghai Institute of Biological Products) used was chosen such that the cross-reactivity against progesterone at 50% displacement was 0.018% for pregnenolone, 1.6% for 17α-hydroxyprogesterone, 0.09% for testosterone, and 0.001% for estradiol and dihydrotestosterone. The cross-reactivity against estradiol was 0.13%, 0.02%, 0.02%, 0.007% and 0.01% for estriol, estrone, cortisol, progesterone and testosterone, respectively. The significance of differences in levels of steroids between sets of incubations was calculated using paired Student's t tests.

Results

Responsiveness of human luteal cells to hCG

Figure 1 shows that, in the mixed population of dispersed human luteal cells, the production of progesterone was stimulated by different concentrations of hCG. The minimum effective dose of hCG was 0.01 i.u./ml and 1 i.u./ml was sufficient to elicit a maximum production. Figure 2 shows that when stimulated by hCG, the small cells responded with a fourfold increase in formation of progesterone, whereas the large cells showed no significant response. Under basal condition the large cells were more active in terms of production of progesterone than the small cells ($p<0.05$). Figure 3 shows that estradiol could be produced by both large and small cells. The levels were much higher in the presence of testosterone, but no further increase was found after addition of hCG. The large cells were active in the production of estradiol with or without testosterone.

The inhibitory effects of estradiol on 3β-HSD

Figure 4 shows that, in the presence or absence of hCG, estradiol markedly inhibited the production of progesterone in a dose-related manner at concentrations from 0.1 μmol/l to 10 μmol/l ($p<0.001$). For a further

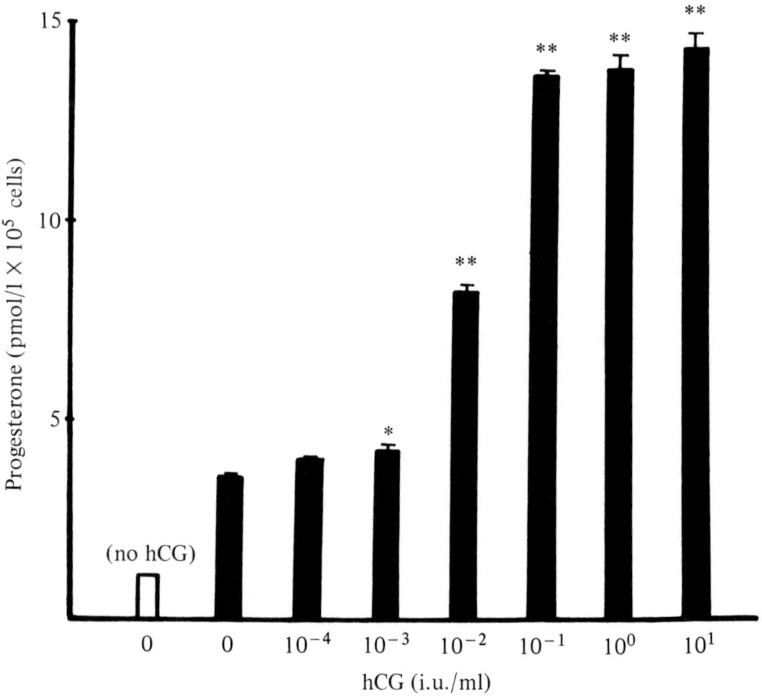

Fig. 1 Effect of human chorionic gonadotropin (hCG) on the production of progesterone by dispersed human luteal cells incubated for 3 hours at 37°C in 95% O_2:5% CO_2. Values represent the mean ± S.E.M. of triplicate incubations. Open bar indicates the level of progesterone before incubation. (*p⟨0.05; **p⟨0.001.)

investigation of the mechanism by which estradiol inhibits production of progesterone, the 3β-HSD activity was measured in intact luteal cells. The activity of 3β-HSD was expressed in terms of conversion rates of pregnenolone to progesterone in 30 minutes per 10^5 cells. The rate of transformation of pregnenolone into progesterone was linear with 10^5 cells up to 30 minutes. In the present cell system, it was not necessary to add nicotinamide-adenine dinucleotide (NAD) to the medium for the transformation (Wang *et al.*, unpublished data).

Lineweaver–Burk analysis revealed that estradiol exerted a non-competitive type of inhibition (Fig. 5). Figure 6 shows that by Dixon plot, estradiol had a K_i of 2 ± 0.45 μmol/l (mean ± s.d.).

Figure 7 shows that under basal conditions, the rate of production of progesterone was higher in large than in small cells. Addition of pregnenolone resulted in a rate of production of progesterone by large cells that was

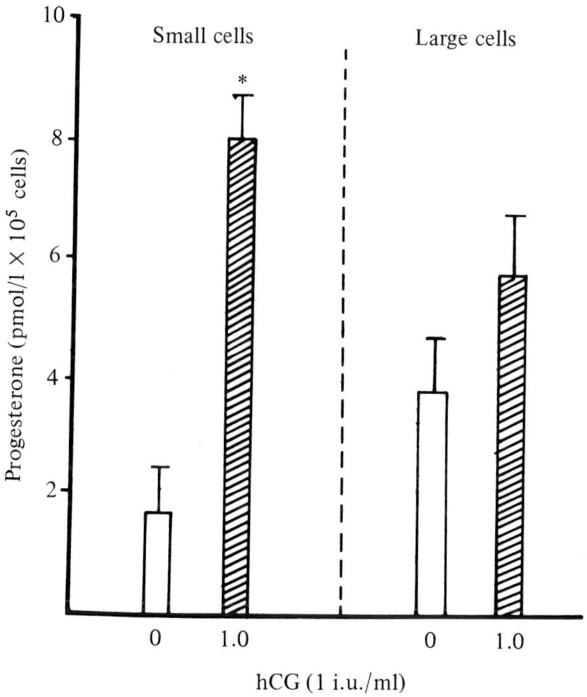

Fig. 2 Effect of hCG (1 i.u./ml) on the production of progesterone by small and large human luteal cells incubated for 3 hours. The values represent the mean ± S.E.M. of results of four separate experiments. hCG significantly increased the amount of progesterone produced by small cells, but its effect was not significant on large cells. (*p⟨0.001.)

approximately twofold higher than that in small cells (p⟨0.05).

Figure 8 shows that estradiol inhibited 3β-HSD in both large and small cells. The extent of inhibition, shown by the decrease in transformation of pregnenolone to progesterone, was greater in small than in large luteal cells (p⟨0.02).

Effect of oxytocin

To account for the discrepancy in results among the various laboratories, two preparations of oxytocin were used in this study, synthetic oxytocin (504 i.u./mg) and pharmaceutical ampoules (10 i.u./2 ml). The results were as follows.

(a) *Synthetic oxytocin.* Figures 9 and 10 show that addition of 2 i.u./ml oxytocin to two preparations of human luteal cells (day 19, day 23) exerted no effect on either the basal production of progesterone or the

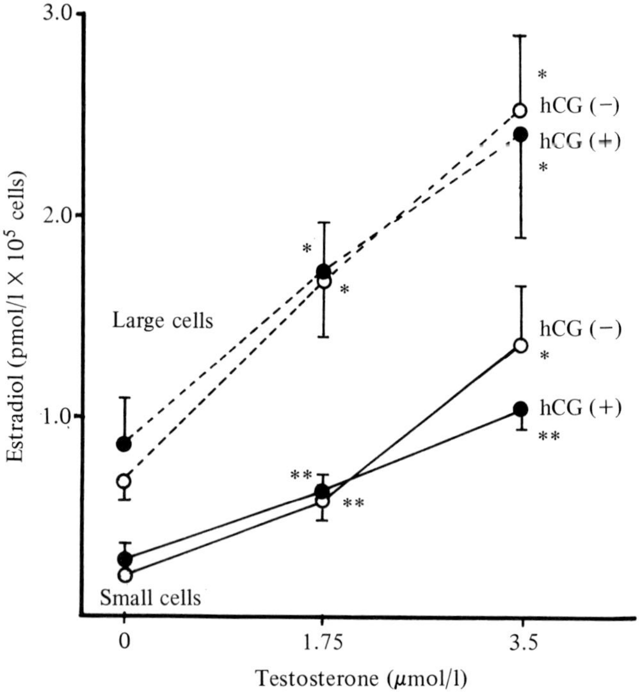

Fig. 3 Production of estradiol by small and large cells incubated for 3 hours in the presence and absence of hCG (1 i.u./ml). The values are the mean ± S.E.M. of results of three experiments. (*$p < 0.05$; **$p < 0.01$.)

response to hCG. Figure 11 shows that addition of a wide range of concentrations of oxytocin (1–1000 mu/ml) also had no effect on either the basal production or the response of human luteal cells to 1 i.u./ml hCG.

(b) *Pharmaceutical oxytocin.* As shown in Figure 12, the pharmaceutical oxytocin at a concentration of 1 i.u./ml suppressed both basal and hCG-induced production of progesterone. However, when the pH of the medium was adjusted to pH 7.0, oxytocin was shown to have no significant action on the production of progesterone.

Discussion

Many studies have demonstrated a stimulatory action of LH/hCG on the production of progesterone by corpora lutea both *in vivo* and *in vitro*. Recently, the results of our successful separation of mixed populations into two types of luteal cell have further revealed that large luteal cells produce

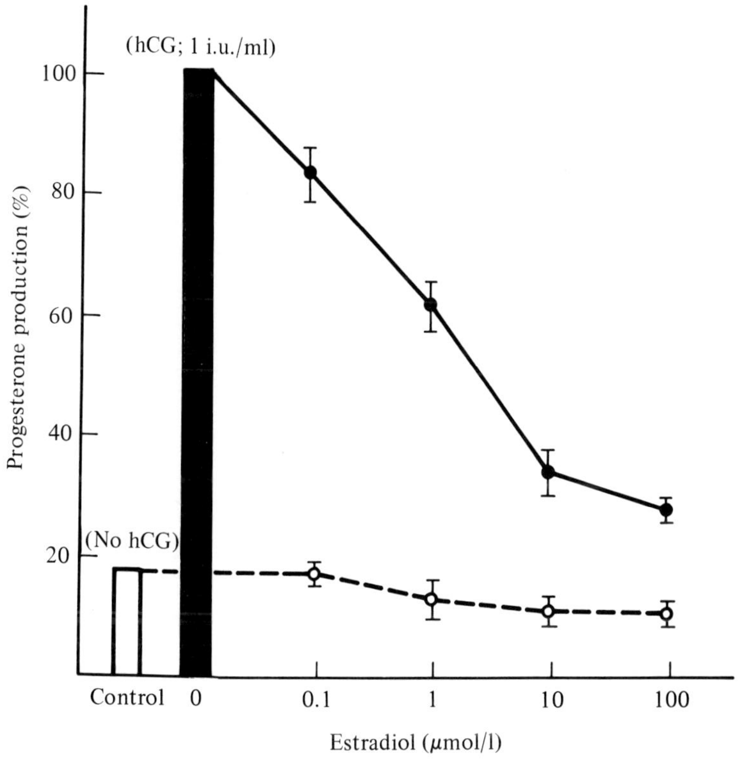

Fig. 4 The inhibitory effect of estradiol on the production of progesterone by dispersed, human luteal cells incubated for 3 hours at 37°C in the presence or absence of hCG. Values represent the mean ± S.E.M. of results of three separate experiments, each with triplicate incubations

more progesterone during the incubation under basal conditions, but they are less responsive to LH/hCG than small cells. Our results are consistent with those of previous studies by Ohara *et al.* (1987) and results for sheep (Rodgers and O'Shea, 1982). Large cells were approximately two times more active than small cells in terms of the basal production either of progesterone or estradiol. However, when stimulated with hCG, only the small cells responded with a four- to tenfold increase in the production of progesterone. Although secretion of progesterone was always a little greater in the presence than in the absence of hCG, this difference may be due to the contamination by small cells in our large-cell fraction.

A reasonable explanation for these different responses is that the specific receptors for LH/hCG are located mainly on the surface of small cells. It is generally accepted that LH interacts with specific receptors on the cell surface

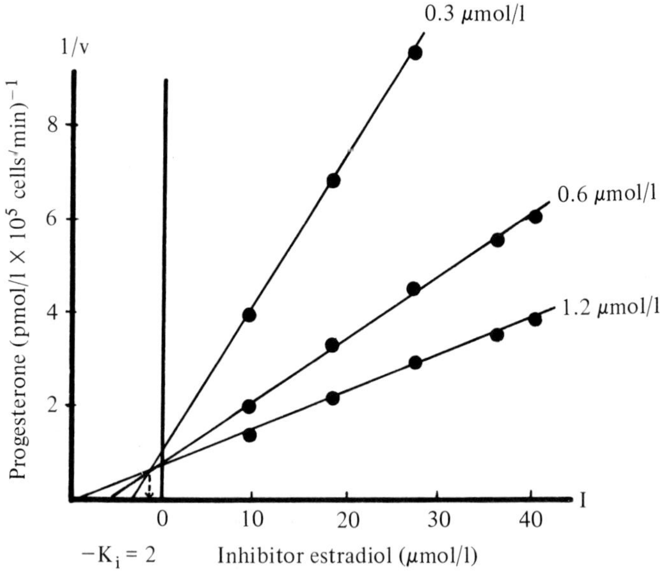

Fig. 5 The inhibition of 3β-HSD in human luteal cells by estradiol is shown as a Dixon plot. $-K_i = 2 \pm 0.45$ μmol/l. The values are the mean ± S.E.M. of results of three separate experiments. The concentrations of the substrate, pregnenolone, are given next to each line.

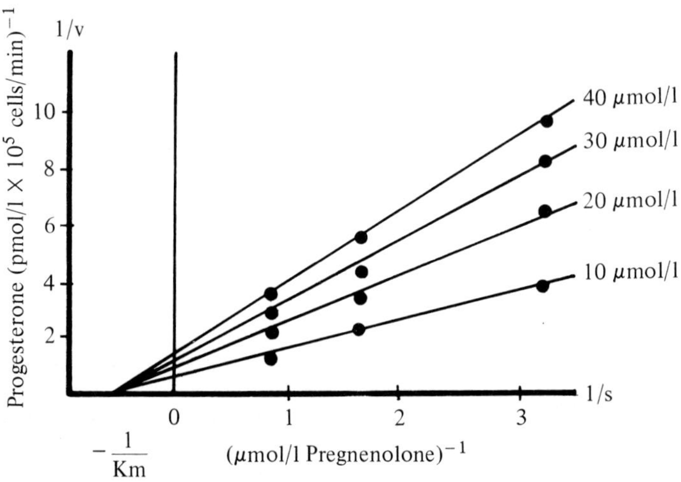

Fig. 6 The non-competitive type of inhibition of 3β-HSD in human luteal cells by estradiol is shown by a Lineweaver–Burk plot. The concentrations of estradiol are given next to each line.

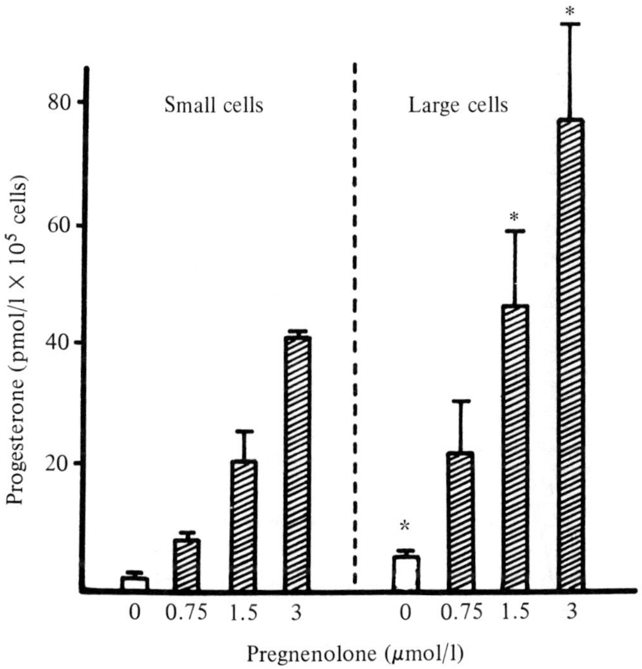

Fig. 7 Production of progesterone in large and small luteal cells, incubated at 37°C. The enzymatic activity is expressed in terms of the rate of conversion of pregnenolone into progesterone per 10^5 cells in 30 minutes. The values represent the mean ± S.E.M. of results of three separate experiments with triplicate incubations. (*$p < 0.05$.)

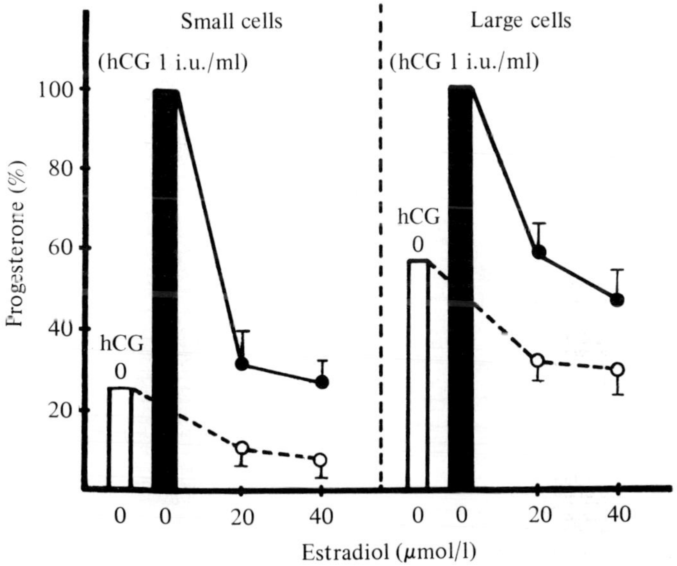

Fig. 8 The inhibition of 3β-HSD activity by estradiol in large and small human luteal cells incubated for 30 minutes at 37°C. The values are the mean ± S.E.M. of results of three separate experiments. The average rate of formation of progesterone was compared with that of the control, which was taken as 100%.

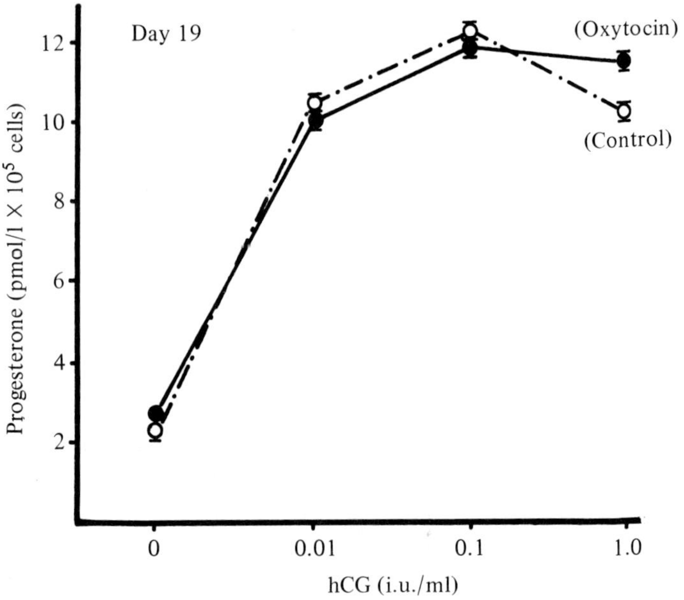

Fig. 9 Effects of various amounts of hCG alone (open circles) or with 2 i.u./ml oxytocin (closed circles) on the production of progesterone by preparations of dispersed cells from human corpus luteum. Values are the mean ± S.E.M. of results from triplicate incubations for 3 hours at 37°C. Oxytocin: Sigma product, 504 i.u./mg.

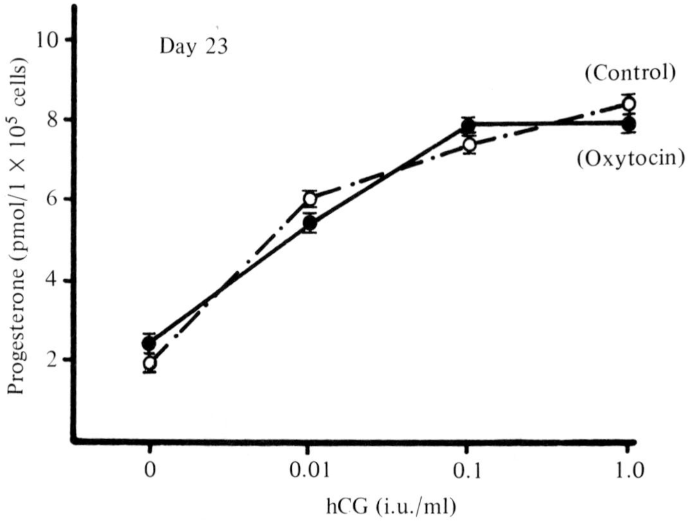

Fig. 10 Effects of various amounts of hCG alone (open circles) or with 2 i.u./ml oxytocin (closed circles) on the production of progesterone by preparations of dispersed cells from human corpus luteum. Values are the mean ± S.E.M. of results from triplicate incubates for 3 hours at 37°C. Oxytocin: Sigma product, 504 i.u./mg.

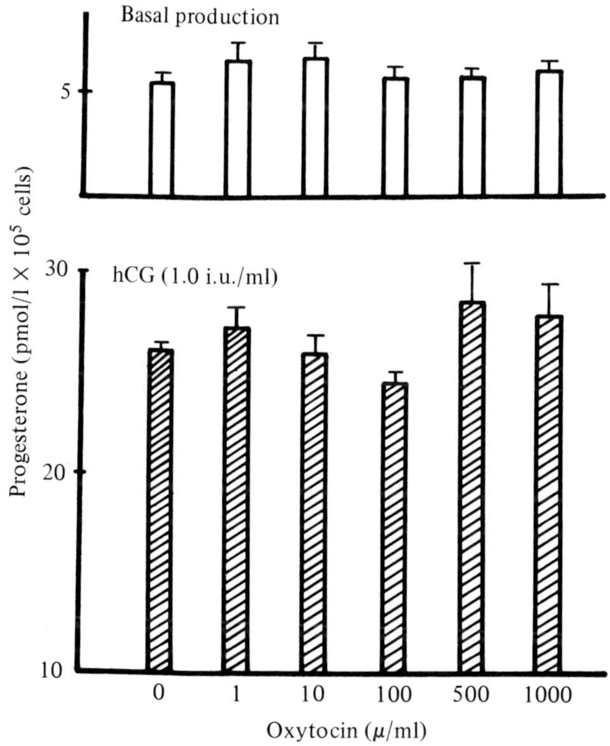

Fig. 11 Effects of various amounts of oxytocin (1–1000 μ/ml) on the production of progesterone by dispersed cells from human corpus luteum, in the presence or absence or hCG. Values are the mean ± S.E.M. of results from three separate experiments with duplicate incubations. Oxytocin: Sigma product, 504 i.u./mg.

in the activation of adenylate cyclase (Cole *et al.*, 1973; Harwood *et al.*, 1978), an event that occurs before the involvement of the intermediate pregnenolone (Savard *et al.*, 1965). From this perspective, one can assume that the small cells may contribute significantly to luteal production of progesterone, particularly during stimulation by LH.

Our results indicated that the activity of 3β-HSD in large cells was more potent than that in small cells. This conclusion derives from results of two experiments. First, the rate of conversion of pregnenolone into progesterone was higher in large cells. The response was dose related. Second, when the inhibitor estradiol was added, the decrease in the production of progesterone was smaller in large cells. We assume that the abundance of 3β-HSD in large cells is responsible for its comparatively higher basal rate of production of progesterone. The activity in the small cells was more easily inhibited.

Preparations of dispersed luteal cells have been used successfully to study

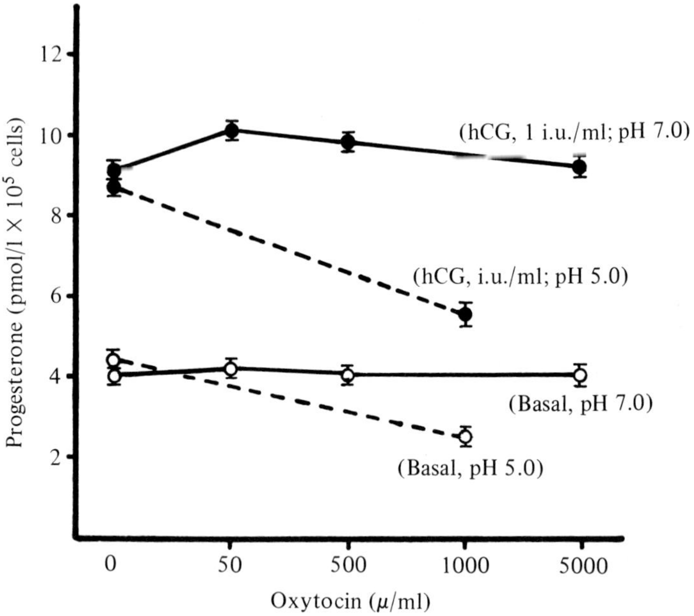

Fig. 12 Effect of pharmaceutical oxytocin before and after adjustment of pH on the production of progesterone by dispersed cells from human corpus luteum. Culture medium was adjusted to pH 7.0 after addition of oxytocin plus vehicle (pH 5.0).

the inhibitory effects of estradiol. The possibility that estradiol-induced luteolysis may be mediated by $PGF_{2\alpha}$, does not appear to exist in human luteal cells (Thibier *et al.*, 1980). It has been suggested that the site of action of estradiol may be at locations after the accumulation of cAMP (Williams *et al.*, 1979). Estradiol may inhibit the activity of 3β-HSD (Depp *et al.*, 1973). In the present study, we examined the activity of 3β-HSD, the enzyme responsible for converting pregnenolone to progesterone, in intact dispersed luteal cells instead of by extraction of the enzyme. Estradiol acted as a potent non-competitive inhibitor in human luteal cells. The effective concentrations of estradiol were similar to endogenous levels seen in human corpus luteum tissue (Swanston *et al.*, 1977). The present results agree with the data that suggest that estradiol may act directly at a site distal to adenylate cyclase.

There are discrepancies between the results from different laboratories on the effects of oxytocin on human luteal function. An inhibitory effect of oxytocin on human luteal cells was reported earlier by Tan and Biggs (1982) and Tan *et al.* (1982), who used pharmacological doses. Recently, Bennegard *et al.* (1987), reported that oxytocin in subpharmacological amounts caused hCG-stimulated synthesis of progesterone and the accumulation of cAMP. In contrast, Richardson and Masson (1984) failed to observe any change in either basal or hCG-stimulated production of progesterone. We obtained the same negative results. When we repeated the experiments using a pharmaceutical preparation instead of the pure powder, we observed a suppression. We found that the vehicle (0.5% chlorobutanol in 0.9% NaCl) that contained the oxytocin was acidic and when the pH of the ampoule was adjusted correctly, no apparent action of oxytocin on the production of progesterone was evident. In addition, similar negative results were also obtained with related peptides, such as vasopressin and vasotocin (unpublished data). Our results indicate that the acidic pH or some contaminating impurity may cause inhibition of the production of progesterone in human luteal cells.

Collectively, in view of the above observations, it is possible to conclude that LH/hCG significantly stimulates small luteal cells in the production of the steroids progesterone, androstenedione and testosterone (Ohara *et al.*, 1987), and that LH/hCG is thereby involved in the maintenance of the biochemical integrity of human corpus luteum. Androstenedione and testosterone contribute to the formation of estradiol in large cells as substrates. 3β-HSD is more potent in large cells which contribute mainly to the basal production of progesterone. Estradiol has been demonstrated to be a potent non-competitive inhibitor of 3β-HSD in both types of intact luteal cell, and the results strongly suggest that estradiol may be involved in the local control of the human corpus luteum, in addition to the hypothalamic pituitary regulation, in its passage toward luteal demise. The role of oxytocin in human luteolysis must be regarded as equivocal.

Acknowledgements

This study received some financial support from the Special Program of Research in Human Reproduction of the World Health Organization and the Shanghai Municipal Commission of Family Planning. We thank Dr J.K. Findlay and Dr J.R. Clarke for their help and encouragement.

References

Auletta, R.J. & Flint, A.P.F. (1988). Mechanisms controlling corpus luteum function in sheep, cows, non-human primates, and women, especially in relation to the time of luteolysis. **Endocrine Reviews** 9:88–105.

Bennegard, B., Hahlin, M. & Dennofors, B. (1987). Antigonadotropic effect of oxytocin on the isolated human corpus luteum. **Fertility and Sterility** 47:431–435.

Cole, F.E., Weed, J.C., Schneider, G.T., Holland, J.B., Geary, W.L. & Rice, B.F. (1973). The gonadotropin receptor of the human corpus luteum. **American Journal of Obstetrics and Gynecology** 117:87–95.

Depp, R., Cox, D.W., Pion, R.J., Conrad, S.H. & Heinrichs, W.L. (1973). Inhibition of the pregnenolone $\Delta^5$3β-hydroxysteroid dehydrogenase-$\Delta^{5,4}$-isomerase systems of human placenta and corpus luteum. **Biology of Reproduction** 23:253–263.

Harwood, J.P., Clayton, R.N. & Catt, K.J. (1980). Ovarian gonadotropin-releasing hormone receptors. 1. Properties and inhibition of luteal cell function. **Endocrinology** 107:407–413.

Karsch, F.J., Krey, L.C., Weik, R.F., Dierschke, D.J. & Knobil, E. (1978). Functional luteolysis in the rhesus monkey: the role of estrogen. **Endocrinology** 92:1148–1152.

Laherty, R.F., Rotter, D., Yamamoto, M. & Jaffe, R.B. (1985). Effects of estradiol and prolactin on progesterone production by rhesus monkey luteal cells *in vitro*. **Acta Endocrinologia** 108:266–272.

Ohara, K., Mori, T., Tall, S., Ban, C. & Narimoto, A. (1987). Functional differentiation in steroidogenesis of two types of luteal cells isolated from mature human corpora lutea of menstrual cycle. **Journal of Clinical Endocrinology and Metabolism** 65:1192–1199.

Richardson, M.C. (1986). Hormonal control of ovarian luteal cells. **Oxford Reviews of Reproductive Biology** 8:342–346.

Richardson, M.C. & Masson, G.M. (1980). Progesterone production by dispersed cells from human corpus luteum: stimulation by gonadotropins and prostaglandin F2α and lack of response to adrenaline and isoprenaline. **Journal of Endocrinology** 87:247–254.

Richardson, M.C. & Masson, G.M. (1985). Lack of direct inhibitory action of oxytocin on progesterone production by dispersed cells from human corpus luteum. **Journal of Endocrinology** 104:149–151.

Rodgers, R.J. & O'Shea, J.D. (1982). Purification, morphology, and progesterone production and content of three cell types isolated from the corpus luteum of the sheep. **Australian Journal of Biological Sciences** 35:441–455.

Savard, K., Marsh, J.M. & Rice, B.F. (1965). Gonadotropins and ovarian steroidogenesis. **Recent Progress in Hormone Research** 21:285–365.

Sheldrick, E.L. & Flint, A.P.F. (1980). Delayed luteal regression in ewes immunized against oxytocin. **Journal of Reproduction and Fertility** 59:37–42.

Shinada, T., Yohota, Y. & Igarashi, M. (1978). Inhibition effect of various gestagens upon the pregnenolone 3β-aldehydrogenase-5,4-isomerase system in human corpora lutea of menstrual cycle. **Fertility and Sterility** 29:84–87.

Stouffer, R.L., Nixon, W.E. & Hodgen, G.D. (1977). Estrogen inhibition of basal and gonadotropin-stimulated progesterone production by rhesus monkey luteal cells *in vitro*. **Endocrinology** 101:1157–1163.

Swanston, I.A., McNatty, K.P. & Baird, D.T. (1977). Concentrations of prostaglandin F and steroids in the human corpus luteum. **Journal of Endocrinology** 73:115–122.

Tan, G.J.S. & Biggs, J.S.G. (1982). Effects of oxytocin on the bovine corpus luteum of early pregnancy. **Journal of Reproduction and Fertility** 66:75–78.

Tan, G.J.S., Tweedale, R. & Biggs, J.S.G. (1982). Oxytocin may play a role in the control of the human corpus luteum. **Journal of Endocrinology** 95:65–70.

Tennant, J.R. (1964). Evaluation of the trypan blue technique for the determination of cell viability. **Transplantation** 2:685–694.

Thibier, M., El-Hassan, X., Clark, M.R., Lematre, W.J. & Marsh, J.M. (1980). Inhibition by estradiol of human chorionic gonadotropin-induced progesterone accumulation in isolated human luteal cells: lack of mediation by prostaglandin. **Journal of Clinical Endocrinology and Metabolism** 50:590–592.

Wang H.Z., Lu, S.H., Shen, W.X., Sun, Z.D., Zhou, W., Wu, Y.F. & Zhou, M.R. (1988). Effect of A-nor steroids and estradiol on progesterone production by human luteal cells. **Journal of Reproduction and Fertility** 83:647–653.

Wathes, D.C. (1984). Possible actions of gonadal oxytocin and vasopressin. **Journal of Reproduction and Fertility** 71:315–345.

Wathes, D.C. & Swann, R.W. (1982). Is oxytocin an ovarian hormone? **Nature** 297:225–227.

Williams, M.T., Roth, M.A., Marsh, J.M. & Le Maire, W.J. (1979). Inhibition of human chorionic gonadotropin-induced progesterone synthesis by estradiol in isolated human luteal cells. **Journal of Clinical Endocrinology and Metabolism** 48:437–440.

III Local regulatory processes

Ovarian insulin-like growth factor 1: basic and clinical implications

E.Y. ADASHI,[1] C.E. RESNICK,[1] E.R. HERNANDEZ,[1] M.E. SVOBODA,[2]
E. HOYT,[3] D.R. CLEMMONS,[4] P.K. LUND,[3] AND J.J. VAN WYK[2]

[1] *Division of Reproductive Endocrinology, Department of Obstetrics and Gynecology, University of Maryland School of Medicine, Baltimore, MD 21201, USA. Departments of Pediatrics,*[2] *Physiology,*[3] *and Medicine,*[4] *University of North Carolina at Chapel Hill, Chapel Hill, NC 27514, USA.*

Keywords

Ovarian insulin-like growth factor 1.

Introduction

The cyclic process of ovarian folliculogenesis is an exponential rather than a linear process and is marked by the dramatic proliferation and differentiation of the developing granulosa cell. Although the central role(s) of gonadotropins and of gonadal steroids in this explosive agenda is well accepted, the variable fate of follicles which have been afforded comparable gonadotropic stimulation suggests the existence of additional intraovarian modulatory systems. Among potential novel intraovarian regulators, insulin-like growth factor 1 (IGF-1) has been the subject of increasingly intense investigation (Adashi *et al.*, 1985). Considered together, the various relevant studies strongly suggest the existence of an intraovarian autocrine control mechanism, wherein IGF-1 may serve as the central signal, with the granulosa cell being the site of its production, reception, and action. In this capacity, IGF-1 may promote the replication and/or cytodifferentiation of the developing granulosa cell, acting largely (but not exclusively) as an amplifier of the action of gonadotropin. In addition, IGF-1 (presumably originating in the granulosa cell) may also provide paracrine input to the adjacent theca–interstitial cell compartment in the interests of coordinated follicular development.

Basic implications

Ovarian production of IGF-1

Ovarian production of IGF-1 was initially suggested by studies that revealed that the level of immunoreactive IGF-1 (iIGF-1) of porcine follicular fluid substantially exceeded that encountered in serum (Hammond, 1981). Further evidence came from the demonstration of cycloheximide-inhibitable, gonadotropin-dependent (and estradiol-dependent) (Hsu and Hammond, 1987) iIGF-1 in serum-free media conditioned by cultured porcine granulosa cells

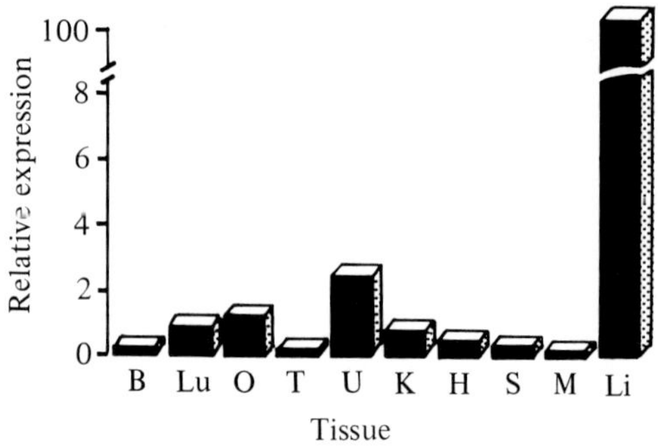

Fig. 1 Relative expression of the IGF-1 gene in various tissues. (L, liver; U, uterus; 0, ovary.) From Murphy *et al.* (1987). **Endocrinology** 120:1279.

(Hammond *et al.*, 1985). Although the level of iIGF-1 in the rat ovary appears to be dependent on growth hormone (Davoren *et al.*, 1986), a direct effect of growth hormone at the level of the rat granulosa cell remains to be demonstrated. Extending these investigations to the transcriptional level, we have recently shown that the adult and immature rat ovary (as well as the isolated, immature granulosa cell) is a site of expression of the IGF-1 gene (Hernandez *et al.*, 1987a) and that it may be subject to gonadotropic regulation. It is significant that, of all adult rat organs tested (Murphy *et al.*, 1987), the ovary displays the third highest level of expression of the IGF-1 gene, the uterus and liver being the most active in this regard (Fig. 1). In contrast, human granulosa cells may be a site of expression of the IGF-2 (Fig. 2) rather than of the IGF-1 gene (Voutilainen and Miller, 1987). These observations and the absence of IGF-2 gene expression in the adult rat ovary (Hernandez *et al.*, 1987a) suggest possible species specificity. However, profound differences in the experimental conditions may favor IGF-2 gene expression as a marker of (fetal) dedifferentiation. Our group has also explored the possibility of ovarian expression of the IGF-1 gene. To this end, polyadenylated RNA from the ovaries of immature (21–23 days old; diethylstilbestrol (DES)-treated) or randomly cycling adult (70–80 days old; non-DES-treated) rats was hybridized with a ^{32}P-labeled rat IGF-1 genomic DNA probe (Fig. 3). As in liver, Northern blot analysis revealed three major RNA species of 1.7, 4.7 and 7.5 kb. Significantly, however, a comparison of hybridization signals indicated substantially greater abundance of specific pre-proIGF-1 RNAs (mostly 7.5 and 1.7 kb) in ovaries of immature DES-treated (lane 2) as compared with adult (lane 1) rats. Given that the ovaries of immature DES-treated rats are comprised largely (>90%) of granulosa cells, these findings suggest measurable expression of the IGF-1 gene at the level of the ovarian granulosa cell. Reprobing of the blots with a ubiquitin cDNA

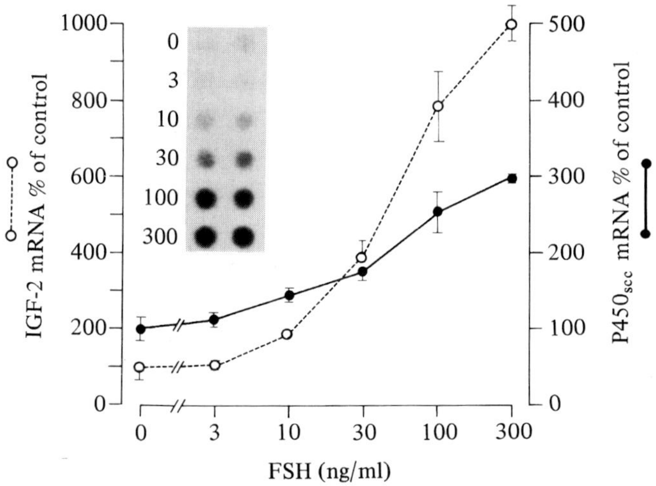

Fig. 2 Expression of the ovarian IGF-2 gene in humans: effect of FSH. Dot blots served as the basis for the relative numerical data. $P450_{scc}$, cholesterol side-chain cleavage enzyme.

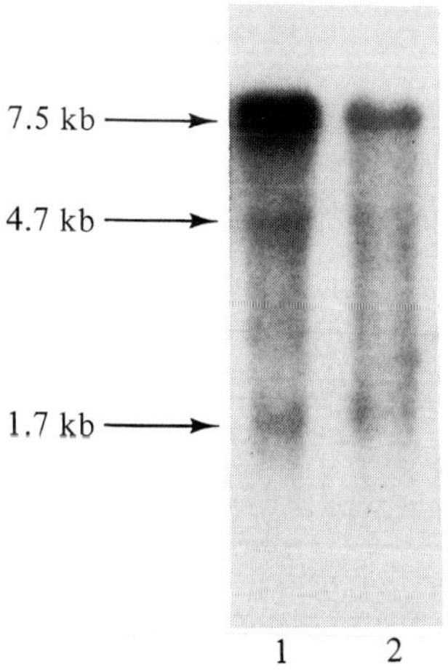

Fig. 3 Expression of the ovarian IGF-1 gene. Samples of polyadenylated RNA (20 μg/lane) are from: (1) immature (21–23 days old), DES-treated, or (2) randomly cycling adult (70–80 days old) rats. Northern blot reflects hybridization with a ^{32}P-labeled rat genomic IGF-1 probe.

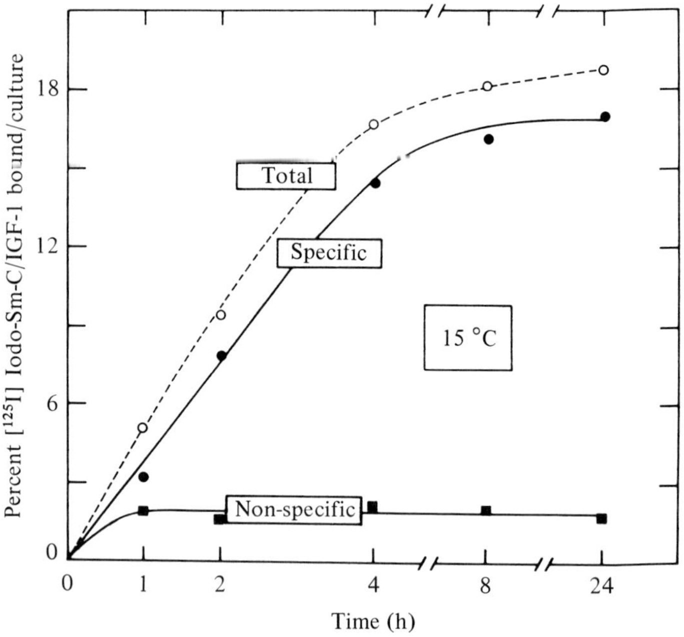

Fig. 4 Binding of [^{125}I]IGF-1 to granulosa cells: time dependence.

probe revealed a similar abundance of ubiquitin mRNA in all samples (not shown), indicating that the observed differences are not due to differences in the load of polyadenylated message. The significance and the translational competence of the multiple, relatively high-molecular-weight RNA transcripts (the smallest of which is of sufficient size to encode pre-proIGF-1) remain uncertain. However, it is likely that these RNA transcripts represent processing variants since pre-proIGF-1 is encoded by a single gene. Regardless of the number of copies of the gene, these observations are in keeping with the notion that the ovary is a site of IGF-1 gene expression and that locally rather than circulatory-derived IGF-1 may play a role in ovarian physiology. However, additional studies are required to determine whether the differences observed between immature and adult rats are, in effect, age dependent or whether DES, applied to immature but not to adult rats, may play a role in this regard.

Receptors for IGF-1 in the ovary

Freshly obtained porcine granulosa cells possess high-affinity (Kd of 0.69–2.1×10^{-9} mol/l), low-capacity binding sites for IGF-1 (Hammond, 1981; Hernandez *et al.*, 1987). Binding to FSH-primed rat granulosa cells proved to be time (Fig. 4), temperature and pH dependent, with optimal steady-state conditions being achieved after an 8-hour incubation at 15°C and at pH 8.0

(Adashi *et al.*, 1987). Although subject to regulation by the cellular density of plating, the binding of [^{125}I]IGF-1 to its receptor proved saturable (apparent Kd of 3.3x10^{-9} mol/l) as well as reversible: complete or partial displacement of tracer was effected by competitive inhibition or dilution, respectively (Adashi *et al.*, 1987). Scatchard and Hill analyses yielded linear plots which were consistent with a single class of non-interacting binding sites. Specificity studies revealed that the competition for binding of [^{125}I]IGF-1 followed a rank order of potency of IGF-1 > MSA (multielevation stimulating activity) > insulin, a pattern compatible with a type 1 receptor for IGF. Limited or no displacement was observed with a series of chemically related and unrelated polypeptides, as well as with an antiserum specific for insulin receptors of human origin (Adashi *et al.*, 1987). Using affinity cross-linking, we have also been able to observe that whole ovarian membranes of untreated (or FSH-treated) immature, hypophysectomized, DES-treated rats are endowed with specific type-1 IGF receptors (Adashi *et al.*, 1985). Similar results have been obtained more recently with isolated granulosa cells from the same experimental model (unpublished).

We have recently reported (Adashi *et al.*, 1986) that FSH and LH are capable of upregulating the binding by granulosa cells of IGF-1, an effect further augmented by growth hormone but not by prolactin. Specifically, we were able to show that FSH is capable of upregulating the binding of IGF-1 in a time- and dose-dependent fashion and that cAMP, its purported intracellular second messenger, may play an intermediary role in this effect (Adashi *et al.*, 1986). Indeed, binding by granulosa cells of IGF-1 was enhanced following elevation of the intracellular level of cAMP by a series of cAMP-generating agonists, inhibition of cAMP-phosphodiesterase activity, or the provision of non-degradable analogs of cAMP. A high dose of forskolin (10^{-5} mol/l), like FSH, proved capable of augmenting the binding of IGF-1 by itself, while an essentially inert dose (10^{-7} mol/l) acted synergistically with FSH to augment binding. It is significant that upregulation of heterologous receptors was not limited to FSH, and similar increments were observed in the case of luteotropic, β_2-adrenergic, but not lactogenic agonists of granulosa cells (Adashi *et al.*, 1987). Related studies *in vivo* using immature, hypophysectomized, DES-treated rats revealed that the ability of FSH to upregulate binding of IGF-1 by granulosa cells: (a) is not strictly an in-vitro phenomenon and can be fully reproduced *in vivo*, (b) is due to enhancement of IGF-1 binding capacity rather than affinity, (c) may be subject to diametrically opposed modulation by somatogenic and GnRH-like agonists of granulosa cells (up- and down-regulation, respectively), and (d) is best maintained by gonadotropins but not by prolactin. Inasmuch as gonadotropin dependence constitutes a unique attribute of the ovarian granulosa cell, our findings further suggest that the granulosa cell receptor for IGF-1 may have thoroughly adapted to its unique environment, providing the first example of a cell type for which the complement of receptors for IGF-1 may be cAMP dependent.

Given the pivotal role of FSH in the induction of granulosa cell receptors for

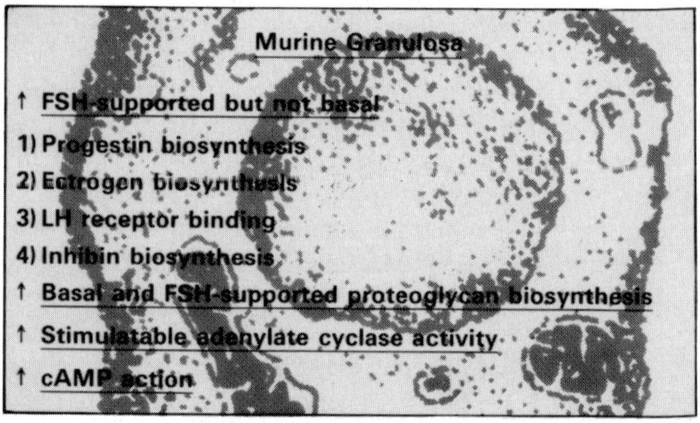

Fig. 5 Reported actions of IGF-1 with reference to the rat granulosa cell.

luteotropic and lactogenic ligands, this finding of cAMP dependence strongly suggests that the acquisition of responsiveness to IGF-1 may be part and parcel of the ontogeny of granulosa cells. Accordingly, gonadotropins may condition the granulosa cell to respond optimally to IGF-1, thereby conferring a selective advantage upon follicles that have been conditioned in this way.

Ovarian action of IGF-1

Studies carried out in the past several years have clearly established the granulosa cell as a site of action of IGF-1 (Adashi *et al.*, 1985). The action of IGF-1 at the level of the rat, but not the porcine, granulosa cell appears largely (but not exclusively) contingent upon its ability to act synergistically with pituitary gonadotropins (Fig. 5). The observed effects are unaccounted for by enhanced cellular viability, plating efficiency, or DNA synthesis. Thus, this ability of IGF-1 to augment differentiated phenotypic expression of the developing granulosa cell may be distinct from its well-established growth-promoting property and can, thus, be considered a novel biologic effect of this polypeptide. In this connection, we have been able to show that IGF-1 is capable of augmenting FSH-supported (but not basal) biosynthesis of progesterone and estrogen as well as the FSH-mediated acquisition of LH receptors. More recently, IGF-1 was also found to augment basal as well as FSH-supported biosynthesis of proteoglycans (May *et al.*, 1985). In this respect, IGF-1 appears to exert its classic 'sulfation factor' activity at the level of the granulosa cell, the very chondrotropic effect that led to its discovery. Fractionation of the major extracellular species of proteoglycans revealed FSH to favor the exclusive production of dermatan sulfate, whereas IGF-1 appears to support the simultaneous biosynthesis of both heparin and dermatan sulfate. These findings suggest that IGF-1 may effect marked quantitative as well as qualitative alterations in proteoglycan economy. Given the possible role of proteoglycans in follicular antrum formation and follicular atresia, these findings raised the possibility that IGF-1, originating in the granulosa cells, may partake in the growth as well as demise of the developing ovarian follicle.

It has been shown that IGF-1 is capable of amplifying the FSH transduction sequence at multiple cellular site(s) both proximal and distal to the generation of cAMP (Adashi *et al.*, 1987). Although it does not affect the breakdown of cAMP, IGF-1 appears to exert a direct stimulatory effect at the level of the adenylate cyclase complex in the face of unaltered levels of receptors for FSH. However, additional studies will be required to distinguish between direct effect(s) of this peptide on the stimulatory or inhibitory regulatory membrane proteins, the catalytic cyclase protein, or combinations thereof. In addition, IGF-1 has been observed to exert a potent stimulatory effect on the action of cAMP, as reflected in the cAMP-supported biosynthesis of progesterone. However, additional studies will be required to determine which of the post cAMP-mediated events may be involved. There is reason to believe, however, that the ability of IGF-1 to enhance the hormonal action of FSH may not be limited to perturbation of intracellular signalling but may also involve enhanced intercellular communication, e.g. clumping of granulosa cells and formation of intercellular gap junctions (May *et al.*, 1985).

Clinical implications

The possibility that intragonadal IGF-1 may be growth-hormone dependent, and that it might amplify the action of gonadotropin, could also have a bearing on the otherwise unexplained puberty-promoting effect of growth hormone. This permissive action of growth hormone has been suggested by observations in growth-hormone-deficient rats, mice, and humans. In each case, an association appears to exist between an isolated deficiency in growth hormone and delayed puberty, a process reversed by systemic administration of the hormone to mice and humans. Although a direct effect of growth hormone on the reproductive axis (e.g. enhanced release of gonadotropin, or enhanced response by target tissues to gonadal steroids) cannot be excluded, it is tempting to speculate that the ability of growth hormone to accelerate pubertal maturation may be due, at least in part, to the generation of intragonadal IGF and the consequent local amplification of the action of gonadotropin. In this connection, the results of recent clinical investigations suggest that the concurrent administration of growth hormone and gonadotropin may in fact result in reduced requirements for gonadotropin, as might be anticipated from the hypothetical intraovarian generation of IGF-1 and the consequent amplification of the action of gonadotropin. Although additional work is required, preliminary information suggests that the addition of growth hormone to ovulation-induction regimens may in fact prove useful in terms of overall outcome, as measured by overall rates of ovulation and conception. In this context, growth hormone may well be useful in the context of chronic anovulatory conditions as well as in the context of in-vitro fertilization procedures.

Summary

We have recently observed that the theca–interstitial cell, like the granulosa cell, may be a site of reception and action of IGF-1, and that physiological concentrations of IGF-1 may participate in the regulation of ovarian biosynthesis of androgens (Hernandez *et al.*, 1987). These observations are in keeping with the view that IGF-1 of granulosal origin may not only play an *autocrine* role but may also serve as one of several signals through which the granulosa cell may communicate in a *paracrine* fashion with the adjacent theca–interstitial cell compartment. In doing so, the granulosa cell may exert some control over its own destiny by enhancing ovarian levels of androgens to suit its aromatizing capabilities and the requirements for estrogen of the developing follicle as a whole. This line of reasoning introduces a level of complexity not previously envisioned, implicating IGF-1 in the orchestration of the coupling of the biosynthesis of androgens to that of estrogen, which would promote coordinated follicular development. Thus, ovarian IGF-1 may subserve at least three central functions.

1. *Amplification* of the hormonal action of gonadotropin – a key requirement, given the exponential nature of follicular development.
2. *Integration* of follicular development – an essential facet concerned with the coordination of granulosa–theca cooperation.
3. *Selection* of dominant follicle(s) – a speculative proposition, assuming timely and selective activation of the IGF-1 system in 'chosen' follicles.

Aside from its possible role(s) in the course of established follicular cycles, IGF-1 (and/or IGF-2) may also participate in the actual formation of the follicular apparatus during the late fetal/early neonatal period. Although the ovary is gonadotropin independent at that time, we have previously shown that IGF-1 may well interact with vasoactive intestinal peptide activity input now implicated in the morphodifferentiation of the follicular apparatus. Similarly, IGF-1 may be concerned with the promotion of juvenile and early pubertal follicular development, a time period characterized by low, ever-declining levels of gonadotropin (FSH) but rising titers of serum growth hormone. At the clinical level, ovarian IGF-1 may have some relevance to the puberty-promoting effect of growth hormone. Indeed, an association appears to exist between isolated deficiency of growth hormone and delayed puberty in both rodents and human subjects, a process reversed by systemic replacement therapy with growth hormone. Given that ovarian IGF-1 and its receptor may be growth-hormone dependent, it is tempting to speculate that the ability of growth hormone to accelerate pubertal maturation may be due, at least in part, to the promotion of ovarian production and of IGF-1 reception with the consequent local potentiation of the action of gonadotropin.

Acknowledgements

This work was supported in part by NIH Research Grant HD-19998 (to E.Y.A.) and USPHS Research Career Development Award l-K04-HD-00697 from the National Institute of Child Health and Human Development, National Institutes of Health (to E.Y.A.).

References

Adashi, E.Y., Resnick, C.E., D'Ercole, A.J., Svoboda, M.E. & Van Wyk, J.J. (1985). Insulin-like growth factors as intraovarian regulators of granulosa cell growth and function. **Endocrine Reviews** 6:400–420.

Adashi, E.Y., Resnick, C.E., Hernandez, E.R., Svoboda, M.E. & Van Wyk, J.J. (1987a). Characterization and regulation of a specific cell membrane receptor for somatomedin-C/Insulin-Like Growth Factor I in cultured rat granulosa cells. **Endocrinology** 122:194–201.

Adashi, E.Y., Resnick, C.E., May, J.V., Knecht, M., Svoboda, M.E. & Van Wyk, J.J. (1987b). Somatomedin-C/Insulin-Like Growth Factor I as an amplifier of follicle-stimulating hormone reaction: studies on mechanism(s) and site(s) of action in cultured rat granulosa cells. **Endocrinology** 122:1583–1592.

Adashi, E.Y., Resnick, C.E., Svoboda, M.E. & Van Wyk, J.J. (1986a). Follicle-stimulating hormone enhances somatomedin-C binding to cultured rat granulosa cells: evidence for cAMP-dependence. **Journal of Biological Chemistry** 261:3923–3926.

Adashi, E.Y., Resnick, C.E., Svoboda, M.E., Van Wyk, J.J., Hascall, V.C. & Yanagish-Ita, M. (1986b). Independent and synergistic actions of somatomedin-C in the stimulation of proteoglycan biosynthesis by cultured rat granulosa cells. **Endocrinology** 118:456–458.

Baranao, J.L.S. & Hammond, J.M. (1984). Comparative effects of insulin and insulin-like growth factors on DNA synthesis and differentiation of porcine granulosa cells. **Biochemical and Biophysical Research Communications** 124:484.

Davoren, J.B., Kasson, B.G., Li, C.H. & Hsueh, A.J.W. (1986). Specific insulin-like growth factor (IGF) I- and II-binding sites on rat granulosa cells: relation to IGF action. **Endocrinology** 119:2155–2162.

Hammond, J.M. (1981). Peptide regulators in the ovarian follicle. **Australian Journal of Biological Sciences** 34:491–504.

Hammond, J.M., Baranao, J.L.S., Skaleris, D., Knight, A.B., Romanus, J.A. & Rechler, M.M. (1985). Production of insulin-like growth factors by ovarian granulosa cells. **Endocrinology** 117:2553–2555.

Hernandez, E.R., Hoyt, E., Van Wyk, J.J. & Adashi, E.Y. (1987a). The somatomedin-C/ insulin-like growth factor I (Sm-C/IGF-1) gene is expressed in the rat ovary.

Presented at the **69th Annual Meeting of the Endocrine Society**, Indianapolis (Abstract no. 821).

Hernandez, E.R., Resnick, C.E., Svoboda, M.E., Van Wyk, J.J., Payne, D.W. & Adashi, E.Y. (1987b). Somatomedin-C/Insulin-Like Growth Factor I (Sm-C/IGF-1) as an enhancer of androgen biosynthesis by cultured rat ovarian cells. **Endocrinology** 122:1583–1592.

Hsu, C.-J. & Hammond, J.M. (1987). Gonadotropins and estradiol stimulate immunoreactive insulin-like growth factor-1 production by porcine granulosa cells *in vitro*. **Endocrinology** 120:198–207.

May, J.V., Schomberg, D.W., Gordon, S. & Amsterdam, A. (1985). Synergistic effect of insulin and follicle-stimulating hormone on biochemical and morphological differentiation of porcine granulosa cells. **Biology of Reproduction** 32, Suppl. 53.

Murphy, L.J., Bell, G.I. & Friesen, H.G. (1987). Tissue distribution of insulin-like growth factor I and II messenger ribonucleic acid in the adult rat. **Endocrinology** 120:1279–1282.

Veldhuis, J.D., Furlanetto, R.W., Juchter, D., Garmey, J. & Veldhuis, P. (1985). Trophic actions of human somatomedin-C/insulin-like growth factor I on ovarian cells: *in vitro* studies with swine granulosa cells. **Endocrinology** 116:1235–1242.

Voutilainen, R. & Miller, W.L. (1987). Coordinate tropic hormone regulation of mRNAs for insulin-like growth factor II and the cholesterol side-chain-cleavage enzyme, P450scc, in human steroidogenic tissues. **Proceedings of the National Academy of Sciences, USA** 84:1590–1594.

Isolation and characterization of growth factors from porcine ovarian follicular fluid

M. YAMAMOTO, N. UENO, M. SHIMONAKA, S. SHIMASAKI AND N. LING

Laboratories for Neuroendocrinology, The Salk Institute, La Jolla, CA 92037, USA.

Keywords

IGF-1, IGF-2, IGF-2 variant, porcine ovary, microsequencing, HPLC.

Introduction

During each ovarian cycle a definite number of follicles undergoes growth and maturation in a sequence that ends in ovulation and formation of a corpus luteum or degenerative atresia (Grady and Smith, 1963). In the developing follicle, the granulosa cells lining the follicular wall can increase in number by more than tenfold and the daughter cells also differentiate and acquire altered responsiveness to hormones (Greenwald, 1974; Richards, 1980). Although it is well known that the primary regulators for the ovarian cycles are the gonadotropins, the detailed mechanism responsible for the growth, differentiation and atretic process is not well understood. Presumably, peptide growth factors are also involved in this process. Indeed, studies with epidermal growth factor, fibroblast growth factor, platelet-derived growth factor, insulin and insulin-like growth factors (IGF) have demonstrated that these polypeptides can regulate the growth and differentiation of cultured granulosa cells (Schomberg *et al.*, 1983; Hsueh *et al.*, 1984; Adashi *et al.*, 1985). However, with the exception of fibroblast growth factor, which has been isolated from the corpus luteum and characterized in terms of its amino acid sequence (Gospodarowicz *et al.*, 1985), none of these growth factors has been purified to homogeneity from the ovary and chemically characterized.

In order to establish the physiological importance of these putative ovarian regulators and to allow detailed studies of their secretion and biological action, we undertook a vigorous program of purification in an attempt to isolate and chemically characterize all the growth factors present in ovarian follicular fluid. Furthermore, since our overall objective was not targeted towards any particular family of mitogenic polypeptides, we selected a rather common bioassay, which quantitates the growth-promoting effect *in vitro* exerted by a mitogen by measuring the incorporation of tritiated thymidine into Balb/c 3T3 cells, to monitor the purification. With this bioassay, we have determined that porcine ovarian follicular fluid contains growth factors with both high (20–40 kDa) and low (5–8 kDa) molecular weights. Furthermore, within the low-molecular-weight category, three IGFs, namely, IGF-1, IGF-

2, and a variant form of IGF-2, have been purified to homogeneity and their structures established by amino-acid sequence analysis.

Materials and methods

Materials

Porcine ovarian follicular fluid was generously supplied by the Contraceptive Development Branch, Center for Population Research, National Institute of Child Health and Human Development. Dulbecco's modified Eagle's medium (DMEM), trypsin-EDTA, penicillin–streptomycin solution, and trypan blue stain were obtained from Grand Island Biological (Grand Island, NY). Tritiated thymidine was obtained from New England Nuclear (Boston, MA). Hyclone (Logan, UT) supplied the fetal bovine serum. Tissue culture plates with 96 wells each were obtained from Costar (Cambridge, MA). Sephacryl S-200 superfine was purchased from Pharmacia (Piscataway, NJ). High performance liquid chromatography (HPLC)-grade acetonitrile was obtained from Baker (Phillipsburg, NJ). All other chemicals were of reagent grade, obtained from the standard suppliers.

Incorporation of tritiated thymidine

The bioassay used to monitor the purification of the growth factors employed Balb/c 3T3 cells obtained from the American Type Culture Collection (Rockville, MD). Stimulation of the uptake of labeled thymidine into the cells by the active fractions was monitored by a method similar to the published procedure (Maciag *et al.*, 1979). Briefly, after the cells were seeded in the 96-well culture plates, they were cultured for 48 hours in 10% fetal bovine serum in DMEM. The cells were then washed and incubated for 24 hours in DMEM that contained 0.75% fetal bovine serum. Incorporation of thymidine into the cells was measured after the addition of aliquots of the column fractions to the serum-starved cells which were incubated for a further 24 hours. Then 0.1 μCi of the labeled nucleotide was added. After a further 5-hour incubation, the amount of radioactivity incorporated into the trichloroacetic acid-precipitated and sodium hydroxide-solubilized DNA was determined in a Beckman scintillation counter (Palo Alto, CA).

Purification of the growth factors

In order to eliminate most of the high-molecular-weight compounds and those proteins that bind to the growth factors, an ammonium sulfate precipitation step, followed by dialysis against 30% acetic acid, was carried out at the beginning of the purification. A sample of 250 ml of porcine follicular fluid (pFF) was mixed with 1 liter of cold water that contained 35 g ammonium sulfate in the cold room for 2 hours, to obtain a 5% saturated solution. The resulting precipitate was removed by centrifugation at 10 000 rpm for 1 hour and the supernatant was dialyzed for 24 hours in the cold room (Spectrapor No. 6 membrane tubing, 28.6 mm cylinder diameter, M^r cutoff 1000; Spectrum Medical Industries, Los Angeles, CA) against 14 liters of 30% (v/v) acetic acid with one change of the acetic acid solution. The retentate was centrifuged at 10 000 rpm to remove a white precipitate and the supernatant (700 ml) was lyophilized. The lyophilized material was dissolved in 200 ml of 30% acetic acid and, after centrifugation to remove the insoluble particles, divided into four equal volumes for loading onto four columns (5 cm i.d.x100 cm) of Sephacryl S-200 superfine. Each column was eluted with 30% acetic acid at a rate of 20 ml/25 minute, and the column fractions were monitored by u.v. absorption at 280 nm and subjected to the bioassay. The bioassay samples were prepared by taking 0.2–1% aliquots of the column fractions and evaporating them in 0.5-ml Eppendorf tubes, each of which had been coated with 50 μg human serum albumin.

The bioactive fractions recovered from each column of Sephacryl S-200 were pooled and, after dilution with 2 volumes of water, filtered through a Millex-HA 0.45 μm Millipore filter (Bedford, MA). The filtrate was applied directly to a HPLC column. After all the filtrate had been loaded, the column was washed with the aqueous solvent A until the u.v. absorption reached the baseline value. The growth factors were separated on a Beckman 322 gradient liquid chromatography system equipped with a Spectroflow 757 UV detector (Kratos Analytical Instruments, Ramsey, NJ), a Soltec 220 recorder (Sun Valley, CA) and a LKB Redirac 2112 fraction collector (Piscataway, NJ).

Two solvent systems for reversed-phase HPLC were used. In the TEAP system, solvent A consisted of 0.1% (v/v) phosphoric acid, 85% (Fisher Scientific, Fair Lawn, NJ) titrated to pH 3.0 with triethylamine, and solvent B was 80% (v/v) acetonitrile in solvent A. In the TFA solvent system, solvent A contained 1 ml of trifluoroacetic acid in 999 ml of water, and solvent B consisted of 1 ml of trifluoroacetic acid in 199 ml of water and 800 ml of acetonitrile. Multiple reversed-phase HPLC steps were used to purify the active factors and the conditions are further described in the text.

Chemical characterization of the growth factors

Determinations of amino acid composition (Böhlen and Schroeder, 1982) and microsequence analysis (Esch, 1985) of the purified growth factors were carried out as previously described.

Results

Each 500-ml bottle of pFF was processed in 250-ml batches to isolate the growth factors. The first step of the purification was an ammonium sulfate precipitation, which was followed by dialysis againt 30% acetic acid. This step greatly expedites the purification procedure because a relatively large volume of pFF can be processed. Furthermore, most of the large proteins that

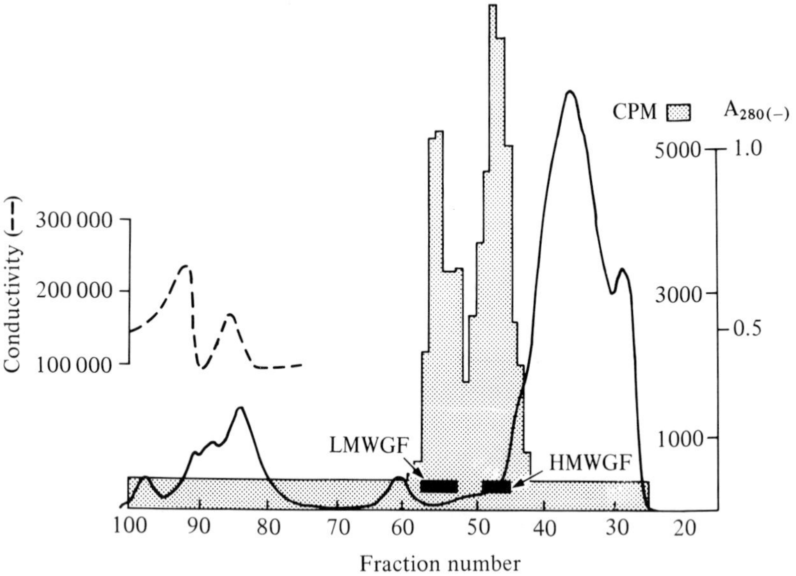

Fig. 1 Gel filtration on Sephacryl S-200 superfine of the 30% acetic acid-soluble proteins from pFF.

aggregate on the gel-filtration column or bind to the growth factors are eliminated. Recovery of the growth-promoting activity after this treatment was at least 90%. The resulting 30% acetic acid-soluble material was gel-filtered through a column of Sephacryl S-200. Figure 1 shows the separation of the mitogenic activity in the column fractions. From the bioassay *in vitro*, there appeared to be two active zones of approximately equal activity, one having an apparent molecular weight of 20–40 kDa, and the other having an apparent molecular weight of 6–8 kDa, as indicated by the two solid bars. These two zones were tentatively labeled as high-molecular-weight growth factors (HMWGF) and low-molecular-weight growth factors (LMWGF), respectively. Since the concentration of protein, as determined by u.v. absorption, was much higher in the HMWGF zone, the LMWGF zone contained much higher specific activity. As a result, this region was selected for further purification by reversed phase HPLC.

After loading of the pooled fraction on an Aquapore RP-300 C8 column (0.7 cm i.d.x25 cm), 7-μm particle size (Brownlee Labs, Santa Clara, CA), the adsorbed proteins were eluted with a linear gradient of 18–36% acetonitrile in 180 minutes in the TFA solvent system with a solvent flow-rate of 3 ml/minute (Fig. 2). Four zones of mitogenic activity, eluting at 21.5%, 24.0%, 27.5%, and 28.5% acetonitrile were detected, as indicated by the solid bars 1, 2, 3, 4 in Figure 2. Since the activity eluting at 27.5% acetonitrile (bar number 3) was

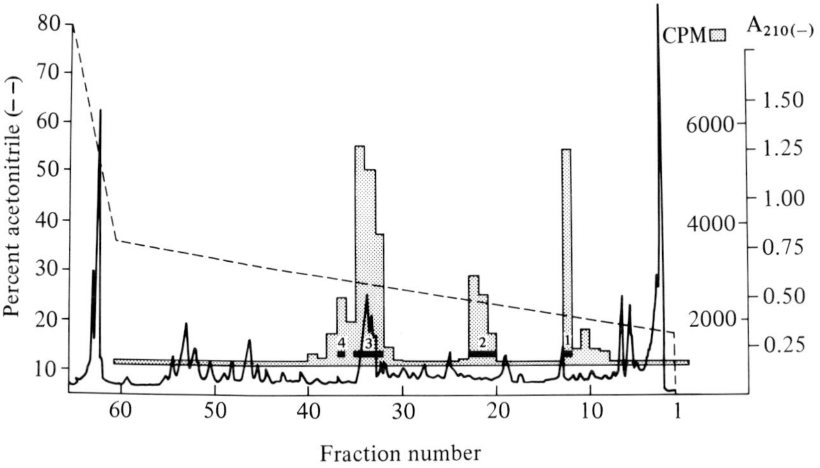

Fig. 2 Purification by reversed-phase HPLC of the low-molecular-weight growth factors recovered after gel filtration. Note that four peaks of mitogenic activity (1–4) were detected.

the strongest, it was selected for further purification. After dilution of the pooled fractions with two volumes of 0.2 N acetic acid, the material was further fractionated on a Vydac C4 column (1 cm i.d.x25 cm), 5-μm particle size (The Separations Group, Hesperia, CA), with the TEAP solvent system and a linear gradient of acetonitrile from 14% to 26% in 120 minutes at a solvent flow-rate of 3 ml/minute, as shown in Figure 3. Again, two zones of growth-promoting activity were detected; one eluting at 22.5% acetonitrile and the other at 23.0% acetonitrile. Both zones were separately pooled as indicated by the bars (3A and 3B in Fig. 3) and further purified on another identical column using the TFA solvent system. The activity was eluted by a linear gradient of acetonitrile from 23% to 32% in 90 minutes at a flow-rate of 1 ml/minute. Figures 4a and 5a show the fractionation by HPLC of the LMWGF3A and 3B, respectively. Since the bioactivity in both chromatograms matched one of the symmetrical u.v.-absorption peaks, the fractions containing these respective peaks from four to eight similar columns were pooled and concentrated by reversed-phase HPLC using an Aquapore RP-300 C8 column (0.46 cm i.d.x25 cm), 10-μm particle size, and the TFA solvent system, with a linear gradient of 0–80% acetonitrile in 80 minutes at a flow-rate of 0.5 ml/minute, as shown in Figures 4b and 5b, respectively.

Amino-terminal sequence analysis of 600 pmol of LMWGF3A revealed a sequence that is identical to the amino terminal of human IGF-2 with the exception of residue 36 (Fig. 6). In the porcine sequence this residue is asparagine; in the human sequence it is serine. Thus, the LMWGF3A isolated from follicular fluid is porcine IGF-2. Amino-acid analysis of the purified

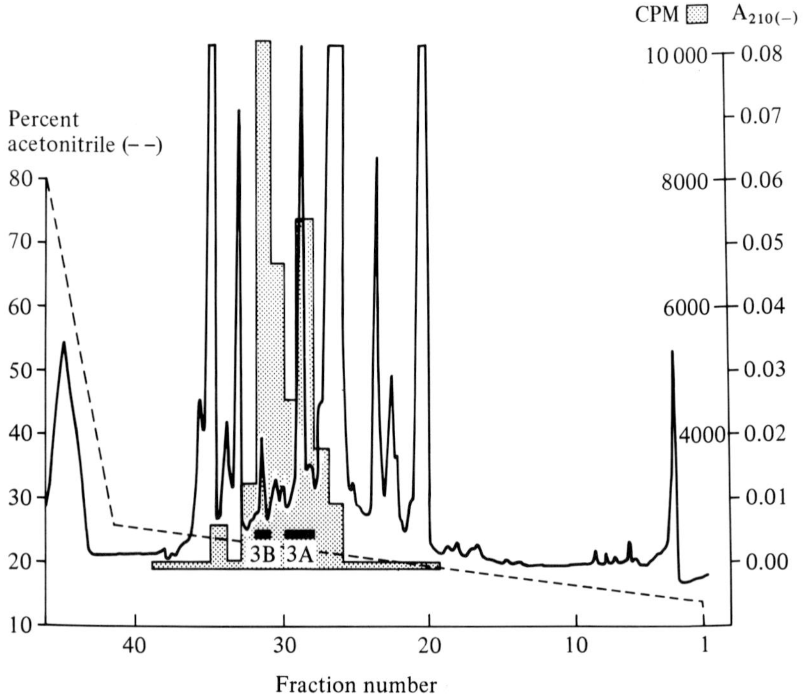

Fig. 3 Purification by reversed-phase HPLC of the activity in peak number 3 in Figure 2. Note that two zones of activity (3A, 3B) were detected.

factor is presented in Table 1 and the composition is in agreement with human IGF-2 (Rinderknecht and Humbel, 1978b) with two exceptions. The porcine peptide contains one more aspartic acid residue, but lacks one serine residue when compared with human IGF-2. Since replacement of the serine at position 36 by asparagine has been determined by sequencing, we are able to account for the amino acid substitution.

Sequence analysis of 200 pmol of the other purified growth factor, LMWGF3B from the amino terminus (Fig. 7), showed that it is completely identical to the amino terminal of human IGF-1 (Rinderknecht and Humbel, 1978a). These results demonstrated that the LMWGF3B isolated from follicular fluid is porcine IGF-1.

Having isolated and characterized the two growth factors located in zone 3 of Figure 2, we next turned our attention to the purification of the mitogenic activity present in zone 4. Using HPLC conditions identical to those used to generate the data in Figure 3, we purified the pooled activity on a Vydac C4 column, as shown in Figure 8a. Only one zone of activity was located eluting at 23% acetonitrile. This activity was pooled (solid bar) and, after dilution,

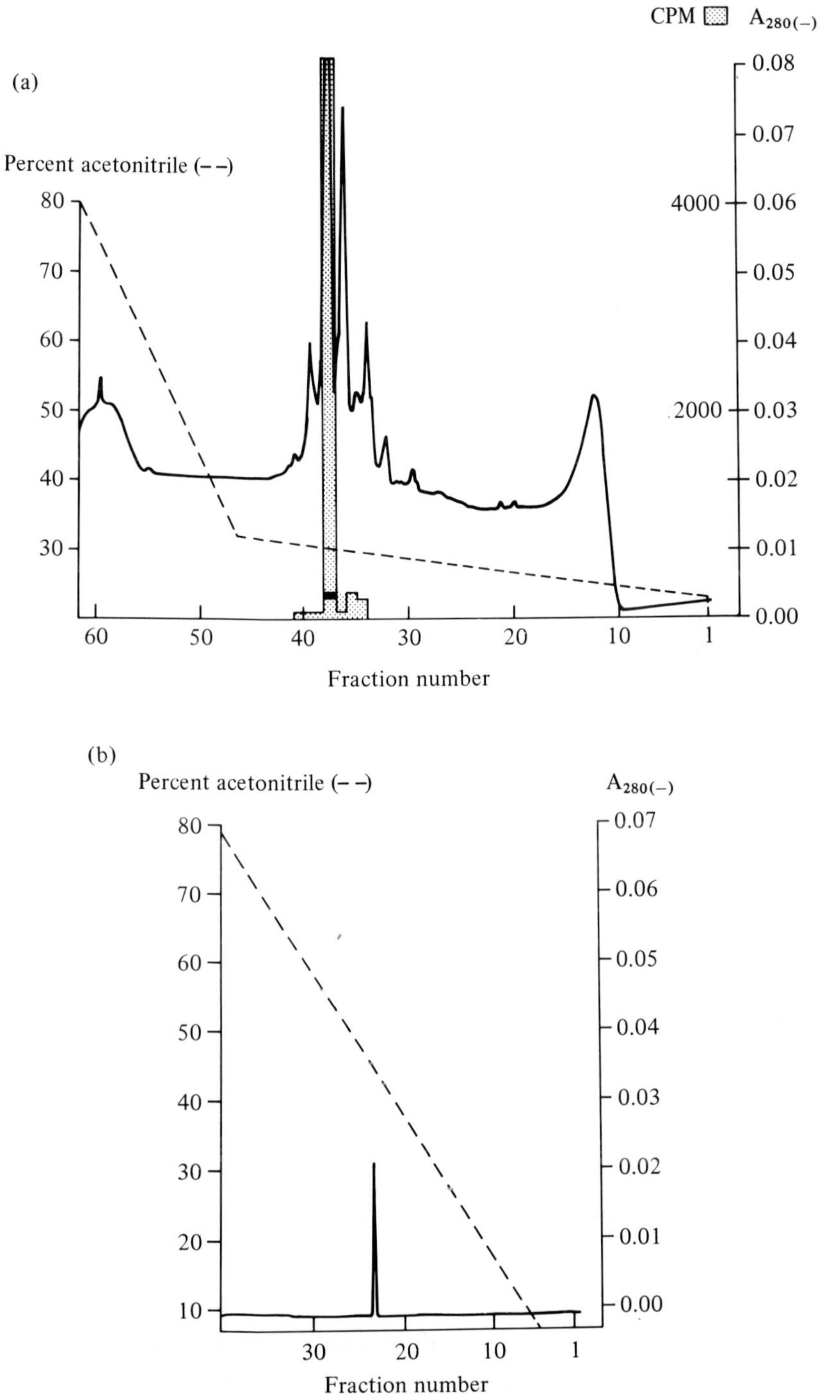

Fig. 4 (a) Purification by reversed-phase HPLC of peak 3A in Figure 3. (b) Concentration of the active peak, denoted by the solid bar in Figure 4a, by HPLC for chemical analysis.

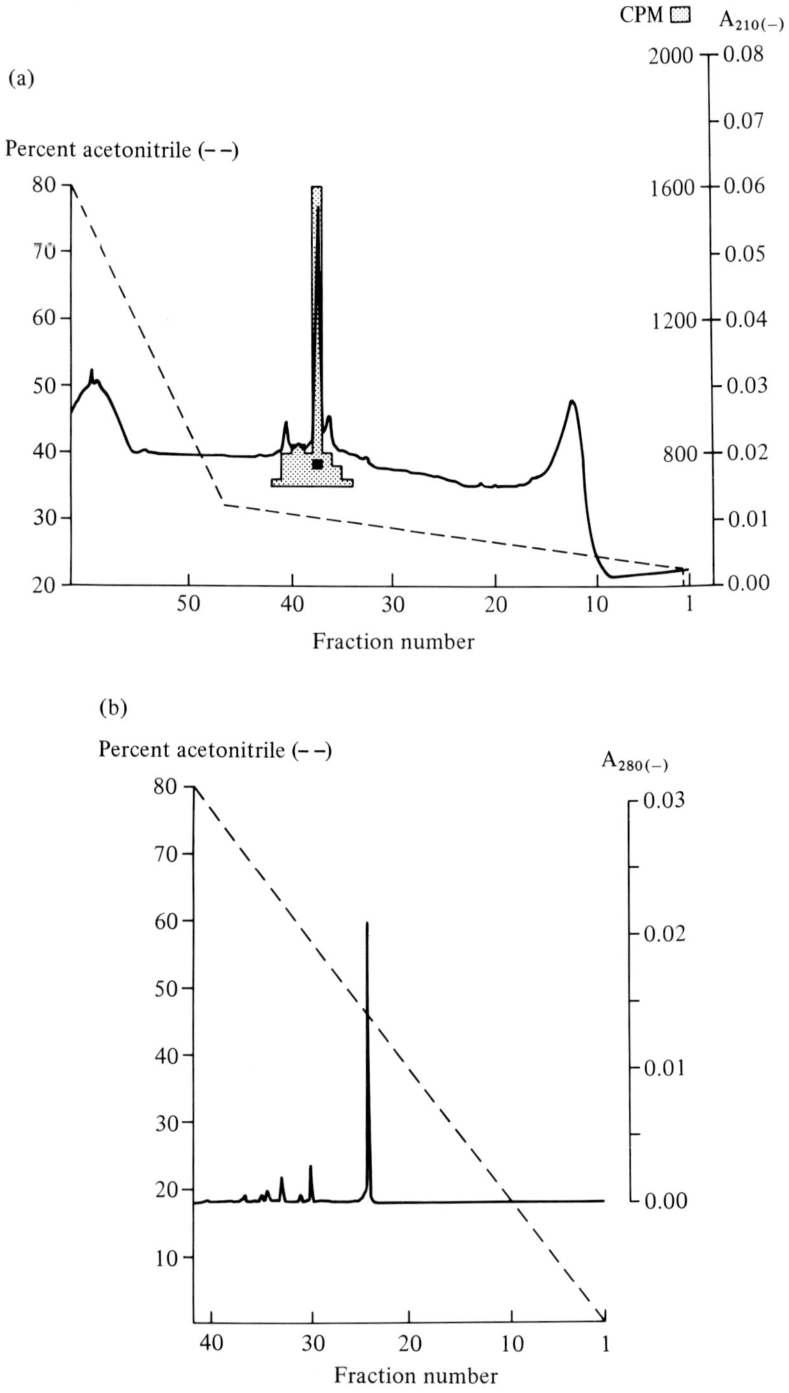

Fig. 5 (a) Purification by reversed-phase HPLC of peak 3B in Figure 3. (b) Concentration of the active peak, denoted by the solid bar in Figure 5a, by HPLC for chemical analysis.

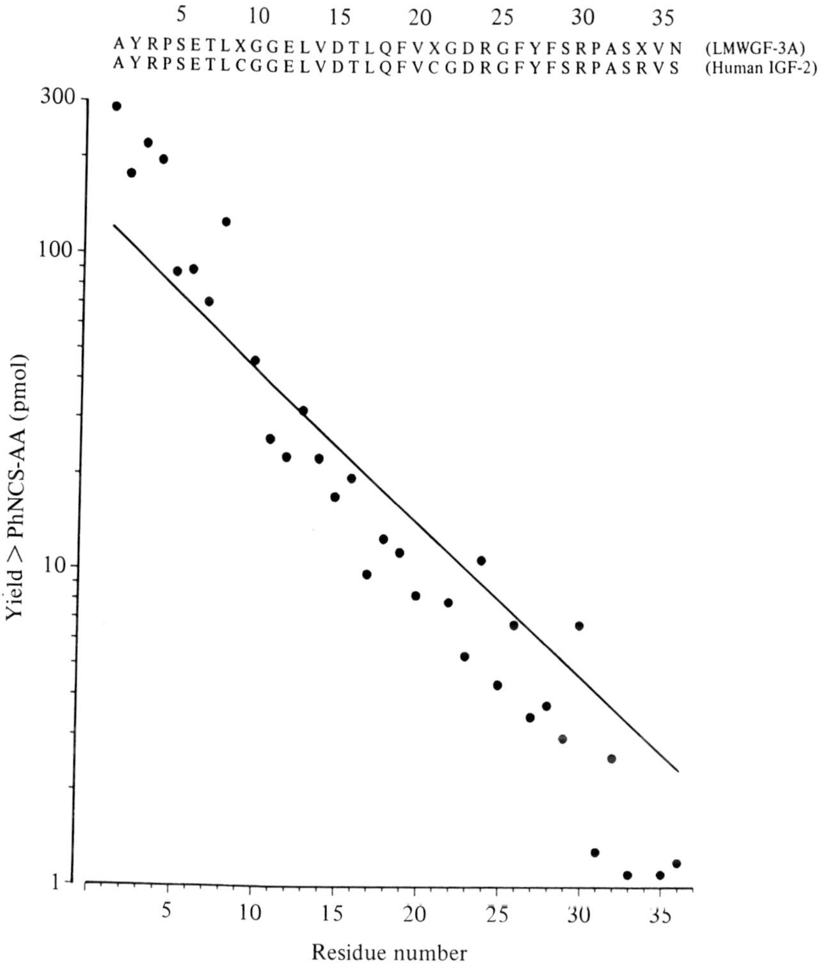

Fig. 6 Amino-terminal sequence analysis of LMWGF3A recovered from the chromatographic step shown in Figure 4b. 〉PhNCS-AA is an abbreviation for the phenylthiohydantoin derivative of the released amino acid from each cycle. The symbol 'x' represents a residue which was not identified.

pumped onto another Vydac C4 column (1 cm i.d.x25 cm), 5-μm particle size, and fractionated with a linear gradient of 21–30% acetonitrile in the TFA solvent system, in 90 minutes, at a flow-rate of 1 ml/minute (Fig. 8b). Because the u.v. absorption peak at the active region was not symmetrical, the active fractions were pooled and further purified with the TEAP solvent system on a Vydac phenyl column (1 cm i.d.x25 cm), 5-μm particle size, with a linear gradient of 18–27% acetonitrile in 90 minutes, at a flow-rate of 1 ml/minute

Table 1. *Amino acid composition of purified LMWGF3A*

Amino acid	LMWGF3A	Human IGF-2[a]
Asx	4.13	3
Thr	3.85	4
Ser	5.87	7
Glx	6.75	7
Gly	5.23	5
Ala	5.00	5
Val	3.77	4
Met	0.00	0
Ile	0.89	1
Leu	5.95	6
Tyr	3.13	3
Phe	4.01	4
His	0.00	0
Trp	0.00	0
Lys	1.04	1
Arg	8.26	8
Cys[b]	5.82	6
Pro	3.18	3

Values represent mean of two analyses normalized to a peptide of 67 residues.
[a]Values are calculated from the amino acid sequence of human IGF-2 published by Rinderknecht and Humbel (1978b).
[b]Determined as cysteic acid after performic acid oxidation.

(Fig. 8c). The active zones from eight such fractionations were pooled and concentrated on a column of Aquapore RP-300 for chemical characterization (Fig. 8d).

Amino-terminal sequence analysis of 200 pmol of the purified LMWGF4 revealed that it is the variant form of human IGF-2 (Fig. 9), whose structure had been predicted by DNA sequence analysis of the cloned liver IGF cDNAs (Jansen *et al.*, 1985). In this variant form, the serine residue at position 29 is replaced by the tetrapeptide arg-leu-pro-gly. In addition, the porcine variant form also includes the substitution of an asparagine for a serine residue at position 39 of the human congener.

Attempts to purify the remaining two LMWGFs indicated in Figure 2, using similar reversed-phase HPLC conditions, have not been successful thus far. The difficulties were caused by the extremely low concentrations of these two compounds in the follicular fluid. More efforts to accumulate enough starting material to accomplish their isolation are in progress.

```
          5         10        15        20        25        30        35        40
GPETLXGAELVDALQFVXGDRGFYFNKPTGYGSSSRRAPQ (LMWGF-3B)
GPETLCGAELVDALQFVCGDRGFYFNKPTGYGSSSRRAPQ (Human IGF-1)
```

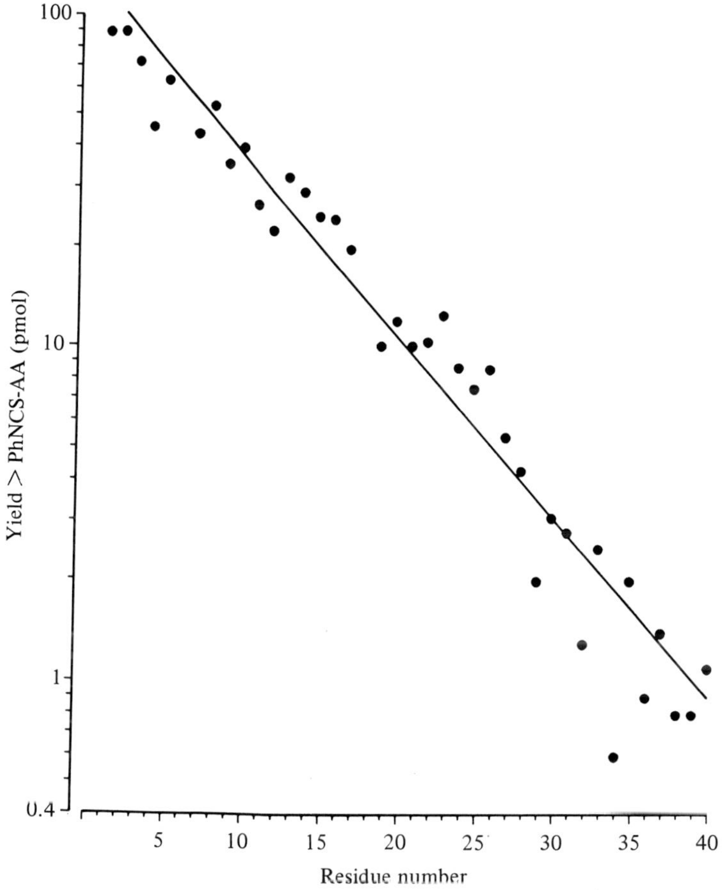

Fig. 7 Amino-terminal sequence analysis of LMWGF3B recovered from the chromatographic step shown in Figure 5b. >PhNCS-AA is an abbreviation for the phenylthiohydantoin derivative of the released amino acid from each cycle. The symbol 'x' represents a residue which was not identified.

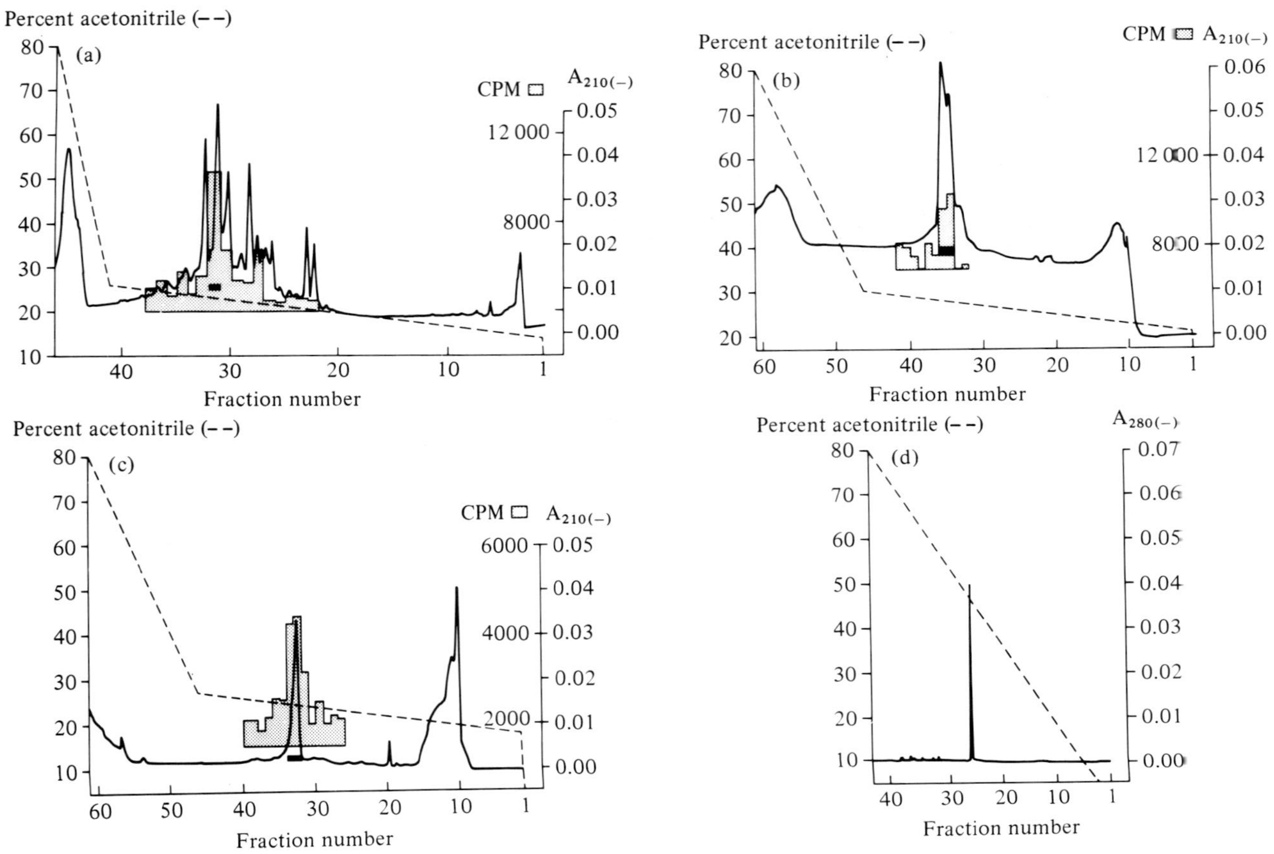

Fig. 8 (a) Purification by reversed-phase HPLC of active peak number 4 in Figure 2. (b) Purification by reversed-phase HPLC of the active peak denoted by the solid bar in Figure 8a. (c) Purification by reversed-phase HPLC of the active peak shown in Figure 8b. (d) Final purification of LMWGF4 by HPLC for chemical analysis

5 10 15 20 25 30 35
A Y R P S E T L X G G E L V D T L Q F V X G D R G F Y F R L P G R P A X R V N (LMWGF-4)
A Y R P S E T L C G G E L V D T L Q F V C G D R G F Y F R L P G R P A S R V S (Human IGF-2 variant)

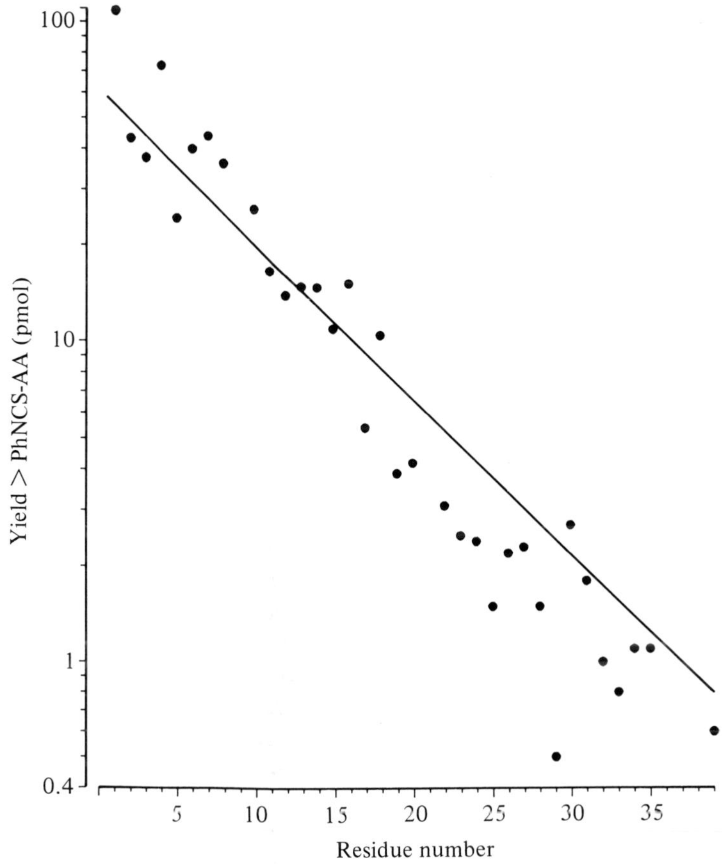

Fig. 9 Amino-terminal sequence analysis of LMWGF4 recovered from the chromatographic step shown in Figure 8d. >PhNCS-AA is an abbreviation for the phenylthiohydantoin derivative of the released amino acid from each cycle. The symbol 'x' represents a residue which was not identified.

Discussion

Three growth factors of molecular weights of 7–8 kDa were isolated from pFF by sequential ammonium sulfate precipitation, dialysis against 30% acetic acid, gel filtration on Sephacryl S-200 and four steps of reversed-phase HPLC. From the amino-acid sequence determination, one of the purified factors was found to be the porcine congener of human IGF-1 while the other two corresponded to porcine IGF-2 and its variant form. Isolation of the porcine IGF-2 variant form from follicular fluid is unexpected since its origin was only predicted by sequence analysis of the cloned IGF-2 DNAs from a human liver cDNA library (Jansen *et al.*, 1985). Isolation of the mature molecule has not been reported. The variant form arises from alternative splicing of the precursor mRNA for IGF-2 (Jansen *et al.*, 1985). Another variant pro-form of IGF-2, containing the substitution of cys-gly-asp for the serine residue at position 33, together with a carboxy-terminal extension of 21 residues of the E peptide, has been reported (Zumstein *et al.*, 1985). The mechanism responsible for generating this variant pro-form is unknown. Like the rat (Dull *et al.*, 1984) and bovine (Honegger and Humbel, 1986) species of IGF-2, porcine IGF-2 contains the substitution of asparagine for serine at residue 36 of the human sequence. This substitution is also preserved in the variant form of porcine IGF-2.

The presence of IGF-1-like and IGF-2-like compounds in follicular fluid has been reported by others (Hammond *et al.*, 1985; Ramasharma *et al.*, 1986). However, the evidence provided to demonstrate the identity of these molecules was based solely on cross-reactivity in radioimmunoassays for IGF or radioreceptor assays. The present work employed the vigorous chemical criteria of amino-acid sequence analysis to establish the identity of the purified factors. Porcine IGF-2 differs from human IGF-2 by one amino acid, but porcine IGF-1 is identical to human IGF-1, as has been reported recently from the results of molecular cloning (Tavakkol *et al.*, 1988). Using the present purification scheme, approximately 18 μg of IGF-2, 7 μg of IGF-2 variant, and 5 μg of IGF-1 can be isolated from 250 ml of porcine follicular fluid. Since our purification procedure is not the most efficient, the final yield of the purified material is probably less than 5%. Thus, the actual amount of IGF peptides present in the original follicular fluid could be similar to that in human plasma (Zapf *et al.*, 1981). This hypothetical result raises the possibility that the peptides could have been transported from the plasma, although other researchers have shown that granulosa cells can synthesize the IGF peptides (Hammond *et al.*, 1985).

Recently, the importance of growth factors in the development and differentiation of ovarian tissue has been pointed out by many workers (Schomberg *et al.*, 1983; Hsueh *et al.*, 1984). In particular, IGF-1 has been shown to act in a paracrine and/or autocrine mode to stimulate the replication and differentiation of granulosa cells (Adashi *et al.*, 1985). It acts synergistically with FSH in the induction of granulosa cell aromatase activity and the production of progesterone. However, only a limited function has been assigned to IGF-2, even though the amount of IGF-2 isolated from porcine follicular fluid is much higher than that of IGF-1. Clearly, more research is needed to elucidate the action of IGF-2 in the ovary.

Acknowledgements

We thank F. Castillo, R. Schroeder, and M. Regno-Lagman for technical assistance and D. Higgins for preparing the manuscript. This work was supported by a contract from the National Institute of Child Health and Human Development, N01-HD-6-2944, National Institutes of Health Program Project Grants HD-09690 and DK-18811, and a grant from the Robert J. and Helen C. Kleberg Foundation.

References

Adashi, E.Y., Resnick, C.E., D'Ercole, A.J., Svoboda, M.E. & Van Wyk, J.J. (1985). Insulin-like growth factors and intraovarian regulators of granulosa cell growth and function. **Endocrine Reviews** 6:400–420.

Böhlen, P. & Schroeder, R. (1982). High-sensitivity amino acid analysis: methodology for the determination of amino acid composition with less than 100 picomoles of peptides. **Analytical Biochemistry** 126:144–152.

Dull, T.J., Gray, A., Hayflick, J.S. & Ullrich, A. (1984). Insulin-like growth factor II precursor gene organization in relation to insulin gene family. **Nature** 310:777–781.

Esch, F. (1984). Polypeptide microsequence analysis with the commercially available gas-phase sequencer. **Analytical Biochemistry** 136:39–47.

Gospodarowicz, D., Cheng, J., Lui, G.M., Baird, A., Esch, F. & Böhlen, P. (1985). Corpus luteum angiogenic factor is related to fibroblast growth factor. **Endocrinology** 117:2283–2391.

Grady, H.G. & Smith, D.E. (1963). **The Ovary**. Baltimore, Williams and Wilkins.

Greenwald, G.S. (1974). Role of follicle-stimulating hormone and luteinizing hormone in follicular development and ovulation. In: Greep, R.O., Astwood, E.B., Knobil, E., Sawyer, W.H. & Geiger, S.R., eds. **Handbook of Physiology**, Vol. IV, Part 2, Section 7, Washington DC, American Physiological Society, pp.293–323.

Hammond, J.M., Baranao, L.S., Skaleris, D., Knight, A.B., Romanus, J.A. & Rechler, M.M. (1985). Production of insulin-like growth factors by ovarian granulosa cells. **Endocrinology** 117:2553–2555.

Honegger, A. & Humbel, R.E. (1986). Insulin-like growth factor I and II in fetal and adult bovine serum. **Journal of Biological Chemistry** 261:569–575.

Hsueh, A.J.W., Adashi, E.Y., Jones, P.B.S. & Welsh, T.H. Jr (1984). Hormonal regulation of the differentiation of cultured ovarian granulosa cells. **Endocrine Reviews** 5:76–127.

Jansen, M., Van Schaik, F.M.A., Van Tol, H., Van Der Brande, J.L. & Sussenbach, J.S. (1985). Nucleotide sequences of cDNAs encoding precursors of human insulin-like growth factor-II (IGF-2) and an IGF-2 variant. **FEBS Letters** 179:243–246.

Maciag, T., Cerundolo, J., Ilsley, S., Kelly, P.R. & Forand, R. (1979). An endothelial cell growth factor from bovine hypothalamus: identification and partial characterization. **Proceedings of the National Academy of Sciences, USA** 76:5674–5678.

Ramasharma, K., Cabrera, C.M. & Li, C.H. (1986). Identification of insulin-like growth factor II in human seminal and follicular fluids. **Biochemical and Biophysical Research Communications** 140:536–542.

Richards, J.S. (1980). Maturation of ovarian follicles: actions and interactions of pituitary and ovarian hormones in follicular cell differentiation. **Physiological Reviews** 60:51–89.

Rinderknecht, E. & Humbel, R.E. (1978a). The amino acid sequence of human insulin-like growth factor I and its structural homology with pro-insulin. **Journal of Biological Chemistry** 253:2769–2776.

Rinderknecht, E. & Humbel, R.E. (1978b). Primary structure of human insulin-like growth factor-II. **FEBS Letters** 89:283–286.

Schomberg, D.W., May, J.V. & Mondschein, J.S. (1983). Interactions between hormones and growth factors in the regulation of granulosa cell differentiation *in vitro*. **Journal of Steroid Chemistry** 19:291–295.

Tavakkol, A., Simmen, F.A. & Simmen, R.C.M. (1988). Porcine insulin-like growth factor-1 (pIGF-1): complementary deoxyribonucleic acid cloning and uterine expression of messenger ribonucleic acid encoding evolutionarily conserved IGF-1 peptides. **Molecular Endocrinology** 2:674–681.

Zapf, J., Waltz, H. & Froesch, E.R. (1981). Radioimmunological determination of insulin-like growth factors I and II in normal subjects and in patients with growth disorders and extrapancreatic tumor hypoglycemia. **Journal of Clinical Investigation** 68:1321–1330.

Zumstein, P.P., Luthi, C. & Humbel, R.E. (1985). Amino acid sequence of a variant pro-form of insulin-like growth factor-II. **Proceedings of the National Academy of Sciences, USA** 82:3169–3172.

Paracrine mechanisms in the regulation of testicular function

D.M. DE KRETSER, G.P. RISBRIDGER, A.E. DRUMMOND, G. GONZALES AND Y.T. SUN

Department of Anatomy, Monash University, Melbourne, Victoria, Australia.

Keywords

Seminiferous tubules, Sertoli cells, Leydig cells.

Introduction

For many years we have considered the testis as comprising two independent compartments which are involved in steroidogenesis and spermatogenesis, but the past decade has produced evidence to link the function of the tubule and intertubular compartments in both normal and pathological states (see reviews by Sharpe, 1984; de Kretser, 1987; Findlay and Risbridger, 1987). It is clear that the germ cells, Sertoli cells and Leydig cells are functionally interrelated and that there are significant modifications of the functions of these types of cell that can occur as a result of changes in the testicular vascular system.

Control of seminiferous tubule function by Leydig cells

The best recognized intracompartmental regulatory mechanism in the testis is the dependence of spermatogenesis on testosterone. It is generally accepted that both FSH and LH are required for spermatogenesis and the absence of receptors for LH in the seminiferous tubules points to an indirect mechanism of action of this hormone (Lostroh, 1969; Odell *et al.*, 1973). That the intermediary is testosterone is best demonstrated by the spermatogenic disruption that results from passive immunization using an LH-specific antiserum (Raj and Dym, 1976) and the restoration of spermatogenesis after hypophysectomy by testosterone (Clermont and Harvey, 1965).

The high doses of testosterone that are required to restore spermatogenesis led to the view that very high, local, intratesticular levels of testosterone were necessary and resulted from the juxtaposition of the Leydig cells and the seminiferous tubules. However, recent studies which have measured intratesticular concentrations of testosterone have shown that spermatogenesis can be restored by levels that represent only 10–15% of normal levels (Cunningham and Huckins, 1979; Huang and Nieschlag, 1986). Although some controversy exists as to the actual intratesticular levels of testosterone, the relatively low levels of testosterone in the testis at which spermatogenesis is restored are greater than the concentrations of peripheral circulating testosterone that are above those found in normal rats (Huang and Nieschlag, 1986; Sun *et al.*, 1989). This observation itself creates a dilemma, since normal circulating levels of testosterone are clearly adequate for activation of the androgen receptors at many sites. Why then are relatively higher levels required to maintain spermatogenesis? Does this mechanism of action of androgens require a receptor with different features to those found in other tissues?

Evidence exists that some actions of androgens on the Sertoli cell may occur via an indirect mechanism that involves receptors on the peritubular cells, through the secretion of an intermediary protein termed P.Mod.S. (Skinner and Fritz, 1985). Furthermore, Verhoeven and Cailleau (1988) demonstrated that androgens induce the formation of additional androgen receptors on Sertoli cells. Further studies are necessary to eludicate all the details of the action of androgens on the spermatogenic process.

Alternative mechanisms exist by which the Leydig cells influence the functions of seminiferous tubules. β-Endorphin is known to be present in Leydig cells, as shown by immunocytochemistry (Tsong *et al.*, 1982a, 1982b), and the mRNA for its precursor protein, pro-opiomelanocortin (POMC), has been shown to occur in Leydig cells by *in-situ* hybridization (Pintar *et al.*, 1984). In turn, receptors for β-endorphin are found on Sertoli cells and administration of this peptide to cultures of Sertoli cells *in vitro* results in a decrease in basal and FSH-stimulated secretion of androgen-binding protein (ABP) (Fabbri *et al.*, 1985). Whether other aspects of Sertoli cell function can be influenced by β-endorphin requires further investigation. Elucidation of the testicular physiology of the POMC peptides has also been complicated by the demonstration of β-endorphin in the germ cells (Cheng *et al.*, 1985; Gizang-Ginsberg and Wolgemuth, 1987).

Our own studies have identified yet another function of the tubule that is influenced by the Leydig cells, namely the secretion of inhibin. Stimulation of the rat testis *in vivo* with human chorionic gonadotropin (hCG) results in a significant increase in serum levels of inhibin 24 hours after the injection (Drummond *et al.*, 1988). This action was shown to involve the Leydig cells since, if they are destroyed by the drug ethane dimethane sulphonate prior to stimulation with hCG, no increase in levels of inhibin occurs. It is likely that this stimulation is not due to secretion of testosterone, since supraphysiological levels (10^{-5} mol/l) of testosterone are required to influence the secretion of inhibin *in vitro* and this action is inhibitory rather than stimulatory (Bicsak *et al.*, 1987; Bardin *et al.*, 1987; Gonzales *et al.*, 1988). The nature of the signal from the Leydig cell that controls the secretion of inhibin is unknown. Since inhibin has the potential to influence mitotic and meiotic activity in germ cells (see below), this action of the Leydig cells may have significant physiological relevance to the control of spermatogenesis.

Germ cell–Sertoli cell interactions

There is considerable evidence, from a structural point of view, to indicate a remarkably close association between the Sertoli cells and the germ cells in the seminiferous epithelium (for review, see de Kretser and Kerr, 1988). The existence of specialized inter-Sertoli cell junctions which prevent intercellular transport, situated luminal to the spermatogonial cell layer, effectively divides the epithelium into a basal and an adluminal compartment (Dym and Fawcett, 1970). The primary spermatocytes, secondary spermatocytes and spermatids in the adluminal compartment are dependent on the Sertoli cells for the transport of metabolites and substrates required for their metabolism. This dependence is best illustrated by the demonstration that the Sertoli cells metabolize glucose to lactate, which is the substrate required by the germ cells but which they are unable to produce (Jutte *et al.*, 1981, 1982; Mita *et al.*, 1982). Furthermore, the production of lactate by the Sertoli cells is under the control of FSH, insulin and IGF-1 (Mita *et al.*, 1982, 1985; Jutte *et al.*, 1983, Borland *et al.*, 1984).

With such a fundamental dependence of the germ cells on the Sertoli cells, the existence of mechanisms by which the germ cells can interact with the Sertoli cells is to be expected. Evidence that such relationships exist came from the studies of Parvinen and colleagues (1982, 1987), who were able to dissect out segments of seminiferous tubules in the rat which were at specific stages of the seminiferous cycle, as originally described by Leblond and Clermont (1952). The studies demonstrated stage-dependent changes in the functions of the Sertoli cell which include: (i) changes in the number of FSH receptors and the responsiveness of the tubule to FSH (Parvinen, 1982); (ii) alterations in the production of a number of proteins such as transferrin, androgen-binding protein (ABP), and ceruloplasmin (Ritzen *et al.*, 1982; Wright *et al.*, 1983); and (iii) changes in the activity of certain enzymes, such as aromatase and plasminogen activator (Lacroix *et al.*, 1981; Boitani *et al.*, 1981). These changes and the stages at which they occur are illustrated diagrammatically in Figure 1.

Other indirect evidence in support of the concept that germ cells influence Sertoli cell function comes from studies of damage to the spermatogenic process. This approach is best illustrated by a series of experiments that involved local heating of rat testes to 43°C for 15 minutes. This treatment resulted in damage to the most heat-sensitive intermediates in spermatogenesis, namely, the pachytene spermatocytes and round spermatids (Chowdhury and Steinberger, 1964). When measurements of Sertoli cell function were performed in conjunction with this heat-induced degeneration, no changes in the testicular content of ABP or inhibin were observed for 7–10 days after the initial injurious stimulus (Fig. 2). Subsequently, both parameters declined and then recovered 28–35 days after the heat treatment (Jégou *et al.*, 1984; Au *et*

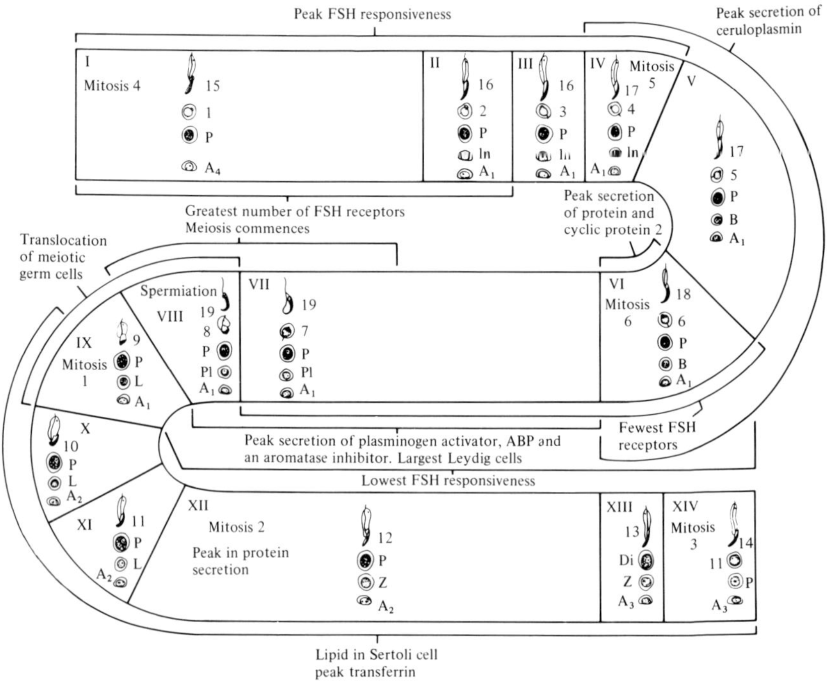

Fig. 1 The changes in several parameters of Sertoli cells during the rat seminiferous cycle are shown. The length of the tubules is a proportional representation of the duration of each stage of the cycle. Reproduced with permission from de Kretser, D.M. (1987). **International Review of Cytology** 10:89–112.

al., 1987). The absence of an immediate change in Sertoli cell function after the heat treatment suggested that the heating *per se* was not the cause of the changes in Sertoli cell function. The pattern of changes strongly suggested that the function of Sertoli cells may be linked to alterations in the population of germ cells that surrounds the Sertoli cells, as a result of the heat treatment. The temporal sequence correlated best with the loss and return of spermatids in the epithelium (Jégou *et al.*, 1984). More recently, a number of experimental studies using different models have supported the concept that destruction of certain types of germ cell can influence Sertoli cell function (Pinon-Lataillade *et al.*, 1988).

Direct evidence for these interactions is also available from the studies of Galdieri and colleagues (1984) who showed that the secretion of ABP by Sertoli cells in culture could be stimulated by contact with primary spermatocytes. Furthermore, Vihko *et al.* (1984) noted that the return of preleptotene primary spermatocytes after testicular irradiation was associated

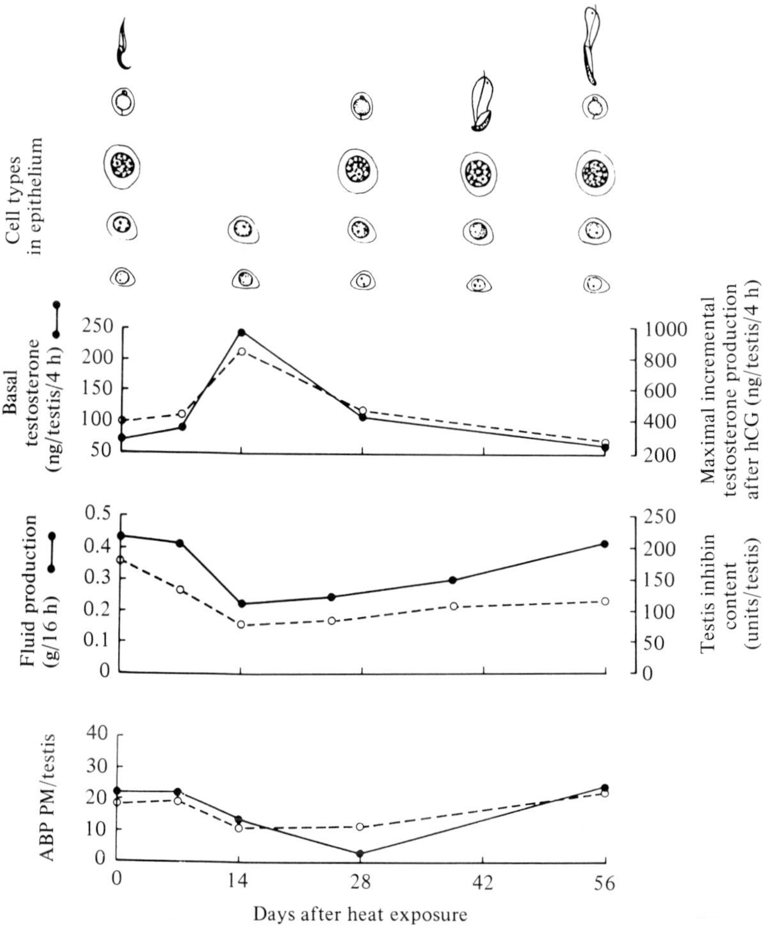

Fig. 2 The changes in spermatogenesis and in the function of Sertoli cells and Leydig cells after treatment of the rat testis with a single exposure to heat, 43°C for 15 minutes, are shown. Reproduced with permission from de Kretser, D.M. (1987). **International Review of Cytology** 10:89–112.

with a stimulation of plasminogen activator activity in segments of seminiferous tubules. Further evidence for such interactions has come from the effects of germ cells *in vitro* on the secretory activity of Sertoli cells recovered from rats at different ages, as judged by the influence of these germ cells on the secretion of ABP (Le Magueresse and Jégou, 1988a). The specific mechanisms by which the germ cells influence the Sertoli cells still remain unknown. However, a recent study by Le Magueresse and Jégou (1988b) produced evidence that at least one of these mechanisms may involve the production of a proteinaceous factor present in the media of cultures of germ cells. Further work is clearly necessary to identify the nature of these signals.

Evidence that the Sertoli cells can significantly influence germ cells can be deduced from several pieces of information. Skinner and Griswold (1982) demonstrated that the secretion of transferrin by Sertoli cells in culture is regulated by FSH, testosterone, retinol and insulin, but Wright and colleagues (1983) noted that the maximal levels of transferrin were found at stages IX and XIV of the seminiferous cycle. This information suggests that hormonal signals are modified by local events to create a cyclic, stage-specific pattern. The importance of the secretion of transferrin to germ cells may be in its utilization in enzymes present within those cells, since transferrin has been shown to bind to primary spermatocytes (Holmes *et al.*, 1983) and has also been shown to transport iron into germ cells (Toebosch *et al.*, 1986). We have recently shown that the secretion of inhibin by the Sertoli cells is maximal between stages II and VI of the cycle and declines dramatically during stages VII and VIII (Gonzales, unpublished data). This cyclic change may have a significant influence on the surrounding germ cells: it has been shown in oocytes that inhibin disrupts the resumption of meiosis, as demonstrated by the inhibition of germinal vesicle breakdown in oocytes (O *et al.*, 1989). Furthermore, Franchimont *et al.* (1981) and van Dissel-Emiliani *et al.* (1988) have demonstrated that impure preparations of inhibin have the ability to inhibit uptake of [^{3}H]-thymidine by germ cells *in vitro*, suggesting that the local secretion of inhibin by the Sertoli cell may influence mitotic activity in adjacent germ cells.

The influence of seminiferous tubules on Leydig cells

The possibility that events within the seminiferous tubules can influence the function of Leydig cells emerged initially from the studies of a number of agents capable of disrupting spermatogenesis. Rich and de Kretser (1977) demonstrated that disruption of spermatogenesis caused by treatment with hydroxyurea, vitamin A deficiency, or irradiation *in utero*, resulted in significant changes in Leydig cell function, as demonstrated by elevated levels of LH and decreased levels of testosterone. Despite these changes, which are suggestive of a functional impairment of Leydig cells, ultrastructural studies demonstrated hypertrophied Leydig cells associated with increased quantities of smooth endoplasmic reticulum and mitochondria (Kerr *et al.*, 1979). Proof that these ultrastructural changes were related to local changes emerged in the study by Aoki and Fawcett (1978), who demonstrated that focal spermatogenic damage resulted in enlargement of Leydig cells in the region surrounding the damaged tubules, while normal Leydig cells continued to surround the tubules in which spermatogenesis proceeded normally. These structural changes supporting the hypothesis of local regulation of Leydig cell function were supported by functional data from the studies of Risbridger *et al.*

(1981a). In these studies, the induction of unilateral cryptorchidism resulted in Leydig cells with an increased content of smooth endoplasmic reticulum and hyper-responsiveness to LH, in terms of production of testosterone in the abdominal testis, while structurally normal Leydig cells remained in the scrotal testis, with a normal response to hCG. These changes were not dependent on the increased temperature of the abdominal testis since it could be shown that other types of testicular damage, such as that caused by unilateral ligation of the efferent duct, could induce the same features. In these studies, the pressure atrophy that results from unilateral ligation of the efferent duct resulted in enlarged Leydig cells and increased hyper-responsiveness in the damaged testis while no changes occurred in the unligated testis (Risbridger *et al.*, 1981b).

Since the testes in both these experiments were exposed to the same circulating factors, the change in function of the Leydig cells in the damaged testes must be related to local changes. Since other experiments in our laboratory have demonstrated a significant impairment of Sertoli cell function after the induction of cryptorchidism (Jégou *et al.*, 1983), we have postulated that the regulatory factor that influences Leydig cell function is a product of the Sertoli cell. Experiments involving a single exposure of the rat testis to heat provided data to suggest that this signal emanated from the Sertoli cells, and that the signal could also be controlled by some influence from germ cells. This possibility was revealed by the fact that changes in Leydig cell function after a brief exposure to heat of the rat testis did not occur immediately but were first detectable 14 days after the heat treatment (Jégou *et al.*, 1984). These data suggested that if the Sertoli cells were the source of the signal, then they did not produce this change immediately but did so later, perhaps in association with changes in the population of germ cells that surround the Sertoli cells.

Evidence that the Leydig cells could be influenced by the seminiferous tubules in normal rats emerged from the morphometric studies of Bergh (1982, 1983), who showed that Leydig cells immediately adjacent to the tubules changed in size according to the stage of the spermatogenic cycle. Bergh was able to demonstrate that the Leydig cells were largest when closely associated with stages VII and VIII of the rat seminiferous cycle. This observation correlated well with the demonstration that stages VII and VIII of the rat seminiferous cycle are the stages that are most sensitive to testosterone deprivation (Russell and Clermont, 1977). It is also of interest to note that the changes in size of Leydig cells do not occur during development until late in puberty when step-19 spermatids appear (Bergh, 1985). This fact correlates with the observation that the changes in Leydig cell function after heat treatment were most closely related to the loss and recovery of spermatids in the epithelium (Jégou *et al.*, 1984).

The circumstantial evidence for the existence of a local regulatory factor(s) that can influence Leydig cell function has been supported by direct evidence from the studies of Sharpe and Cooper (1984), who showed that fluid traversing the peritubular lymphatic sinusoids in the rat testis, termed interstitial fluid, contained factors that stimulated Leydig cell function. They demonstrated a dose-dependent increase in basal or maximally hCG-stimulated secretion of testosterone by Leydig cells associated with the addition of interstitial fluid. The active agent appeared to be proteinaceous in nature since it was heat labile and could be destroyed by digestion with pepsin. Evidence that this material was not LH came from studies that showed that antisera raised against LH could not prevent the action of this material on steroidogenesis in Leydig cells. The factor in interstitial fluid was shown to act prior to pregnenolone in its capacity to stimulate steroidogenesis but, to date, it has not been further characterized biochemically (Risbridger *et al.*, 1987b).

From the results of a number of studies, Sharpe and colleagues proposed that this unidentified factor increased in states in which intratesticular concentrations of testosterone had declined, suggesting that its role may be in the maintenance of stable intratesticular levels of testosterone (Sharpe and Bartlett, 1985; Sharpe *et al.*, 1986). Furthermore, we demonstrated that levels of this factor rose and fell after heat-induced spermatogenic damage (Fig. 2), in parallel with the capacity of Leydig cells to respond in an exaggerated manner to hCG (Ishida *et al.*, 1987). More recent data, however, have suggested that the levels of this factor are more closely related to the state of the seminiferous epithelium (Sharpe *et al.*, 1986; Drummond *et al.*, 1989).

Other investigators have attempted to characterize the nature of this stimulator of Leydig cells by incubations of segments of seminiferous tubules in culture or, alternatively, by the use of culture medium from Sertoli cells. Confusing results have emerged since co-incubation of Leydig cells with tubules at stages VII and VIII of the cycle or the use of media from such incubations has resulted in an inhibition of the production of testosterone by crude preparations of Leydig cells, but the same materials caused a stimulation of secretion of testosterone by Percoll-purified Leydig cells (Parvinen *et al.*, 1984; Syed *et al.*, 1985). Media from cultures of immature Sertoli cells have shown the capacity to stimulate the secretion of testosterone by Leydig cells (Verhoeven and Cailleau, 1985; Janecki *et al.*, 1985). However, contradictory findings have also been reported by Benahmed and colleagues (1986).

Clearly, further progress in this area requires that the factor or factors involved in the stimulation of Leydig cells by the seminiferous tubules should be characterized biochemically. Such characterization is clearly difficult since the volume of interstitial fluid obtained from the rat testis is of the order of 35–75 μl per testis. The demonstration that bovine follicular fluid contains a similar steroidogenic stimulatory factor raises the possibility that this fluid may provide a useful source for the purification of this factor(s) (Risbridger *et al.*, 1987a). More recently, Khan and colleagues (1988) have shown that human follicular fluid also has the ability to stimulate the production of testosterone by Leydig cells from human, rat, mouse and hamster testes. These studies have provided further evidence that this material is a protein with a pI between 8.8 and 9.5.

The action of the family of proteins that are related to TGF-β and inhibin on Leydig cells has recently attracted increasing interest. Transforming growth factor-β (TGF-β) has been shown to have a predominantly inhibitory effect on steroidogenesis in Leydig cells (Avallet *et al.*, 1987; Lin *et al.*, 1987). Hsueh and colleagues (1987) showed that inhibin caused a stimulation of the production of testosterone in Leydig cells, while activin, the dimer of the β subunits of inhibin, caused an inhibition of steroidogenesis. However, studies in our own laboratory have failed to show any action of inhibin or activin on the secretion of testosterone by Percoll-purified Leydig cells or by crude preparations of intertubular cells. The reasons for these differing results require further exploration.

Conclusions

The complex nature of spermatogenesis creates the need for the elaboration of regulatory molecules in a sequential manner. This need is most likely to be met by the creation of a microenvironment, which, because of the presence of the blood–testis barrier, is regulated by the Sertoli cell. The cyclic nature of the spermatogenic process results in the requirement that the microenvironment change in a cyclic manner. Our exploration of these regulatory mechanisms is in its earliest stages, but an elucidation of the mechanisms will represent a significant advance in our understanding of normal and pathological testicular function.

References

Aoki, A. & Fawcett, D.W. (1978) Is there a local feedback from the seminiferous tubules affecting activity of the Leydig cell? **Biology of Reproduction** 19:144–158

Avallet, O., Vigier, M.., Perrard-Sapori, M. & Saez, J.M. (1987). Transforming growth factor β inhibits Leydig cell function. **Biochemical and Biophysical Research Communications** 146:575–581.

Au, C.L., Robertson, D.M. & de Kretser, D.M. (1987). Changes in testicular inhibin after a single episode of heating of rat testes. **Endocrinology** 120:973–977.

Bardin, C.W., Morris, P.L., Chen, C.L., Shaha, C., Voglmayr, J., Rivier, J., Spiess, J. & Vale, W.W. (1987). Testicular inhibin: structure and regulation by FSH, androgens and EGF. In: Burger, H.G., de Kretser, D.M., Findlay, J.K. & Igarashi, M., eds. **Inhibin – Non Steroidal Regulation of Follicle-Stimulating Hormone Secretion, Serono Symposia**, New York, Raven Press, pp.179–190.

Benahmed, M., Moreraam, D. & Chauvn, M.A. (1986). Evidence for a Sertoli cell, FSH-suppressible inhibiting factor(s) of testicular steroidogenic activity. **Biochemical and Biophysical Research Communications** 139:169–178.

Bergh, A. (1982). Local differences in Leydig cell morphology in the adult rat testis: evidence for a local control of Leydig cells by adjacent seminiferous tubules. **International Journal of Andrology** 5:325–330.

Bergh, A. (1983). Paracrine regulation of Leydig cells by the seminiferous tubules. **International Journal of Andrology** 6:57–65.

Bergh, A. (1985). Development of stage-specific paracrine regulation of Leydig cells by the seminiferous tubules. **International Journal of Andrology** 8:80–85.

Bicsak, T., Vale, W.W., Vaughan, J., Tucker, E., Cappel, S. & Hsueh, A.J.W. (1987). Hormonal regulation of inhibin production by cultured Sertoli cells **Molecular and Cellular Endocrinology** 49:211–217.

Boitani, C., Ritzen, E.M. & Parvinen, M. (1981). Inhibition of rat Sertoli cell aromatase by factor(s) selected specifically at spermatogenic stages VII and VIII. **Molecular and Cellular Endocrinology** 23:11–12.

Borland, K., Mita, M., Oppenheimier, C.L., Blinderman, L.-A., Massague, J., Hall, P.F. & Czech, M.P. (1984). The actions of insulin-like growth factors I and II on cultured Sertoli cells. **Endocrinology** 114:240–246.

Cheng, M.C., Clements, J.A., Smith, A.I., Lolait, S.J. & Funder, J.W. (1985). N-acetyl endorphin in rat spermatogonia and primary spermatocytes. **Journal of Clinical Investigation** 75:832–835.

Chowdhury, A.K. & Steinberger, E. (1964). A quantitative study of the effects of heat on the germinal epithelium of rat testes. **American Journal of Anatomy** 115:509–524.

Clermont, Y. & Harvey, S.G. (1965). Duration of the cycle of the seminiferous epithelium of normal hypophysectomized and hypophysectomized–hormone treated albino rats. **Endocrinology** 76:80–89.

Cunningham, G.R. & Huckins, C. (1979). Persistence of complete spermatogenesis in the presence of low intratesticular concentrations of testosterone. **Endocrinology** 105:177–186.

Drummond, A.E. & Risbridger, G.P., O'Leary, P.C. & de Kretser, D.M. (1988). Alterations in mitogenic and steroidogenic activities in rat testicular interstitial fluid after administration of ethane dimethane sulphonate. **Journal of Reproduction and Fertility** 83:141–147.

Drummond, A.E., Risbridger, G.P. & de Kretser, D.M. (1989). The involvement of Leydig cells in the regulation of inhibin secretion by the testis. **Endocrinology** 125:510–515.

Dym, M. & Fawcett, D.W. (1970). The blood–testis barrier in the rat and the physiological compartmentation of the seminiferous epithelium. **Biology of Reproduction** 3:308–326.

Fabbri, A., Tsai Morris, C.H., Luna, S.., Fraioli, F. & Dufau, M. (1985). Opiate receptors are present in the rat testis. Identification and localization in Sertoli cells. **Endocrinology** 17:2544–2546.

Findlay, J.K. & Risbridger, G.P. (1987). Intragonadal control mechanisms. In: Burger, H.G. ed., **Bailliere's Clinical Endocrinology and Metabolism**, Vol. 1, London, W.B. Saunders, pp.223–243.

Franchimont, P., Croze, F., Demoulin, A., Bologne, R. & Hustin, J. (1981). Effect of inhibin on rat testicular desoxyribonucleic acid (DNA) synthesis *in vivo* and *in vitro*. **Acta Endocrinologica** 98:312–320.

Galdieri, M., Monaco, L. & Stefanini, M. (1984). Secretion of androgen binding protein by Sertoli cells is infuenced by contact with germ cells. **Journal of Andrology** 5:409–415.

Gizang-Ginsberg, E. & Wolgemuth, D.J. (1987). Expression of the proopiomelanocortin gene is developmentally regulated and effected by germ cells in the male mouse reproductive system. **Proceedings of the National Academy of Sciences, USA** 84:1600–1604.

Gonzales, G.F., Risbridger, G.P., Ishida, H., Hodgson, Y.H., Pollanen, P. & de Kretser, D.M. (1989). Stage-specific inhibin synthesized by rat seminiferous tubules. **Reproduction, Fertility and Development** 1:275–279.

Holmes, D., Bucci, L.R., Lipshultz, L.I. & Smith, R.G. (1983). Transferrin binds specifically to pachytene spermatocytes. **Endocrinology** 113:1916–1918.

Hsueh, A.J., Dahl, K.D., Vaughan, J., Tucker, E., Rivier, J., Bardin, C.W. & Vale, W. (1987). Heterodimers and homodimers of inhibin subunits have different paracrine action in the modulation of luteinizing hormone-stimulated androgen biosynthesis. **Proceedings of the National Academy of Sciences, USA** 84:5082–5086.

Huang, H.F.S. & Nieschlag, E. (1986). Suppression of the intratesticular testosterone is associated with quantitative changes in spermatogonial populations in intact adult rats. **Endocrinology** 118:619–627.

Ishida, H., Risbridger, G.P. & de Kretser, D.M. (1987). Variation in the effect of a non-gonadotrophic Leydig cell stimulating factor in testicular interstitial fluid (IF) after exposure of the testis to a single episode of heat treatment. **Journal of Andrology** 8:247–252.

Janecki, A., Jakubowiak, A. & Lukaszyk, A. (1985). Stimulatory effect of Sertoli cell secretory products on testosterone secretion by purified Leydig cells in primary culture. **Molecular and Cellular Endocrinology** 42:235–243.

Jégou, B., Risbridger, G.P. & de Kretser, D.M. (1983). Effects of experimental cryptorchidism on testicular function in adult rats. **Journal of Andrology** 4:88–94.

Jégou, B., Laws, A.O. & de Kretser, D.M. (1984). Changes in testicular function induced by short-term exposure of the rat testis to heat: further evidence for interaction of germ cells, Sertoli cells and Leydig cells. **International Journal of Andrology** 7:244–257.

Jutte, N.H.P.M., Grootegoed, J.A., Rommerts, F.F.G. & Van der Molen, H.J. (1981). Exogenous lactate is essential for metabolic activity in isolated rat spermatogenesis and spermatids. **Journal of Reproduction and Fertility** 62:399–405.

Jutte, N.H.P.M., Jansen, R., Grootegoed, J.A., Rommerts, F.F.G., Clausen, O.P.F. & Van der Molen, H.J. (1982). Regulation of survival of rat pachytene spermatocytes by lactate supply from Sertoli cells. **Journal of Reproduction and Fertility** 65:431–438.

Jutte, N.H.P.M., Jansen, R., Grootegoed, J.A., Rommerts, F.F.G. & Van der Molen, H.J. (1983). FSH stimulation of the production of pyruvate and lactate by rat Sertoli cells may be involved in hormonal regulation of spermatogenesis. **Journal of Reproduction and Fertility** 68:219–226.

Kerr, J.B., Rich, K.A. & de Kretser, D.M. (1979). Alterations of the fine structure and androgen secretion of the interstitial cells in the experimentally cryptorchid rat testis. **Biology of Reproduction** 20:409–422.

Khan, S.A., Hall, P., Bartlett, J., Degeyter, C.H. & Nieschlag, E. (1988). Characterization of a factor from human ovarian follicular fluid which stimulates Leydig cell testosterone production. **Acta Endocrinologica** 118:283–293.

de Kretser, D.M. (1987). Local regulation of testicular function. **International Review of Cytology** 10:89–112.

de Kretser, D.M. & Kerr, J.B. (1988). The cytology of the testis. In: Knobil, E. & Neill, J.D., eds. **The Physiology of Reproduction**, New York, Raven Press, pp.837–932.

Lacroix, M., Parvinen, M. & Fritz, I.B. (1981). Localization of testicular plasminogen activator in discrete portions (states VII and VIII) of the seminiferous tubule. **Biology of Reproduction** 25:143–146.

Leblond, C.P. & Clermont, Y. (1952). Spermiogenesis of rat, mouse, hamster and guinea pig as revealed by the 'periodic and -fuchsin sulphurous acid' technique. **American Journal of Anatomy** 90:167206.

Lin, T., Blaisdell, J. & Haskell, J.F. (1987). Transforming growth factor β inhibits Leydig cell steroidogenesis in primary culture. **Biochemical and Biophysical Research Communications** 146:387–394.

Lostroh, A.J. (1969). Regulation of FSH and ICSH (LH) of reproductive function in the immature male rat. **Endocrinology** 85:438–445.

Le Magueresse, B. & Jégou, B. (1988a). *In vitro* effects of germ cells on the secretory activity of Sertoli cells recovered from rats of different ages. **Endocrinology** 22:1672–1680.

Le Magueresse, B. & Jégou, B. (1988b). Paracrine control of immature Sertoli cells by adult germ cells in the rat (an *in vitro* study). Cell–cell interactions within the testis. **Molecular and Cellular Endocrinology** 58:65–72.

Mita, M., Borland, K., Price, J.M. & Hall, P. (1985). The influence of insulin and insulin-like growth factor-1 on hexose transport by Sertoli cells. **Endocrinology** 116:987–992.

Mita, M., Price, J.M. & Hall, P.F. (1982). Stimulation by FSH of synthesis of lactate by Sertoli cells from rat testis. **Endocrinology** 110:1535–1541.

O, W.S., Robertson, D.M. & de Kretser, D.M. (1989). Inhibin as an oocyte meiosis inhibitor. **Molecular and Cellular Endocrinology** 62:307–311.

Odell, W.D., Swerdloff, R.S., Jacobs, H.S. & Hescox, M.A. (1973). FSH induction of sensitivity to LH: one cause of sexual maturation in the male rat. **Endocrinology** 92:160–165.

Parvinen, M. (1982). Regulation of the seminiferous epithelium. **Endocrine Reviews** 3:404–417.

Parvinen, M., Nikula, H. & Huhtaniemi, I. (1984). Influence of rat seminiferous tubules on Leydig cell testosterone production *in vitro*. **Molecular and Cellular Endocrinology** 37:331–336.

Parvinen, M., Vihko, K.K. & Toppari, J. (1987). Cell interactions during the seminiferous epithelial cycle. **International Review of Cytology** 104:115–151.

Pinon-Lataillade, G., Velez de la Calle, J.F., Viguier-Martinez, M.C., Garnier, D.H., Maas, J. & Jégou, B. (1988). Influence of germ cells upon Sertoli cells during continuous low-dose rate gamma-irradiation of adult rats. **Molecular and Cellular Endocrinology** 58:51–63.

Pintar, J.E., Schachter, B.S., Herman, A.B., Durgerian, S. & Krieger, D.T. (1984). Characterization and localization of proopiomelanocortin messenger RNA in the adult rat testis. **Science** 225:632–634.

Raj, H.G.M. & Dym, M. (1976). The effects of selective withdrawal of FSH or LH on spermatogenesis in the immature rat. **Biology of Reproduction** 14:489–494.

Rich, K.A. & de Kretser, D.M. (1977). Effect of differing degrees of destruction of the rat seminiferous epithelium on levels of serum FSH and androgen binding protein. **Endocrinology** 101:959–974.

Risbridger, G.P., Kerr, J.B. & de Kretser, D.M. (1981a). An evaluation of Leydig cell function and gonadotrophin binding in unilateral and bilateral cryptorchidism. Evidence for local control of Leydig cell function by the seminiferous tubule. **Biology of Reproduction** 24:534–540.

Risbridger, G.P., Kerr, J.B., Peake, R.A. & de Kretser, D.M. (1981b). An assessment of Leydig cell function after bilateral or unilateral efferent duct ligation: further evidence for local control of Leydig cell function. **Endocrinology** 109:1234–1241.

Risbridger, G.P., Averill, S. & de Kretser, D.M. (1987a). Does bovine follicular fluid stimulate Leydig cell steroidogenesis? In: Spera, G. & de Kretser, D.M., eds. **Morphological Basis of Human Reproductive Function**, New York, Plenum Press, pp.63–64.

Risbridger, G.P., Jenkin, G.J. & de Kretser, D.M. (1987b). The interaction of hCG, hydroxysteroids and interstitial fluid on Leydig cell steroidogenesis *in vivo*. **Journal of Reproduction and Fertility** 76:331–338.

Ritzen, E.M., Boitani, C., Parvinen, M., French, F.S. & Feldman, M. (1982). Stage-dependent secretion of ABP by rat seminiferous tubules. **Molecular and Cellular Endocrinology** 25:25–33.

Russell, L.D. & Clermont, Y. (1977). Degeneration of germ cells in normal, hypophysectomised and hormone-treated hypophysectomized rats. **Anatomical Record** 187:347–366.

Sharpe, R.M. (1984). Intratesticular factors controlling testicular function. **Biology of Reproduction** 30:29–49.

Sharpe, R.M. & Bartlett, J.M.S. (1985). The intratesticular distribution of testosterone and the relationship to the levels of a peptide that stimulates testosterone production. **Journal of Reproduction and Fertility** 73:223–236.

Sharpe, R.M. & Cooper, I. (1984). Intratesticular secretion of a factor(s) with major stimulatory effects on Leydig cell testosterone secretion *in vivo*. **Molecular Cellular Endocrinology** 37:159–168.

Sharpe, R.M., Doogan, D.G. & Cooper, I. (1986a). Intratesticular factors and testosterone secretion: the role of luteinizing hormone in relation to changes during puberty and experimental cryptorchidism. **Endocrinology** 119:2089–2096.

Sharpe, R.M., Kerr, J.B., Cooper, I. & Bartlett, J.M.S. (1986b). Intratesticular factors and testosterone secretion: the effect of treatment with ethane dimethane sulphonate (EDS) and the induction of seminiferous tubule damage. **International Journal of Andrology** 9:285–298.

Skinner, M.K. & Fritz, I.B. (1985). Testicular intertubular cells secrete a protein under androgen control that modulates Sertoli cell function. **Journal of Cell Biology** 82:114–118.

Skinner, M.K. & Griswold, M.D. (1982). Secretion of testicular transferrin by cultured Sertoli cells is regulated by hormones and retinoids. **Biology of Reproduction** 27:211–221.

Sun, Y.T., Irby, D.C., Robertson, D.M. & de Kretser, D.M. (1989). The effects of exogenously administered testosterone on spermatogenesis in intact and hypophysectomized rats. **Endocrinology** 125:1000-1010.

Syed, V., Khan, S.A. & Ritzen, E.M. (1985). Stage-specific inhibition of interstitial cell testosterone secretion by rat seminiferous tubules *in vitro*. **Molecular and Cellular Endocrinology** 40:257–264.

Toebosch, A.M.W, Grootegoed, J.A. & Kroos, M.S. (1986). Transport of iron into rat Sertoli cells and spermatids. **Proceedings of Testis Workshop**, Nashville, TN, USA, p.53.

Tsong, S.D., Phillips, D.M., Halmi, N., Krieger, D.T. & Bardin, C.W. (1982a). β-endorphin is present in male reproductive tract of five species. **Biology of Reproduction** 27:759–764.

Tsong, S.D., Phillips, D.M., Halmi, N., Liotta, A.S., Margioris, A., Bardin, C.W. & Krieger, D.T. (1982b). ACTH and β-endorphin-related peptides are present in multiple sites in reproductive tract of the male rat. **Endocrinology** 110:2204–2206.

Van Dissel-Emiliani, F.M.F., Grootenhuis, A.J., de Jong, F.H. & de Rooij, D.G. (1988). Local action of 'inhibin' in the testis. **Proceedings of the European Workshop on Molecular and Cellular Endocrinology of the Testis**, A10.

Verhoeven, G. & Cailleau, J. (1985). A factor in spent media from Sertoli cell-enriched cultures that stimulates steroidogenesis in Leydig cells. **Molecular and Cellular Endocrinology** 40:57–68.

Verhoeven, G. & Cailleau, J. (1988). Follicle-stimulating hormone and androgens increase the concentration of the androgen receptor in Sertoli cells. **Endocrinology** 122:1541–1550.

Vihko, K.K., Suominen, J.J.O. & Parvinen, M. (1984). Cellular regulation of plasminogen activator secretion during spermiogenesis. **Biology of Reproduction** 31:383–389.

Wright, W.W., Parvinen, M., Musto, N.A., Gunsalus, G.I., Phillips, D.M., Mather, J.P. & Bardin, C.W. (1983). Identification of stage-specific proteins synthesized by rat seminiferous tubules. **Biology of Reproduction** 29:257–270.

Stage-specific regulation of spermatogenesis

M. PARVINEN, P. MALI, Z. KRAWCZYK,[1] K.K. VIHKO,[2] T.-L. PENTTILA, A. KAIPIA, M. KANGASNIEMI AND J. TOPPARI

Departments of Anatomy and [2] Physiology, Institute of Biomedicine, University of Turku, SF-20520 Turku, Finland; and [1] Department of Tumor Biology, Institute of Oncology, 44-100 Gliwice, Poland.

Keywords

Testis, spermatogenesis, testosterone, follicle-stimulating hormone, plasminogen activators, protamine, heat-shock protein, gene expression.

Introduction

The spermatozoon represents one of the most differentiated cells of the body with its haploid, tightly packed, inactive chromosomes, a small amount of cytoplasm, and a flagellum for independent movement. In the seminiferous epithelium of the testis, spermatogenic cells develop through spermatogonial proliferation and renewal, meiosis and terminal differentiation during spermiogenesis. Sertoli cells, the somatic components of the seminiferous epithelium, are essential for spermatogenesis. They completely surround spermatocytes and spermatids after the onset of meiosis.

Follicle-stimulating hormone (FSH) and testosterone regulate spermatogenesis through their specific action on Sertoli cells (Steinberger, 1971; Fritz, 1978; Ritzen *et al.*, 1981; Bardin *et al.*, 1988). According to present understanding, the development of the spermatogenic cells is dependent on factors produced by Sertoli cells under stimulation by these hormones. This local paracrine type of cell interaction is poorly understood at the molecular level. Some advances, made by analyses of the physiology of the seminiferous epithelial cycle and by activation of specific genes during spermatogenesis, are summarized below.

Sertoli cells and spermatogenic cells studied together at defined stages of the seminiferous epithelial cycle

Because of the histological complexity of the testis, special methods are needed for the isolation of cells at different stages of development. For studies of interactions between Sertoli cells and germ cells, we have taken advantage of the constant associations of stages of spermatogenic cells in the seminiferous epithelium (Leblond and Clermont, 1952) which follow each other along the seminiferous tubules in a wave-like fashion (Perry *et al.*, 1961). When a freshly isolated, unstained rat seminiferous tubule is transilluminated under a stereomicroscope at 10–40-fold magnification, the point of spermiation at stage VIII of the cycle can easily be recognized as an abrupt disappearance of the dark-absorbing center of the tubule. A pale zone follows and is visible during stages IX–XII. Weak spots due to the arrangement of elongated spermatids in dense bundles, concomitant with the condensation of their nuclei, are characteristic of stages XIII–I. The density of the spots increases markedly at stages II–V. At stage VI, the bundle arrangement disappears and the late spermatids form a dense layer at the top of the seminiferous epithelium, resulting in a dark, homogeneous, central area in the transilluminated seminiferous tubules at stages VII and VIII (Parvinen and Vanha-Perttula, 1972; Parvinen and Ruokonen, 1982). Experiments with pooled segments of seminiferous tubules from defined stages of the cycle have revealed a cyclic variation in levels of several endocrine and biochemical parameters, suggesting that the function of Sertoli cells is influenced by associated spermatogenic cells (Parvinen, 1982; Parvinen *et al.*, 1986).

Local hormonal influences in the seminiferous epithelium

Since FSH-stimulated production of cAMP decreases at puberty (Steinberger *et al.*, 1978; Ritzen *et al.*, 1981) and since spermatogenesis can be qualitatively maintained in adult hypophysectomized animals by administration of testosterone alone (Ahmad *et al.*, 1973), FSH may be essential only at the onset of spermatogenesis. However, recent observations confirm the findings of Clermont and Harvey (1967) that FSH is needed for the maintenance of quantitatively normal spermatogenesis in adults (Matsumoto *et al.*, 1986; Toppari *et al.*, unpublished observation).

The local action of this hormone in the seminiferous epithelium suggests that some cellular events at stages XIII–V may be more dependent on stimulation by FSH than those at other stages (Parvinen, 1982). The cellular events in the seminiferous epithelium in which the actions of FSH and cAMP are mainly involved have been further investigated after depletion of spermatogonia by x-irradiation, and by assays of the FSH-stimulated production of cAMP at specific time intervals in the selective absence of defined populations of germ cells. Pachytene spermatocytes and round spermatids seem to have the most profound regulatory action on the FSH responsiveness of the Sertoli cells (Kaipia and Kangasniemi, unpublished observation).

Sertoli cells also are the main, if not the only, targets of androgens in the seminiferous epithelium (Bardin *et al.*, 1988). Paradoxically, although androgens are essential for normal spermatogenesis, the molecular mechanisms of the action of androgens in the seminiferous epithelium have remained poorly understood. However, several indirect observations suggest that androgens exert a local, stage-specific effect in the seminiferous epithelium. In addition to morphological observations of selective degeneration of cells at stages VII and VIII of the cycle after hypophysectomy (Russell and Clermont,

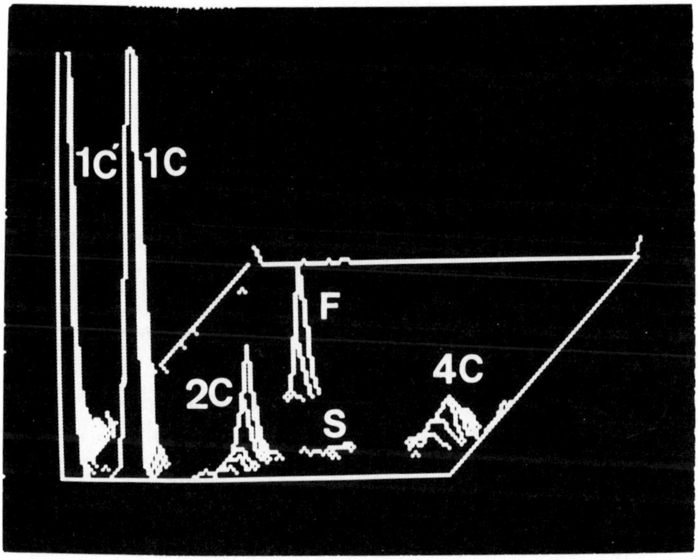

Fig. 1 Three-dimensional flow cytometric pattern of spermatogenic cells at stage VIII of the rat seminiferous epithelial cycle, indicating DNA-fluorescence (propidium iodide, x-axis), cell numbers (z-axis) and cell size (y-axis). The haploid cells form two populations since the nuclei of condensed step-19 spermatids have a lower capacity to bind the fluorochrome (1C') than the round spermatids (1C). The 2C group consists of spermatogonic and Sertoli cells, and the 4C group consists of mid-pachytene primary spermatocytes. Preleptotene spermatocytes are engaged in DNA synthesis, detected as a small S-peak between the 2C and 4C regions. The other peak at the 2C region is raised by the standard fluorescent particles (F).

1977), there are data to indicate that endogenous concentration of testosterone, secretion of androgen-binding protein and local concentration of nuclear androgen receptors are high at the same or adjacent stages (Parvinen, 1982; Parvinen *et al.*, 1986).

DNA flow cytometric analysis of defined segments of seminiferous tubules before and after culture under various conditions

Flow cytometric analysis of DNA provides a practical tool for quantification of spermatogenic cells at defined stages of the seminiferous epithelial cycle (Fig. 1), since each stage has a characteristic histogram (Toppari *et al.*, 1985). Microdissection techniques and quantitative DNA flow cytometry allow the determination of the numbers of defined spermatogenic cells per unit length of seminiferous tubule (Toppari *et al.*, 1986a, 1988b) in studies of spermatogenesis after treatment with irradiation, cytotoxic drugs, hypophysectomy, and hormonal supplementation (Toppari *et al.*, 1988a; Toppari, unpublished observation). Furthermore, cultured seminiferous tubules can be examined quantitatively (Toppari *et al.*, 1985, 1986a, 1986b).

In vitro, spermatogonia proliferate and spermatocytes develop through meiosis to give rise to haploid spermatids (Parvinen *et al.*, 1983; Toppari and Parvinen, 1985). Early spermiogenesis, up to step 7, occurs in cultured seminiferous tubules, but these cells do not elongate and mature to spermatozoa (Toppari *et al.*, 1986a, 1986b). Addition of several hormones and factors did not influence the survival or differentiation of the tubular segments, possibly because of their endogenous levels (Parvinen *et al.*, 1983). Similar results were attained when spermatogenesis was quantified by DNA flow cytometry (Toppari *et al.*, 1986b). The intact physiological contacts between Sertoli and spermatogenic cells during the culture were an essential prerequisite for differentiation.

Role of plasminogen activators in spermatogenesis

Plasminogen activators (PA) are specific serine proteinases that are involved in the remodelling of tissue and the migration of cells in both normal and malignant conditions (Dano *et al.*, 1985). In the rat seminiferous epithelium, PA is specifically secreted during stages VII and VIII of the cycle (Lacroix *et al.*, 1981). The activity of PA in culture medium was decreased when preleptotene spermatocytes were reduced in number 8 days after x-irradiation, but the activity returned to almost normal levels concomitant with the reappearance of a new generation of preleptotene spermatocytes 37 days after irradiation (Vihko *et al.*, 1984). PA-induced proteolysis may, therefore, play a role in the release of preleptotene spermatocytes from the basal lamina of the seminiferous tubule at the onset of meiosis. The cellular composition of the seminiferous epithelium also modulates the stimulation of secretion of PA by retinoic acid and FSH. The former has an effect at stages I–VII_{ab} whereas the action of FSH occurs at stages VII_{cd}–XI of the cycle (Vihko *et al.*, 1989). The locations of two known types of PA, urokinase (u-PA) and tissue-type PA (t-PA) were analyzed immunohistochemically. The former was localized in Sertoli cells at stages VII and VIII, whereas t-PA immunoreactivity was confined to mid- and late pachytene and to diakinetic primary spermatocytes of stages VII–XIII of the cycle (Vihko *et al.*, 1988). To ascertain whether retinoic acid and FSH specifically influence the activities of either of the genes for PA, the steady-state levels of mRNA in segments of staged seminiferous tubules were analyzed by Northern blot hybridization with cRNA probes for u-PA and t-PA (Vihko *et al.*, 1989). Segments at stages VII and VIII contained more u-PA mRNA than those at other stages, whereas more t-PA mRNA was found in segments at stages IX–I than in those at stages II–VIII. FSH and the second-messenger analog, dibutyryl-3',5'-adenosine monophosphate, increased the level of t-PA mRNA, while retinoic acid had a specific effect on levels of u-PA mRNA. Both effects occurred at the same stages as stimulation of the respective catalytic activities of the plasminogen activators. Data from immunocytochemical analysis also support these findings (Penttila, unpublished observation). Therefore, spermatogenic cells seem to modulate the action of FSH and retinoic acid on the secretion of PA at the level of the specific mRNAs in a stage-dependent fashion.

Regulation of gene expression during spermatogenesis

Spermatogenesis is an excellent model for studies of gene expression during cell differentiation, namely, during the haploid phase (Hecht, 1988). The mRNAs of two variants of mouse protamine have been found to be synthesized in round spermatids, and to be stored (Kleene *et al.*, 1983, 1984; Hecht and Penschow, 1987), i.e. translation in elongating spermatids occurs approximately one week after synthesis of mRNA has been initiated. We have determined the exact stages of spermiogenesis at which the transcription and translation of protamine mRNA occur. In-situ hybridization experiments showed that transcription of the P1 protamine mRNA starts in the middle of step 7 of spermiogenesis during substage VIIc. The mRNA levels remain high in step 7 to step 14 spermatids (Figs. 2a, 2b) but decrease during steps 15–16 (Figs. 2c, 2d) and are virtually undetectable in steps 17–19. Northern blot analyses of RNAs isolated from microdissected pools of seminiferous tubules revealed a Pl protamine mRNA of about 580 nucleotides during stages VII_c–XIV of the cycle and a mRNA of 450 nucleotides during stages XIII–XIV and I–VI, suggesting an initiation of translation of protamine 1 in spermatids at steps 13–14. In stages II–VI (spermatids at steps 16–18), only the smaller size of protamine 1 mRNA was detectable. A digestion experiment with RNase H suggested that a small poly(A) fragment remains in this RNA during and after translation. The protamine 1 mRNA obviously undergoes post-transcriptional processing, but the regulation of the synthesis of protamine mRNA in spermatids remains to be investigated. Its translation and storage occur in spermatids that have the poorest ability to differentiate *in vitro* (Toppari and Parvinen, 1985), and which are most sensitive to the effects of hypophysectomy (Russell and Clermont, 1977). It is, therefore, possible that the steps of spermiogenesis that involve nucleoprotein transitions are critical with respect to optimal culture conditions, hormonal stimulation, and interaction with the Sertoli cells.

Expression of a testis-specific RNA related to a heat-shock gene

The function of heat-shock proteins (hsp) is poorly understood, although recent observations suggest that they may be involved in stabilization and assembly of nascent proteins, in the recovery of cellular structures from injuries, and in cellular growth and differentiation (Kao *et al.*, 1985; Milarski

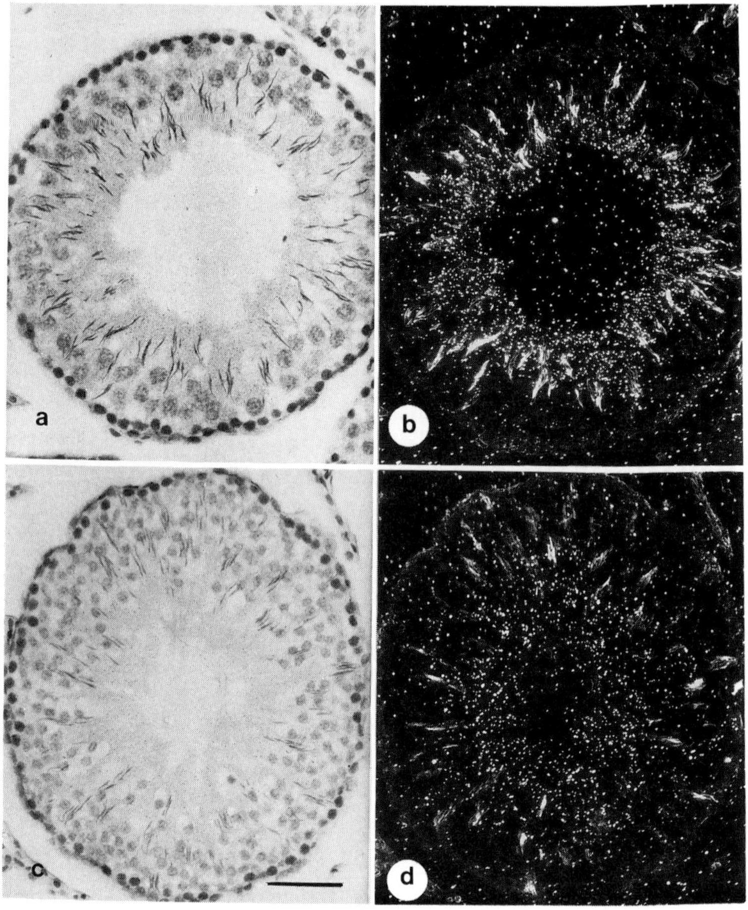

Fig. 2 Normal (a and c) and corresponding dark-field (b and d) photomicrographs of a hematoxylin-stained paraffin section of rat testis to show the in-situ hybridization of the cDNA probe for protamine 1. Stage XIII (a and b) shows strong hybridization over step-13 spermatids. The radioactivity is decreasing over step-16 spermatids at stage II (c and d). Bar = 50 μm.

and Morimoto, 1986; Pelham, 1986; Kaczmarek *et al.*, 1987). The testes of the adult rat and mouse contain abundant amounts of the transcript related to the hsp70 gene (Krawczyk *et al.*, 1987). The appearance and amount of the transcript are developmentally regulated; the predominant temporal localization has been proposed as being the haploid phase of spermatogenesis (Zakeri and Wolgemuth, 1987). To analyze more accurately the cellular expression of the hsp70 mRNA in the rat seminiferous epithelium, we have utilized the technique of slot-blot hybridization of RNA isolated from microdissected

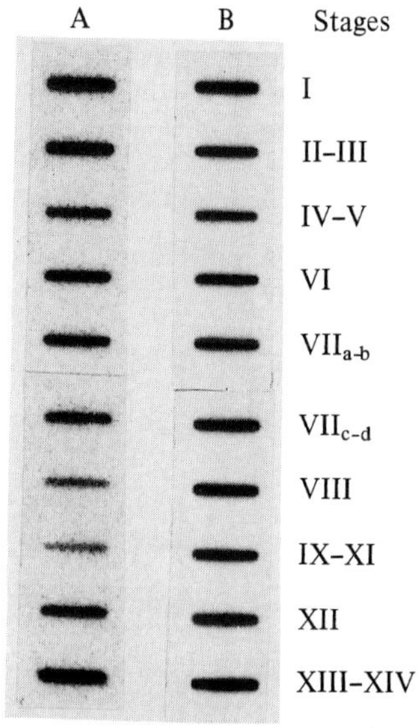

Fig. 3 Slot-blot hybridization analyses of hsp70 RNA (A) and 28S rRNA (B) of pools of segments of rat seminiferous tubules collected from defined stages of the epithelial cycle by transillumination-assisted microdissection. Stages VIII and XI–IX exhibit lower levels of hsp70 RNA than other stages, whereas the level of the ribosomal 28S RNA is more evenly distributed in different stages.

segments of seminiferous tubules at defined stages of the epithelial cycle (Krawczyk *et al.*, 1988).

Slot-blot hybridization revealed a lower level of hsp70 RNA during stages VIII and IX–XI than during other stages (Fig. 3). The hybridization of successive, accurately identified 2-mm segments showed a similar pattern: the signal was high during stages I–VI, decreased at stages VII–VIII, and was low at stages IX–XI (Fig. 4). In segments containing stage XII of the epithelial cycle, the level of the hsp70 RNA increased constantly (Fig. 5). If the same filters were rehybridized to detect levels of ribosomal 28S RNA, no significant differences between stages were found (Figs. 3, 4b). The results of in-situ hybridization were in agreement with the slot-blot analyses and showed, specifically, that late-pachytene primary spermatocytes (stage XII), diakinetic and dividing spermatocytes (stages XIII and XIV) and early round spermatids (stages I–VI) contained most of the label. Therefore, the gene coding for the hsp70 RNA is activated and transcribed premeiotically. The function of the translational product of the hsp70 mRNA remains obscure but, from these observations, it appears that it may be involved in the differentiation of spermatocytes into spermatids.

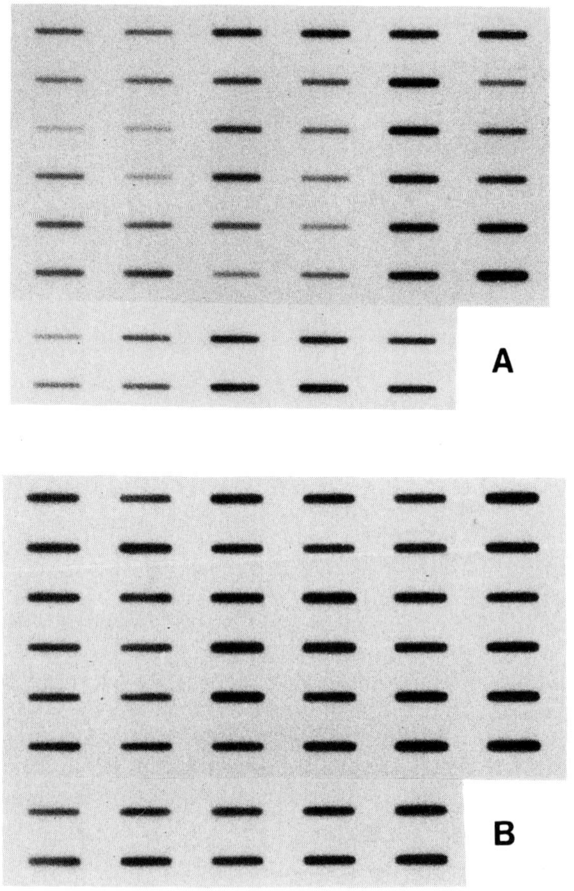

6-7b	7a-7b	2-4	2-5a	1-1	7a-7b
7b-7d	7c-7d	4-6	5a-7a	1-1	9-10
7d-8	7d-8	6-7b	7c-7d	1-2	10-12
11-13	9-11	7b-7d	7d-8	2-3	12-14
13-1	11-12	7d-8	9-10	3-5b	14-1
1-3	12-1	9-12	10-11	5b-5c	1-1
3-6	1-1	12-1	11-13	5c-6	
6-7a	1-2	1-2	13-1	6-7a	

C

Fig. 4 Slot-blot hybridization analyses of hsp70 RNA (A) and 28S rRNA (B) with corresponding stage-map with Arabic numerals (C) from sequentially isolated 2-mm segments of rat seminiferous tubules in which the stages were identified accurately by intermediate squash preparations. The level of hsp70 RNA is repeatedly low in segments that are associated with stages VIId, VIII, and IX–XI, whereas segments associated with stage XII show a constant increase in the level of the transcript. The level of 28S RNA shows less variation.

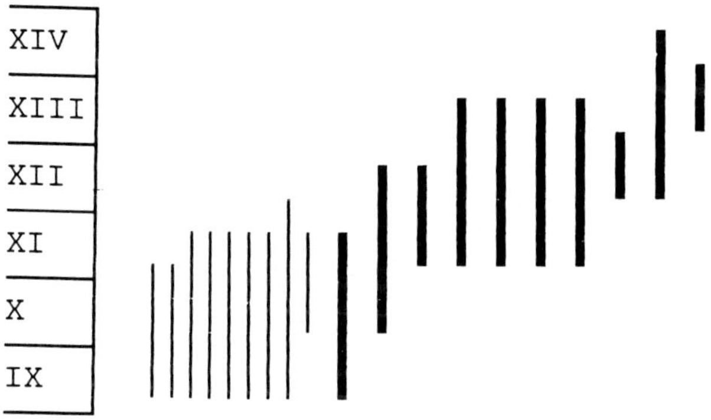

Fig. 5 The activation of the hsp70 gene during stages XI–XIV of the cycle, as evaluated from densitometric traces of data shown in Fig. 4. The level of hsp70 RNA was the same or lower (thin lines) in most segments associated with stages IX–XI but increased (thick lines) in those associated with stages XII–XIV, when compared with the preceding segment of tubule.

Future research directions

The stage-dependent variations in several hormonal and biochemical parameters in the seminiferous epithelium suggest that paracrine regulation is important in the seminiferous epithelium. The nature of factors involved is obscure, but some suggestions have been made. Testicular GnRH-like peptide (Sharpe, 1984), pro-opiomelanocortin-derived peptides (Tsong *et al.*, 1982; Chen *et al.*, 1984) and growth factors (Saez *et al.*, 1987) may have a role in interactions between seminiferous tubules and Leydig cells. In the seminiferous epithelium itself, it has been suggested that growth factors exert a local regulatory effect (Feig *et al.*, 1980; Tres *et al.*, 1986; Veno *et al.*, 1987). Development of recombinant DNA techniques, such as single-cell mRNA phenotyping by the polymerase chain reaction (Rappolee *et al.*, 1988), are opening new possibilities for studies in this area.

Acknowledgements

This project has received long-term support from the Academy of Finlamd. We thank Soili Huhta and Lars-Henrik Wikgren for technical assistance during the preparation of this manuscript.

References

Ahmad, N., Haltmeyer, G.C. & Eik-Nes, K.B. (1973). Maintenance of spermatogenesis in rats with intratesticular implants containing testosterone or dihydrotestosterone (DHT). **Biology of Reproduction** 8:411–419.

Bardin, C.W., Cheng, C.Y., Musto, N.A. & Gunsalus, G.L. (1988). The Sertoli cell. In: Knobil, E., Neill, J.D., Ewing, L.L., Greenwald, G.S., Markert, C.L. & Pfaff, D.W., eds. **The Physiology of Reproduction**, Vol. 1, New York, Raven Press, pp.933–974.

Chen, C.L.C., Mather, J.P., Morris, P.C. & Bardin, C.W. (1984). Expression of proopiomelanocortin-like gene in the testis and epididymis. **Proceedings of the National Academy of Sciences, USA** 81:5672–5675.

Clermont, Y. & Harvey, S.C. (1967). Effects of hormones on spermatogenesis in the rat. **Ciba Foundation Colloquium of Endocrinology** 16:173–196.

Danoa, K., Andreasen, P.A., Grondahl-Hansen, J., Kristensen, P., Nielsen, L.S. & Skriver, L. (1985). Plasminogen activators, tissue degradation and cancer. **Advances in Cancer Research** 44:139–266.

Feig, L.A., Bellvé, A.R., Horbach-Erickson, N. & Klagsbrun, M. (1980). Sertoli cells contain a mitogenic polypeptide. **Proceedings of the National Academy of Sciences, USA** 77:4774–4778.

Fritz, I.B. (1978). Sites of action of androgens and follicle-stimulating hormone on cells of the seminiferous tubule. In: Litwack, G., ed. **Biochemical Actions of Hormones**, Vol. 5, New York, Academic Press, pp.249–281.

Hecht, N.B. (1988). Haploid gene expression and the regulation of post-meiotic structural genes. In: Parvinen, M., Huhtaniemi, I. & Pelliniemi, L.J., eds. **Development and Function of the Reproductive Organs, Serono Symposia**, Review No. 14, Ares-Serono Symposia, Rome, pp.325–334.

Hecht, N.B. & Penschow, J.D. (1987). *In situ* localization of mRNAs coding for mouse testicular structural genes. **Experimental Cell Research** 173:274–281.

Kaczmarek, L., Calabretta, B., Kao, H., Heintz, N., Nevins, J. & Baserga, R. (1987). Control of the hsp70 RNA in human lymphocytes. **Journal of Cell Biology** 14:183–187.

Kao, H.T., Capusso, O., Heintz, N. & Nevins, J.R. (1985). Cell cycle control of the human Hsp70 gene: implications for the role of a cellular E1A-like function. **Molecular and Cellular Biology** 5:628–633.

Kleene, K.C., Distel, R.J. & Hecht, N.B. (1983). cDNA clones encoding cytoplasmic poly(A)$_+$ RNAs which first appear at detectable levels in haploid phases of spermatogenesis in the mouse. **Developmental Biology** 98:455–464.

Kleene, K.C., Distel, R.J. & Hecht, N.B. (1984). Translational regulation and deadenylation of a protamine mRNA during spermiogenesis in the mouse. **Developmental Biology** 105:71–79.

Krawczyk, Z., Mali, P. & Parvinen, M. (1988). Expression of a testis-specific hsp70 gene-related RNA in defined stages of rat seminiferous epithelium. **Journal of Cell Biology** 107:1317–1323.

Krawczyk, Z., Szymik, N. & Wisniewski, J. (1987). Expression of hsp70-related gene developing and degenerating rat testis. **Molecular Biology Reports** 12:35–41.

Lacroix, M., Parvinen, M. & Fritz, I.B. (1981). Localization of testicular plasminogen activator in discrete portions (stages VII and VIII) of the seminiferous tubule. **Biology of Reproduction** 25:143–146.

Leblond, C.P. & Clermont, Y. (1952). Definition of the stages of the cycle of the seminiferous epithelium in the rat. **Annals of the New York Academy of Sciences** 55:548–573.

Mali, P., Sandberg, M., Vuorio, A., Yelick, P., Hecht, N.B. & Parvinen, M. (1988). Localization of protamine 1 mRNA in different stages of the cycle of the rat seminiferous epithelium. **Journal of Cell Biology** 107:407–412.

Matsumoto, A.M., Karpas, A.E. & Bremner, W.J. (1986). Chronic human chorionic gonadotropin administration in normal men: evidence that follicle-stimulating hormone is necessary for the maintenance of quantitatively normal spermatogenesis in man. **Journal of Clinical Endocrinology and Metabolism** 62:1184–1192.

Milarski, K.L. & Morimoto, R.I. (1986). Expression of human hsp70 during the synthetic phase of the cell cycle. **Proceedings of the National Academy of Sciences, USA** 83:9517–9521.

Parvinen, M. (1982). Regulation of the seminiferous epithelium. **Endocrine Reviews** 3:404–417.

Parvinen, M. & Ruokonen, A. (1982). Endogenous steroids in rat seminiferous tubules. Comparison of the stages of the epithelial cycle isolated by transillumination-assisted microdissection. **Journal of Andrology** 3:211–222.

Parvinen, M. & Vanha-Perttula, T. (1972). Identification and enzyme quantitation of the stages of the seminiferous epithelial wave in the rat. **Anatomical Record** 174:435–450.

Parvinen, M., Vihko, K.K. & Toppari, J. (1986). Cell interactions during the seminiferous epithelial cycle. **International Review of Cytology** 104:115–151.

Parvinen, M., Wright, W.W., Phillips, D.M., Mather, J.P., Musto, N.A. & Bardin, C.W. (1983). Spermatogenesis *in vitro*: completion of meiosis and early spermiogenesis. **Endocrinology** 112:1150–1152.

Pelham, H.R.B. (1986). Speculations on the function of the major heat shock and glucose-regulated proteins. **Cell** 46:959–961.

Perry, B., Clermont, Y. & Leblond, C.P. (1961). The wave of the seminiferous epithelium in the rat. **American Journal of Anatomy** 108:47–77.

Rappolee, D.A., Mark, D., Banda, M.J. & Werb, Z. (1988). Wound macrophages express TGF-α and other growth factors *in vivo*: analysis by mRNA phenotyping. **Science** 241:708–712.

Ritzen, E.M., Hansson, V. & French, F.S. (1981). The Sertoli cell. In: Burger, H. & deKretser, D., eds., **The Testis. Comprehensive Endocrinology**, New York, Raven Press, pp.171–194.

Russell, L.D. & Clermont, Y. (1977). Degeneration of germ cells in normal, hypophysectomized and hormone-treated hypophysectomized rats. **Anatomical Record** 187:347–365.

Saez, J.M., Perrard-Sapori, M.H., Chatelain, P.G., Tabone, E. & Rivarola, M.A. (1987). Paracrine regulation of testicular function. **Journal of Steroid Biochemistry** 27:317–329.

Sharpe, R.M. (1984). Intratesticular factors controlling testicular function. **Biology of Reproduction** 30:29–49.

Steinberger, A., Hintz, M. & Heindel, J.J. (1978). Changes in cyclic AMP responses to FSH in isolated rat Sertoli cells during sexual maturation. **Biology of Reproduction** 19:566–572.

Steinberger, E. (1971). Hormonal control of mammalian spermatogenesis. **Physiological Reviews** 51:1–22.

Toppari, J., Bishop, P.C., Parker, J.W. & DiZerega, G.S. (1988b). DNA flow cytometric analysis of mouse seminiferous epithelium. **Cytometry** 9:456–462.

Toppari, J., Eerola, E. & Parvinen, M. (1985). Flow cytometric DNA analysis of defined stages of rat seminiferous epithelial cycle during *in vitro* differentiation.

Journal of Andrology 6:325–333.

Toppari, J., Mali, P. & Eerola, E. (1986a). Rat spermatogenesis *in vitro* traced by quantitative flow cytometry. **Journal of Histochemistry and Cytochemistry** 34:1029–1035.

Toppari, J. & Parvinen, M. (1985). *In vitro* differentiation of rat seminiferous tubular segments from defined stages of the epithelial cycle. Morphologic and immunolocalization analysis. **Journal of Andrology** 6:334–343.

Toppari, J., Parvinen, M., Eerola, E., Bishop, P.C., Parker, J.W. & DiZerega, G.S. (1988a). Local regulation of the seminiferous epithelium as evaluated by flow cytometry. In: Parvinen, M., Huhtaniemi, I. & Pelliniemi, L.J., eds. **Development and Function of the Reproductive Organs, Serono Symposia**, Review No. 14, Ares-Serono Symposia, Rome, pp.103–112.

Toppari, J., Vihko, K.K., Rasanen, K.G.E., Eerola, E. & Parvinen, M. (1986b). Regulation of stages VI and VIII of the rat seminiferous epithelial cycle *in vitro*. **Journal of Endocrinology** 108:417–422.

Tres, L.L., Smith, E.P., Van Wyk, J.J. & Kierszengaum, A.L. (1986). Immunoreactive sites and accumulation of somatomedin C in rat Sertoli–spermatogenic cell cocultures. **Experimental Cell Research** 162:33–50.

Tsong, S.D., Phillips, D.M., Bardin, C.W., Halmi, N., Liotta, A.J., Margioris, A. & Krieger, D.T. (1982). ACTH and β-endorphin-related peptides are present in multiple sites in the reproductive tract of the rat. **Endocrinology** 110:2204–2206.

Veno, N., Baird, A., Esch, F., Ling, N. & Guillemin, R. (1987). Isolation and partial characterization of basic fibroblast growth factor from bovine testis. **Molecular and Cellular Endocrinology** 49:189–194.

Vihko, K.K., Kristensen, P., Dano, K. & Parvinen, M. (1988). Immunohistochemical localization of urokinase-type plasminogen activator in Sertoli cells and tissue-type plasminogen activator in spermatogenic cells in the rat seminiferous epithelium. **Developmental Biology** 126:150–155.

Vihko, K.K., Pentilla, T.L., Toppari, J., Parvinen, M. & Belin, D. (1989). Regulation of urokinase- and tissue-type plasminogen activator gene expression in the rat seminiferous epithelium. **Molecular Endocrinology** 3:52–59.

Vihko, K.K., Suominen, J.J.O. & Parvinen, M. (1984). Cellular regulation of plasminogen activator secretion during spermatogenesis. **Biology of Reproduction** 31:383–389.

Vihko, K.K., Toppari, J. & Parvinen, M. (1987). Stage-specific regulation of plasminogen activator secretion in the rat seminiferous epithelium. **Endocrinology** 120:142–145.

Zakeri, Z.F. & Wolgemuth, D.J. (1987). Developmental-stage-specific expression of the hsp70 gene family during differentiation of the mammalian male germ line. **Molecular and Cellular Biology** 7:1791–1796.

Multiple regulation of Leydig cell functions

F.F.G. ROMMERTS, R. MELSERT, K.J. TEERDS[1] AND D.G. DE ROOIJ[1]

Department of Biochemistry, Division of Chemical Endocrinology, Erasmus University Rotterdam, Rotterdam, The Netherlands; [1] Department of Cell Biology, Medical School, State University of Utrecht, The Netherlands.

Keywords

Leydig cells, gonadotropins, luteinizing hormone, paracrine regulation, albumin, testosterone, spermatogenesis.

Introduction

Growth and development of the testis are regulated by gonadotropins from the pituitary. When pituitary secretion of gonadotropins is deficient, the development of the testes is arrested or delayed, such that their size and histology remain similar to those of fetal testes. In humans this deficiency occurs in patients with Kallman's syndrome. This delayed development, which can persist until long after puberty, shows that circulating growth factors are not sufficient to induce growth of the testis. After administration of gonadotropins, complete restoration of testicular functions can be obtained (Burris *et al.*, 1988). Although these studies clearly illustrate that luteinizing hormone (LH) and follicle-stimulating hormone (FSH) are the major stimuli for growth and development of the testis, locally produced factors may mediate some of the growth effects, especially with respect to types of cell that are not target cells for gonadotropins. A good example of such a factor is testosterone, which is produced by Leydig cells, acts on Sertoli cells, and indirectly supports the development of germinal cells.

Studies on hormonal regulation of growth of testicular cells have been carried out almost exclusively *in vivo*. In-vitro systems have mainly been used for investigations of short-term regulation of cellular activities, such as the production of steroids and secretion of proteins. The studies with isolated cells have shown that locally produced factors can, indeed, regulate cell functions or modify the effects of gonadotropins. However, in most of the studies, short-term effects of such paracrine factors were studied with reference to maintenance or activation of cell functions and it is, as yet, unknown whether these locally produced factors are also important for regulation of cell growth.

In this chapter we summarize our current results and hypotheses on the hormonal regulation of the growth, development and functions of Leydig cells, and the possible contributions of locally operating regulatory systems. Most of our experimental data have been published and the reader is referred to these publications for details and for references to investigations by other research groups.

Materials and methods

Methods for treatment of animals, chemicals, details of morphological studies, methods for the counting, isolation, and incubation of cells, and analytical methods have been described extensively in the original research papers which are cited as references where appropriate.

Results and discussion

Control of Leydig cell growth in prepubertal rats

The growth-promoting effects of LH and FSH on the immature testis are well known. Stimulatory effects of LH or human chorionic gonadotropin (hCG) on Leydig cell growth have been reported by Chemes *et al.* (1976) and Christensen and Peacock (1980). Since LH receptors are exclusively located on Leydig cells and FSH receptors are only present on Sertoli cells, part of the growth-promoting effect of LH must be mediated by a direct hormonal effect on the Leydig cell. FSH can also exert a stimulatory effect on Leydig cell functions, as is evident after treatment of immature hypophysectomized rats with FSH for several days (Odell and Swerdloff, 1976; van Beurden *et al.*, 1976; Purvis *et al.*, 1979). Furthermore, Kerr and Sharpe (1985) have reported that the number of Leydig cells was increased after treatment with FSH. The effect of FSH on the number of Leydig cells can be explained by the effect of small amounts of LH which are present as contaminants in preparations of FSH, but it may also reflect an indirect effect of FSH on Leydig cells via products secreted from Sertoli cells. In view of this uncertainty, we have reinvestigated the effects of pure FSH and LH on the growth and functions of Leydig cells in immature hypophysectomized rats (Teerds *et al.*, 1989).

Existing purified preparations of porcine FSH and human LH were further purified by gel filtration and immunoadsorption until contamination by hormones, such as FSH, thyroid-stimulating hormone (TSH), prolactin and growth hormone (GH), was less than 0.002% by weight (Closset and Hennen, 1989). Immature rats were hypophysectomized at the age of 18 days, and daily treatment with purified hormones (64 μg porcine FSH or 10 μg human LH per rat) was started 4–5 days later. Treatment with FSH for 7 days caused a four- to fivefold increase in the number of recognizable Leydig cells as compared to numbers in hypophysectomized 29-day-old controls (Table 1). After administration of LH, a 17-fold increase in the number of Leydig cells was observed. The endogenous steroidogenic capacities of these testes, as measured by plasma testosterone levels 2 hours after administration of 10 i.u. of hCG per rat, were also affected by the hormone treatments. Compared to values in hypophysectomized controls, plasma testosterone levels increased approximately five- to sixfold after treatment with FSH or LH (Table 1). These results show that, in immature rats, LH has a major effect on the proliferation of Leydig cells. Locally produced factors regulated by FSH have a minor effect

Table 1. *Effect of seven daily injections of porcine FSH (64 μg) or of human LH (10 μg), in immature male rats hypophysectomized at day 18, on the number of Leydig cells and testicular production of steroids*

	Number of Leydig cells per 1000 Sertoli cells	Plasma testosterone levels (nmol/l) 2 hours after injection of 10 i.u. hCG
Intact control	262 ± 14	9.9 ± 1.7
Hypophysectomized	11 ± 3	1.2 ± 0.1
Hypophysectomized, treated with FSH	50 ± 8	9.4 ± 1.1
Hypophysectomized, treated with LH	187 ± 15	7.4 ± 0.4

Mean values ± S.E.M. of results from 4–11 animals are shown. All values were significantly different from values for hypohysectomized rats ($p < 0.01$). (Student's t-test.)

on the division and differentiation of cells, but they exert a strong stimulatory effect on the steroidogenic activities of the relatively low number of Leydig cells. These observations, made with very pure hormones, are similar to those reported earlier when less pure preparations of FSH were used (Odell and Swerdloff, 1976; Kerr and Sharpe, 1985). It can, therefore, be concluded that the very small amounts of LH in currently used preparations of FSH are not a major problem in supplementation studies *in vivo*.

Although local factors produced by Sertoli cells (under the influence of FSH) may not be very important for the regulation of the number of Leydig cells, they may be necessary as permissive factors in the development of Leydig cell functions. To investigate this possibility, the growth and development of Leydig cells should be investigated in testes in which the secretory functions of Sertoli cells are inhibited or, for preference, in the absence of Sertoli cells. Since it is difficult to establish such conditions in testicular tissue, we have explored several techniques for the transplantation of pure interstitial cells after isolation and for the examination of their morphological and functional properties. Male Wistar rats of 21–25 days of age were used. Bilateral orchidectomy was carried out under ether anesthesia through an incision in the lower abdominal region. Testes were decapsulated and Leydig cells were isolated by dispersion with collagenase according to methods described previously (Rommerts *et al.*, 1985b). Portions of the suspensions of cells were used for transplantations (10×10^6 cells per animal) on gelatin sponges (Spongostan, UpJohn Co.) which had been cut into small pieces ($10 \times 10 \times 5$ mm^3) with a scalpel. The castrated rats, from whom the testes had been removed, were used for implantations. Two sponges were placed subcutaneously between the scapulae of each rat after an incision of 1 cm had been made in the neck. Immediately after placement of the sponges, Leydig cells

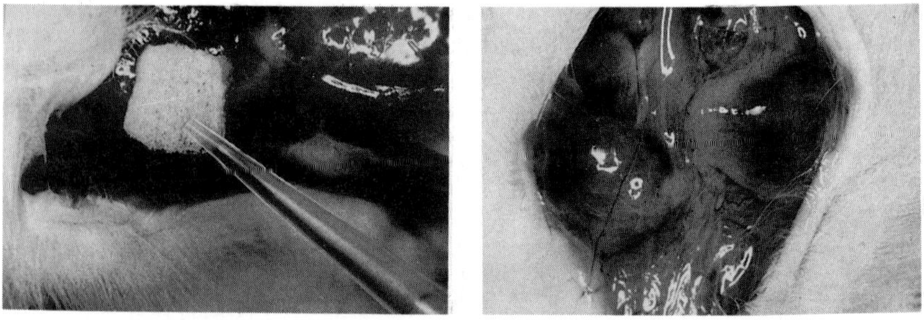

Fig. 1 Implantation of Leydig cells in gelatin sponges. Left: a suspension of cells applied to the sponge located between the scapulae. Right: spongeous tissue 7 days after transplantation of Leydig cells.

($5x10^6$) were applied to each sponge in 100 μl of culture medium (Fig. l). Each incision was sutured after the cells had been absorbed in the sponge. After 7 days the sponges were clearly vascularized and were surrounded by a fibrous capsule (Fig. 1), and numerous Leydig cells could be recognized in the spongeous tissue. The technique appears to be useful for studies of the development of transplanted Leydig cells from immature rats in the absence of Sertoli cells or after co-transplantation of Sertoli cells, but we have not yet carried out specific studies using this system.

Control of the growth of Leydig cells in adult rats

After puberty, the number of Leydig cells and Sertoli cells in the testis does not increase any further. Moreover, under normal conditions, the turnover of these cells is very low. Hence, the growth of Leydig cells and Sertoli cells in mature rats is insignificant while, by contrast, numerous germinal cells develop. The cellular population dynamics in the testis are in sharp contrast with those in the ovary. In the ovary, the number of germinal cells decreases after puberty and only a few germinal cells develop per cycle, whereas the somatic cells show a pronounced growth and development during each cycle. After long-term deprivation of gonadotropin, the volume of Leydig cells and Sertoli cells in rats decreases and many changes in functional properties have been observed. The number of Sertoli cells in adult rats does not change after hypophysectomy but there are uncertainties concerning the stability of the number of Leydig cells. It has been reported that, following hypophysectomy, the number of Leydig cells decreases to approximately 50% of that in controls (Ewing and Zirkin, 1983). However, Leydig cells lose many morphological characteristics after deprivation of LH and the number of Leydig cells is bound to be underestimated if regressed Leydig cells are not included in the cell counts. We have encountered such difficulties when counting Leydig cells in hypophysectomized rats.

Functional activities of Leydig cells are also diminished. For example, cholesterol side-chain cleavage activity per 10^6 Leydig cells, as measured by the production of pregnenolone in the presence of 22R-hydroxycholesterol, was decreased by more than 30-fold, 33 days after hypophysectomy. However, after two injections of hCG (one injection per day) many more Leydig cells could be recognized and the enzymatic activity was almost completely restored. In this period, we were unable to measure any proliferative activity of Leydig cells by labeling rats with ^{3}H-thymidine. Moreover, this trophic effect of hCG was absent when rats were pretreated with ethylene dimethane sulfonate (EDS) which selectively destroys Leydig cells (Molenaar *et al.*, 1985).

The above-mentioned data indicate that, in hypophysectomized rats, many Leydig cells remain and the functional properties of these cells can very rapidly be restored by treatment with hCG/LH. It appears, thus, that in normal adult rats, and even in gonadotropin-deficient rats, the differentiated Leydig cells form a stable population of cells. It was surprising to observe that all these non-dividing Leydig cells could be destroyed by administration of EDS without any noticeable effects on other testicular cells (Molenaar *et al.*, 1985). Even more surprising was the observation that approximately 3–4 weeks after this destructive process, a new generation of Leydig cells was formed (Molenaar *et al.*, 1986). Apparently, precursors to Leydig cells are not destroyed by treatment with EDS and these cells can give rise to new Leydig cells. This development of Leydig cells in adult rats also offers the possibility of studies of the regulation of growth and differentiation in an animal that is fully developed. In such a system, the effects of complicating interactions between different developing systems, as are present in the immature rat, can be reduced.

The molecular mechanisms that form the basis for the specific cytotoxic effects of EDS on rat Leydig cells are unknown, although attempts have been made to study details of the actions of EDS on isolated cells (Rommerts *et al.*, 1985a, 1988). It has been shown that EDS alkylates many proteins, but correlations between alkylation of specific proteins and cytotoxicity were not found. From studies *in vitro* and *in vivo*, it has been concluded that the toxic effects of EDS are limited to Leydig cells of mature and fetal rats. Leydig cells in 21-day-old rats are resistant to the cytotoxic effects of EDS but, in these cells, EDS completely inhibits cholesterol side-chain cleavage activity (Rommerts *et al.*, 1988). Although the mechanism of action of EDS remains an enigma, the compound is very useful for destroying existing Leydig cells in rats and for studies of testicular function in Leydig cell-deficient animals. This system provides a good example of a deletion study at the cellular level which can be extended by investigations of effects of administration of various hormones, e.g. testosterone. The same principles have been used in classical endocrinology to study the functions of specific organs, and they are used today at the cellular and molecular level to study the roles of specific molecules or of functional areas within molecules. EDS is also useful for initiation of the proliferation and differentiation of cells which ultimately lead to a new population of Leydig cells. This developmental process can be studied under a variety of experimental conditions in adult rats.

In normal rats, plasma LH and FSH levels rise gradually after administration of EDS as a result of the destruction of Leydig cells and the absence of the negative feedback action of testosterone. The levels of FSH and LH remain elevated for approximately 2–3 weeks and return to normal when Leydig cells repopulate the testis (Molenaar *et al.*, 1986). The development of the new Leydig cells takes place in the presence of elevated levels of FSH and LH. To investigate whether, as is the case in immature rats, FSH is required in addition to LH for complete development of Leydig cells in mature rats, we have carried out developmental studies with hypophysectomized rats treated with hCG or FSH. Active Leydig cells could be detected only in rats treated with hCG for 35 days. No Leydig cells could be recognized after treatment of these rats with FSH (Molenaar *et al.*, 1986). These results show that FSH, prolactin, and other pituitary hormones are not required for repopulation of Leydig cells after the administration of EDS. However, the absence of effects of FSH does not exclude the possibility that local factors produced by Sertoli cells may play a permissive role. Similarly, the initiation of the development of germinal cells in immature rats requires FSH and LH, whereas in adult rats this process can be maintained by supplementation with testosterone (Fritz, 1978). It may be possible that, in adult rats, locally produced permissive factors are continuously secreted by fully differentiated Sertoli cells. Thus, only developing rats require stimulation by FSH to support the differentiation and secretory activities of Sertoli cells.

Since hCG (LH) appears to be the major growth-promoting hormone for the development of Leydig cells, we wondered about the nature of the intermediate stages of development of cells from which the new population of Leydig cells is generated. It has been reported that high doses of LH/hCG can stimulate growth of Leydig cells in normal rats, but details of kinetic changes in cell populations were not investigated in these studies (Chemes *et al.*, 1976; Christensen and Peacock, 1980). We have, therefore, compared the initial growth events that occur after repeated injections with hCG with those that occur after a single injection of EDS (Teerds *et al.*, 1988). The stimulatory effects of hCG and EDS on cell division were monitored by counting the numbers of Leydig cells and of interstitial cells which could not be identified (presumed to be precursors to Leydig cells) that incorporated ^{3}H-thymidine after treatment with EDS or with hCG for several days. The effects of hCG on cell proliferation or differentiation were determined by comparing the number of nuclei with characteristics of nuclei of Leydig cells with the number of Sertoli cells (Fig. 2). It appears that hCG and EDS have similar effects on the cell divisions of the (putative) precursor cells. When rats were treated with EDS and hCG together, the effects on cell divisions were additive. This result

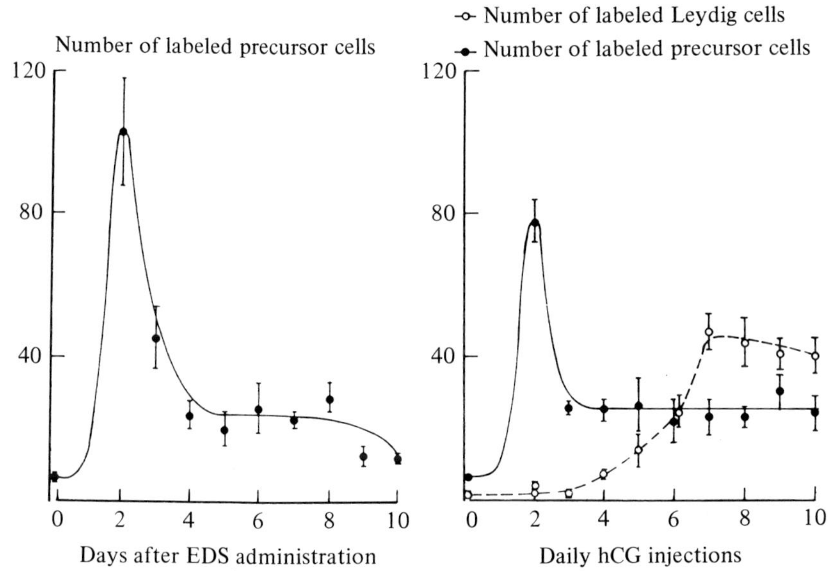

Fig. 2 Number of labeled Leydig cells or precursors to Leydig cells during the first 10 days after administration of EDS (left) or during daily injections of 100 i.u. hCG (right). All numbers are expressed per 1000 Sertoli cells. No labeled Leydig cells were observed after administration of EDS (from Teerds *et al.*, 1988).

suggests that EDS and hCG may act via different mechanisms or on different cells. In contrast to the rapid effect of hCG on the precursor cells, the stimulatory effect on the proliferation of Leydig cells is delayed for approximately 5 days. As can be expected from the increased frequency of division of the precursor cells, the total number of precursor cells increased during the first few days of the experiment. However, we were surprised to see that the number of Leydig cells also increased significantly within 2 days (Fig. 3), while during this period mature Leydig cells do not undergo cell division (see Fig. 2). This result indicates that, under the influence of hCG, advanced precursor cells rapidly differentiate into Leydig cells. When the various sets of different data are considered together, it appears that the number of Leydig cells in a rat can be controlled at three different levels, if not more. Control can be exerted: through rapid differentiation of advanced precursor cells; through rapid divisions of differentiated Leydig cells; or through a long-term process of development from early precursor cells.

The rapid increase in the number of labeled precursor cells and Leydig cells after administration of hCG shows again that cell divisions of testicular cells can be controlled by LH/hCG. A similar increase in cell divisions of precursor cells was observed soon after administration of EDS during a period when the

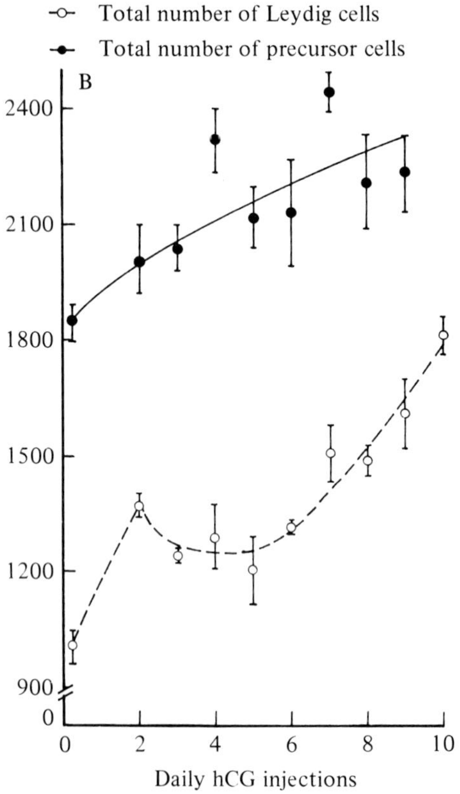

Fig. 3 Total number of precursors to Leydig cells (labeled and unlabeled) and total number of Leydig cells (labeled and unlabeled) during daily treatments with 100 i.u. hCG, expressed per 1000 Sertoli cells (from Teerds *et al.*, 1988).

level of LH is only slightly elevated (Molenaar *et al.*, 1986). This observation suggests that in the period immediately after administration of EDS, locally produced factors were most probably involved in the stimulation of proliferation, and it is possible that locally produced factors also support some aspects of cell development. To examine these possibilities, we have studied the proliferation and development of cells after administration of EDS to hypophysectomized rats. During the first days after treatment of hypophysectomized rats with EDS, a wave of cell proliferation was observed similar to that in unoperated animals (Fig. 4). Confirming earlier observations (Molenaar *et al.*, 1986), we were unable to detect Leydig cells in the hypophysectomized animals 35 days after treatment with EDS. Since the initial steps of the EDS-triggered process of renewal of Leydig cells occurred

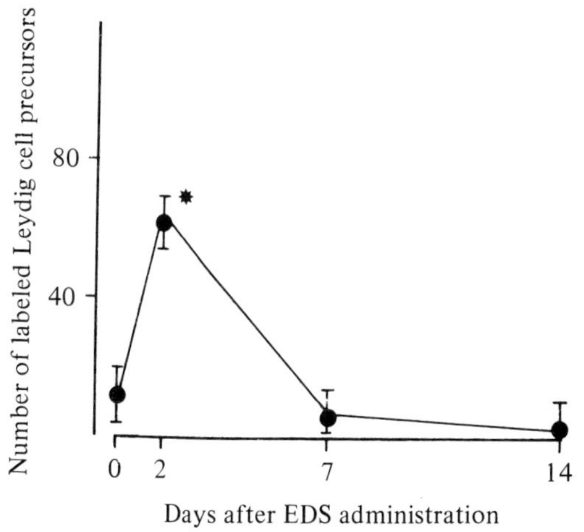

Fig. 4 Incorporation of ^{3}H-thymidine into the precursors to Leydig cells. The number of labeled precursor cells is shown for several days after administration of EDS to hypophysectomized rats. Cell numbers are expressed per 1000 Sertoli cells. *Significantly different from the control, $p < 0.01$; means ± S.E.M.

independently of LH, we tried to determine which developmental steps could take place without LH and which steps require the hormone. To probe cells that have developed independently of LH, rats were injected with hCG 26 days after administration of EDS in order to establish hormonal conditions for the completion of development. We found that, after seven daily injections of hCG (100 i.u. per rat), the number of Leydig cells increased to approximately 5% of the level in intact controls (48 ± 11 per 1000 Sertoli cells; mean ± S.E.M. of results for four animals) and plasma testosterone levels were 15-fold greater than levels in the hypophysectomized controls.

These results show that, under our experimental conditions (no LH), termination of the development of Leydig cells requires elevated levels of LH/hCG, while the initial steps can proceed independently of LH. When EDS-induced development of Leydig cells was studied in rats with an intact pituitary and a testosterone implant, used to prevent the surge of LH after the destruction of the Leydig cells, we found that Leydig cells did not develop within 35 days, although levels of LH were maintained at normal values. When these rats were treated daily with 100 i.u. of hCG, starting 28 days after treatment with EDS, numerous Leydig cells (88 ± 17 per 1000 Sertoli cells) could already be detected after 2 days. When injections of hCG were started immediately after administration of EDS, no Leydig cells were found on day 7, but considerable numbers of Leydig cells (79 ± 11 per 1000 Sertoli cells) were detected on day 14. Thus, significant numbers of Leydig cells cannot develop within 35 days after treatment with EDS in the presence of normal levels of LH, whereas many cells are already present 14 days after treatment with EDS when high doses of hCG are given. It appears from these data not only that the final steps of the development of Leydig cells require high doses of LH/hCG but also that the rate of cell development may depend on the concentration of LH/hCG. It is not known at the present time whether this result implies that all steps in the developmental process are continuously regulated by LH or whether there is discontinuous regulation, such that only late steps (advanced precursor cells) require relatively high concentrations of hormones before completion of development can take place. From the available data it appears that both mechanisms may be operative. Further support for the existence of 'arrested precursor cells' is provided by the observation, mentioned above, that the number of Leydig cells in normal rats can increase by approximately 30% within only 2 days after administration of high doses of hCG without noticeable division of Leydig cells. Similarly, the division of differentiated Leydig cells also appears to be arrested since, in normal rats, significant numbers of mitotic figures or the incorporation of thymidine have not been reported. However, 5 days after administration of hCG, many dividing cells can be detected (Teerds *et al.*, 1988).

Both observations indicate that, in adult rats, the development of Leydig cells may be 'desensitized' or arrested by chalones at normal levels of LH. An important question to be answered concerns the way in which, in immature rats, normal development can occur if such inhibitory systems may operate. It is obvious that more information is required on the various types of precursor cell (morphology, (immuno)histochemical markers, etc.) and their growth properties (kinetics) and on the regulatory elements (hormones and locally produced factors) before the molecular aspects of control of the developmental process can be investigated.

Local control of Leydig cell functions

As discussed earlier, there are many indications that, in addition to LH, other circulating hormones such as FSH and prolactin, as well as locally produced factors, can regulate specific functions of Leydig cells. Attempts are now being made in many laboratories to isolate and characterize these paracrine regulators. Since Sertoli cells may be a major source of such locally produced factors, Sertoli cell-conditioned culture medium has often been used as a starting preparation for assays and purification procedures. It was determined that rat interstitial fluid, but not rat serum, could further enhance the production of steroids that may already be maximally stimulated by LH (Sharpe and Cooper, 1984), and there were indications that this effect was mediated by particular but unidentified biochemical mechanisms (Rommerts *et al.*, 1986). The stimulation of production of steroids obtained with interstitial fluid may reflect the action of locally produced factors. Therefore,

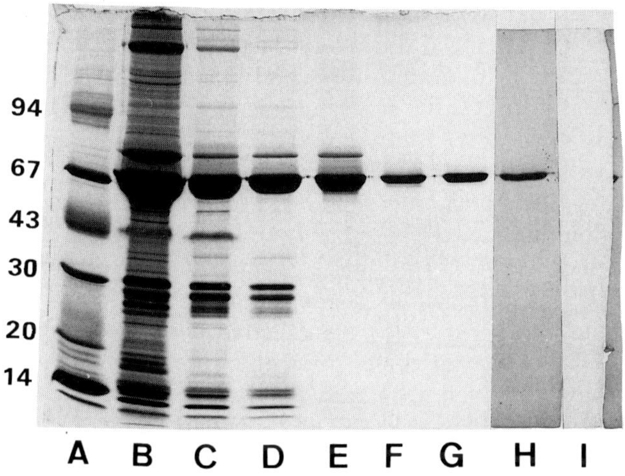

Fig. 5 Silver-stained gel after electrophoresis of testicular fluid and fractions thereof. Lanes A through G contain the following: (A) molecular weight markers (kDa); (B) rat testicular fluid (rTF); (C) ammonium sulfate fraction (50–80% saturated); (D) blue Sepharose GL6B fraction; (E) fraction after anion-exchange chromatography on ZetaPrep 15; (F) pH 5 fraction after chromatofocusing on Mono P; (G) Mono P fraction heated for 16 hours at 60°C. Lane H is a Western blot of fraction G stained after incubation with antibodies raised against rat albumin. Lane I is Western blot of fraction G stained without incubation with antibodies raised against rat albumin.

we decided to isolate and characterize the factors that give rise to this biological activity. From a comparative study of different biological fluids (rat serum and testicular fluid, bovine serum and follicular fluid, and fetal calf serum), it appeared that the biological activities present in rat testicular fluid could also be found in follicular fluid and fetal calf serum, whereas rat and bovine serum had inhibitory effects on the production of steroids (Melsert and Rommerts, 1987). These data suggested that the biological activity may not be organ or species specific. In subsequent studies we found that the activity was always detected in albumin-enriched fractions (Melsert *et al.*, 1988). Results from our most recent experiments have shown that the biological activity is retained in preparations of albumin in which no contaminants were revealed by polyacrylamide gel electrophoresis and silver-staining (Figs. 5 and 6). Moreover, heating of preparations at 60°C, which inactivates many growth factors, did not destroy the biological activity (results not shown). These data strongly support the hypothesis that rather high, but physiological, concentrations of albumin (40 mg/ml) in interstitial fluid can enhance LH-stimulated production of steroids. This effect of testicular fluid is considered to be stimulatory when compared to the effects of rat serum. However, the same data may also be interpreted differently. Since albumin is present both in serum and testicular fluid, the results also indicate that inhibitory factors are present in serum. Whatever the correct explanation, albumin is probably not an important molecule in the establishment of cell-to-cell communication. The result merely reinforces the common knowledge that the responses of isolated cells can be influenced by the conditions of culture *in vitro*. In this respect, there are no indications that our cells are damaged or show a limited response and that albumin 'cures' the cells (Rommerts *et al.*, 1985). Furthermore, albumin also stimulated the production of testosterone when intact testes were perfused (Ewing *et al.*, 1976). Thus, albumin may be considered as one of the external factors, such as ionic composition or temperature, that exert a static control on cell function. Hence, the presence of albumin may be essential when physiological aspects of the regulation of Leydig cells are investigated *in vitro*.

Although we have not been able to detect the presence, in interstitial fluid, of other compounds that can amplify LH-stimulated production of steroids, we cannot exclude the possible presence of factors that can stimulate or inhibit the basal production of steroids. However, the conditions of our bioassay system did not allow us to examine this possibility. In most of the currently used bioassay systems, short-term effects of fluids or extracts on the production of steroids or cAMP or on the number of LH receptors are measured. Although using such assays we will continue to learn more about the molecules and the mechanisms that contribute to the short-term regulation of the production of steroids, it remains to be demonstrated whether local modulation of steroid production is physiologically important when external control by LH via a feedback system predominates. Locally produced factors may still play an important role when they act independently of the LH–testosterone feedback system. We have previously shown in studies *in vivo* that, during the development of Leydig cells, locally produced factors under the influence of FSH may play a role independent of LH. However, since bioassay systems for the assay of Leydig cell growth are not yet available, it is difficult to study this important aspect of local control of Leydig cell functions *in vitro*.

Local control of testicular functions by Leydig cells

The physiological importance of Leydig cells is to supply peripheral and testicular, androgen-dependent cells with androgens. The activity of the Leydig cells is mainly controlled by LH. Spermatogenesis takes place in an environment with high concentrations of testosterone and there are conflicting opinions as to whether spermatogenesis requires a high and accurately controlled level of testosterone or whether the high testicular levels of testosterone are arbitrary and a direct consequence of the local production of this hormone (Rommerts, 1988). Although in many studies of the hormonal requirements of spermatogenesis it has been concluded that local levels of testosterone must be high and carefully regulated by locally produced factors,

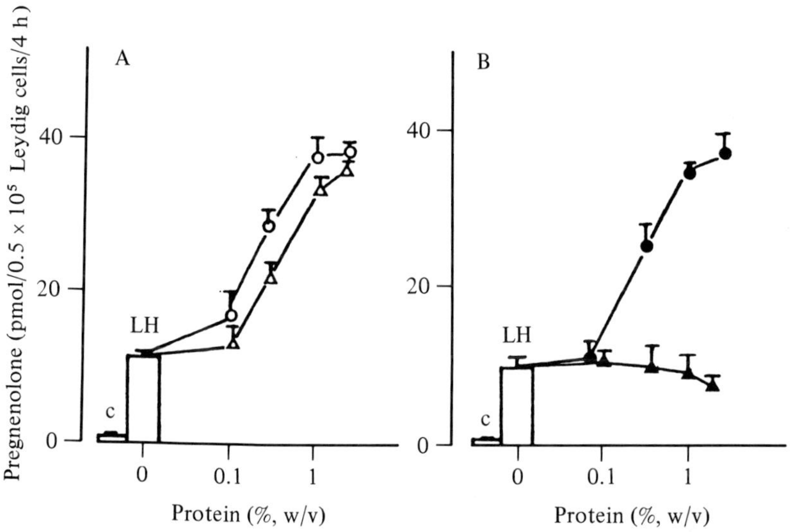

Fig. 6 (A) Dose-dependent effect of rat testicular fluid (open triangles) and the purified albumin fraction G (open circles) (see legend to Fig. 5) on the production of pregnenolone by Leydig cells maximally stimulated with 100 ng LH/ml. (B) As in (A), but for rat serum (closed triangles) and a chromatographically purified albumin fraction from rat serum (closed circles).

results of recent experiments indicate that spermatogenesis can be maintained with approximately 20% of the normal testicular levels of testosterone (Rea *et al.*, 1986). This result indicates that, from a physiological point of view, fine control of the production of steroids by locally produced factors may not be necessary. It remains possible that factors other than steroids produced by Leydig cells may play a role in the regulation of testicular function. These factors could include prostaglandins, which may act on blood vessels and control blood flow (van Vliet *et al.*, 1988), or peptides such as oxytocin, which could regulate tubular contractions (Nicholson *et al.*, 1987), or even compounds that act on the Leydig cells themselves (autocrine regulation). In support of this possibility is the observation that Leydig cells mediate the vascular responses – reduction of blood flow and increases in vascular permeability (Setchell and Rommerts, 1985; van Vliet *et al.*, 1988) – that occur after administration of high doses of hCG (100 i.u. per rat). There may even be many more possibilities for actions of Leydig cells on other testicular cells, which involve other compounds such as opiates, angiotensins, etc. Rather than extending the list of other possible local actions of Leydig cells, it seems more appropriate to pay some attention to results of experiments that indicate that Leydig cells may not be essential for the maintenance of testicular function.

It has been shown that, during the first few days after the specific destruction of Leydig cells by EDS, spermatogenesis, vascular permeability and blood flow remain normal (Molenaar *et al.*, 1985; Setchell and Rommerts, 1985; van Vliet *et al.*, 1988). This observation indicates that Leydig cells and their secretion products are not essential during this period. During the subsequent days after administration of EDS, disturbances in spermatogenesis are seen to increase, probably as the result of a lack of testosterone. Administration of testosterone every 3 days by injections of testosterone esters completely prevents this deterioration of spermatogenesis, even when testicular levels of testosterone are approximately 30% of the normal value (Sharpe *et al.*, 1988). This important observation shows, once again, that the most important function of the Leydig cell is to produce testosterone and that control by LH is sufficient to supply the testis with an excess of testosterone. Other secretion products from Leydig cells are most probably not essential for maintenance of testicular function within the time frame of several weeks. It is theoretically possible that the few developing cells that are precursors of the mature Leydig cells could secrete these factors. However, there is no experimental evidence to support this hypothesis.

In conclusion, locally operating regulatory systems are of paramount importance for the development of germinal cells, since germinal cells have few or no receptors for hormones and growth factors. Regulation of development of Leydig cells may also involve paracrine factors in an important role, especially as 'coordination molecules'. Many scientists have been attracted to studies of paracrine control systems using Leydig cells. This fashionable topic of research has probably become so popular because it is technically feasible to measure, *in vitro*, the short-term modulation of the production of steroids. However, as argued above, the short-term paracrine regulation of the production of steroids appears to be the least important area of paracrinology and studies on long-term paracrine regulation seem to be more relevant. Such studies on the paracrine regulation of development of Leydig cells are hampered by the lack of suitable in-vitro and in-vivo systems. However, numerous observations have demonstrated that LH has major effects on the growth of Leydig cells and on the maintenance and activation of their functions. Since our knowledge of trophic effects of LH is also limited, more detailed studies on this subject are necessary, particularly at the molecular level. In this respect, it seems also of importance to study the physiological relevance of the many pleiomorphic forms of LH secreted by the pituitary. It is possible that the different forms of LH can mediate a 'pituitary-directed' fine regulation of Leydig cell functions which complements the regulation by locally operating systems.

References

Beurden, W.M.O. van, Roodnat, B., de Jong, F.H., Mulder, E. & van der Molen, H.J. (1976). Hormonal regulation of LH stimulation of testosterone production in isolated Leydig cells of immature rats: the effect of hypophysectomy, FSH and estradiol-17 beta. **Steroids** 28:847–855.

Burris, A.S., Rodbard, H.W., Winters, S.J. & Sherins, R.J. (1988). Gonadotropin in therapy in men with isolated hypogonadotropic hypogonadism: the response to human chorionic gonadotropin is produced by initial testicular size. **Journal of Clinical Endocrinology and Metabolism** 66:1144–1151.

Chemes, H.E., Rivarola, M.A. & Bergada, C. (1976). Effect of hCG on the interstitial cells and androgen production in the immature rat testis. **Journal of Reproduction and Fertility** 46:279–282.

Christensen, A.K. & Peacock, K.C. (1980). Increase in Leydig cell number in testes of adult rats treated chronically with an excess of human chorionic gonadotropin. **Biology of Reproduction** 22:383–391.

Closset, J. & Hennen, G. (1989). Biopotency of highly purified porcine follicle-stimulating hormone and human luteinizing hormone on gonadal function. **Journal of Endocrinology** 120:89–96.

Ewing, L.L., Chubb, C.E. & Robaire, B. (1976). Macromolecules, steroid binding and testosterone secretion by rabbit testes. **Nature** 264:84–86.

Ewing, L.L. & Zirkin, B. (1983). Leydig cell structure and steroidogenic function. **Recent Progress in Hormone Research** 39:599–635.

Fritz, I.B. (1978). Sites of action of androgens and follicle-stimulating hormone on cells of the seminiferous tubule. In: Litwack, G., ed. **Biochemical Actions of Hormones**, 5, New York, Academic Press, pp.249–281.

Kerr, J.B. & Sharpe, R.M. (1985). Follicle-stimulating hormone induction of Leydig cell maturation. **Endocrinology** 116:2592–2604.

Melsert, R. & Rommerts, F.F.G. (1987). Leydig cell steroid production in the presence of LH is further stimulated by rat testicular fluid, fetal calf serum and bovine follicular fluid, but not by rat and bovine serum. **Journal of Endocrinology** 115:R17–R20.

Melsert, R., Hoogerbrugge, J.W. & Rommerts, F.F.G. (1988). The albumin fraction of rat testicular fluid stimulates steroid production by isolated Leydig cells. **Molecular and Cellular Endocrinology** 59:221–231.

Molenaar, R., de Rooij, D.G., Rommerts, F.F.G., Reuvers, P.J. & van der Molen, H.J. (1985). Specific destruction of Leydig cells in mature rats after *in vivo* administration of ethane dimethyl sulphonate (EDS). **Biology of Reproduction** 33:1213–1222.

Molenaar, R., de Rooij, D.G., Rommerts, F.F.G. & van der Molen, H.J. (1986). Repopulation of Leydig cells in mature rats after selective destruction of the existent Leydig cells with ethylene dimethane sulfonate is dependent on luteinizing hormone and not follicle-stimulating hormone. **Endocrinology** 118:2546–2554.

Nicholson, H.D., Worley, R.T.S., Guldenaar, S.E.F. & Pickering, B.T. (1987). Ethane-1,2 dimethanesulphonate reduces testicular oxytocin content and seminiferous tubule movements in the rat. **Journal of Endocrinology** 112:311–316.

Odell, W.D. & Swerdloff, R.S. (1976). Etiology of sexual maturation: a model system based on the sexually maturing rat. **Recent Progress in Hormone Research** 32:245–288.

Purvis, K., Clausen, O.P.F. & Hansson, V. (1979). LH contamination may explain FSH effects on rat Leydig cells. **Journal of Reproduction and Fertility** 56:657–665.

Rea, M.A., Marshall, G.R., Weinbauer, G.F. & Nieschlag, E. (1986). Testosterone maintains pituitary and serum FSH and spermatogenesis in gonadotrophin-

releasing hormone antagonist suppressed rats. **Journal of Endocrinology** 108:101–107.
Rommerts, F.F.G. (1988). How much androgen is required for maintenance of spermatogenesis? **Journal of Endocrinology** 116:7–9.
Rommerts, F.F.G., Grootenhuis, A.J., Hoogerbrugge, J.W. & van der Molen, H.J. (1985a). Ethane dimethane sulphonate (EDS) specifically inhibits LH stimulated steroidogenesis in Leydig cells isolated from mature rats but not in cells from immature rats. **Molecular and Cellular Endocrinology** 42:105–111.
Rommerts, F.F.G., Hoogerbrugge, J.W. & van der Molen, H.J. (1986). Stimulation of steroid production in isolated rat Leydig cells by unknown factors in testicular fluid differs from the effects of LH or LH-releasing hormone. **Journal of Endocrinology** 109:111–117.
Rommerts, F.F.G., Molenaar, R. & van der Molen, H.J. (1985b). Preparation of isolated Leydig cells. In: Birnbaumer, L. & O'Malley, B.W., eds. **Methods in Enzymology**, Vol. 109, pp.275–288.
Rommerts, F.F.G., Teerds, K.J. & Hoogerbrugge, J.W. (1988). *In vitro* effects of ethylene-dimethane sulfonate (EDS) on Leydig cells: inhibition of steroid production and cytotoxic effects are dependent on species and age of rat. **Molecular and Cellular Endocrinology** 55:87–94.
Setchell, B.P. & Rommerts, F.F.G. (1985). The importance of the Leydig cells in the vascular response to hCG in the rat testis. **International Journal of Andrology** 8:436–440.
Sharpe, R.M. & Cooper, I. (1984). Intratesticular secretion of factor(s) with major stimulatory effects on Leydig cell testosterone secretion *in vitro*. **Molecular and Cellular Endocrinology** 37:159–168.
Sharpe, R.M., Donahie, K. & Cooper, I. (1988). Re-evaluation of the intratesticular level of testosterone required for quantitative maintenance of spermatogenesis in the rat. **Journal of Endocrinology** 117:19–26.
Teerds, K.J., Closset, J., Rommerts, F.F.G., de Rooij, D.G., Stocco, D.M., Colenbrander, B., Wensing, C.J.G. & Hennen, G. (1989). Effects of pure FSH and LH preparations on the number and function of Leydig cells in immature hypophysectomized rats. **Journal of Endocrinology** 120:97–106.
Teerds, K.J., de Rooij, D.G., Rommerts, F.F.G. & Wensing, C.J.G. (1988). The regulation of the proliferation and differentiation of Leydig cell precursors after EDS administration or daily hCG treatment. **Journal of Andrology** 9:343–351.
Vliet, J. van, Rommerts, F.F.G., de Rooij, D.G., Buwalda, G. & Wensing, C.J.G. (1988). Reduction of testicular blood flow and focal degeneration of tissue in the rat after administration of human chorionic gonadotrophin. **Journal of Endocrinology** 117:51–57.

Stimulation of Leydig cell steroidogenesis by a factor from human ovarian follicular fluid

S.A. KHAN, C. KECK AND E. NIESCHLAG

Clinical Research Unit for Reproductive Medicine of the Max Planck Society and Institute of Reproductive Medicine of the University, Münster, Federal Republic of Germany.

Keywords

Leydig cells, human follicular fluid, interstitial cell-stimulating activity, luteinizing hormone, human chorionic gonadotropin, steroidogenesis.

Introduction

Several studies in recent years have indicated the presence of paracrine and autocrine regulatory factors in the gonads which either inhibit or enhance the function of follicle-stimulating hormone (FSH) and luteinizing hormone (LH) according to the local requirements (Sharpe, 1986; Hsueh, 1986; Tonetta and di Zerega, 1986). These factors either inhibit the binding of FSH and LH to their respective receptors, thereby inhibiting their action, or they enhance the effects of these hormones by stimulating an alternative transducing mechanism (Reichert and Abou-Issa, 1977; di Zerega *et al.*, 1983; Sharpe and Cooper, 1984; Rommerts *et al.*, 1986; Sluss *et al.*, 1987; Risbridger *et al.*, 1987). Rat ovarian extracts have been shown to contain at least two factors that modulate the action of LH. One of these factors was found to inhibit binding of LH to its ovarian receptors and, in turn, to inhibit production of progesterone by ovarian slices *in vitro*; another factor was found to stimulate steroidogenesis by rat Leydig cells *in vitro* (Yang *et al.*, 1979). A factor which stimulates Leydig cell steroidogenesis has also been found in bovine follicular fluid (Risbridger *et al.*, 1987).

In a recent study, human ovarian follicular fluid obtained from preovulatory follicles was found to contain much higher LH bioactivity than LH immunoreactivity (in a ratio of approximately 40:1) (Cha *et al.*, 1986). The LH bioactivity was determined by measurements of the stimulation of production of testosterone by preparations of mouse testicular interstitial cells *in vitro*. The results indicate either that the bioactivity of the LH molecule increases tremendously in these follicles without any significant changes in its immunoreactivity or that the ovarian cells secrete an additional factor with LH-like bioactivity which might be immunologically distinct from the pituitary LH. Our studies, reviewed below, were performed to assess the second possibility and have shown that, indeed, the ovary secretes a factor with LH-like bioactivity, which is distinct from both LH and human chorionic gonadotropin (hCG) (Khan *et al.*, 1988).

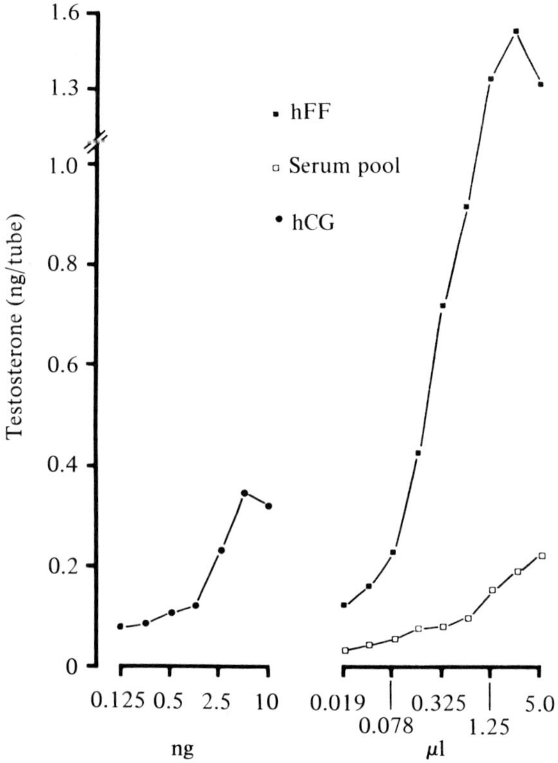

Fig. 1 Influence of human chorionic gonadotropin (hCG; closed circles), a pool of human follicular fluid (hFF; closed squares) and a pool of human serum (open squares) on production of testosterone *in vitro* by rat interstitial cells (taken from Khan *et al.*, 1988).

Effects of human follicular fluid on Leydig cells

Human follicular fluid (hFF) and serum samples were obtained from women who were participating in an in-vitro fertilization programme. These women had previously been treated with human menopausal gonadotropins (hMG) and hCG to stimulate follicular maturation and induce ovulation. When testicular interstitial cells obtained from adult rats (Syed *et al.*, 1985) were incubated with various doses of hFF, serum or hCG for 3 hours, all preparations caused a stimulation of the production of testosterone. However, stimulation obtained with hFF was about 30-fold higher than that obtained with serum from the same patients when used at equivalent doses (Fig. 1). The huge differences in the LH-like bioactivity of hFF and serum suggested an ovarian origin for the interstitial-cell stimulatory activity (ICSA). Moreover, the stimulation with hFF was two- to threefold higher than that obtained with maximum doses of hCG, indicating that the hFF enhanced Leydig cell steroidogenesis by a mechanism different from that associated with LH/hCG. This possibility was further supported by the fact that, in the presence of maximum doses of hCG, hFF further stimulated the production of testosterone (Khan *et al.*, 1988). When the Leydig cells were purified on Percoll gradients (Bartlett and Sharpe, 1987) the hFF had similar effects. Thus, it appears that hFF influenced the Leydig cells directly and that these effects were not mediated by any other type of cell. Furthermore, a preparation of interstitial cells from 10-day-old rats, which was devoid of germ cells and macrophages, responded in a similar fashion to hFF (Khan *et al.*, unpublished data).

Since the follicular fluid used in these studies was obtained from women who had been treated with high doses of hCG (10 000 i.u.) for the induction of ovulation, the hFF may have contained hCG. To ascertain that the effects of hFF on Leydig cells were not due to hCG, we incubated cells in the presence of a specific antiserum raised against hCG. The results showed that, although the antiserum blocked the effects of a maximum dose (1 μg) of a highly purified preparation of hCG, there was very little, if any, effect on the bioactivity of hFF (Khan *et al.*, 1988).

Species specificity

To study the species specificity of hFF factor(s), interstitial cells obtained from human, rat, mouse and hamster testes were incubated with various doses of hFF and hCG. The hFF stimulated steroidogenesis in the cells from four species in a similar fashion (Khan *et al.*, 1988) suggesting that the stimulatory factors in hFF lack species specificity. In this respect, the hFF factor seems to be different from luteinizing hormone releasing hormone (LHRH)-like factors which stimulate steroidogenesis in the rat Leydig cells but are not active when added to mouse Leydig cells (Hunter *et al.*, 1982). Moreover, a pool of bovine ovarian follicular fluid also stimulated production of testosterone by rat Leydig cells, suggesting the presence of a similar factor in the ovaries of other species (Khan *et al.*, unpublished data).

Physicochemical characterization of the active substance(s)

To characterize the active substance(s), aliquots of hFF were heated at different temperatures, dialyzed, precipitated with ammonium sulfate, treated with charcoal, and extracted with organic solvents.

The results showed that the active substance was resistent to heating at 30°C and 60°C for 10 minutes but lost all bioactivity when heated at 80°C or higher temperatures for more than 2–3 minutes (Khan *et al.*, 1988). The activity in hFF was retained after dialysis for 48 hours inside membranes with a molecular-weight limit of 10 kDa. Precipitation with 80% ammonium sulfate and subsequent dialysis showed that the activity could be precipitated by

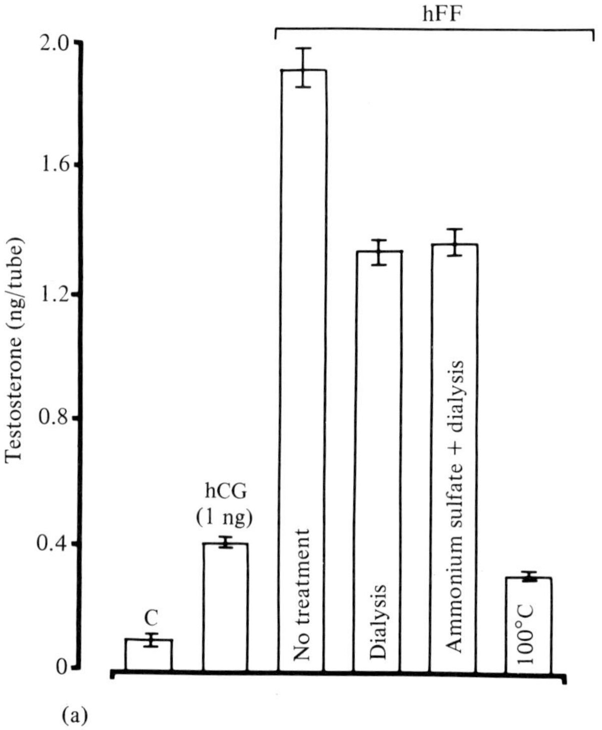

Fig. 2 (a) Influence of dialysis, ammonium sulfate precipitation and heating on the interstitial-cell stimulatory activity of hFF. Testosterone produced in the absence (C) and presence of hCG (1 ng/tube) is also shown. Data shown are means ± S.D. of triplicate determinations. (b) Dialyzed human follicular fluid was treated with ether, ethanol, or acetone to precipitate proteins. The influence of redissolved proteins (from treatment with acetone or ethanol) or the aqueous phase (from treatment with ether) on the production of testosterone by rat interstitial cells is shown (Khan *et al.*, 1988).

ammonium sulfate (Fig. 2a). Although these findings suggested that the active substance might be a high-molecular-weight and heat-sensitive factor (protein?), the activity of hFF was lost after treatment with charcoal. The sensitivity to treatment with charcoal suggested that the activity could be due to a steroid precursor of testosterone bound to a macromolecule which could have been removed by charcoal. This possibility was further explored by treatment of hFF with organic solvents to remove all the possible steroids. The results showed that extraction with ether, ethanol, or acetone caused only a partial loss of activity in the organic phase (Fig. 2b) and indicated that the

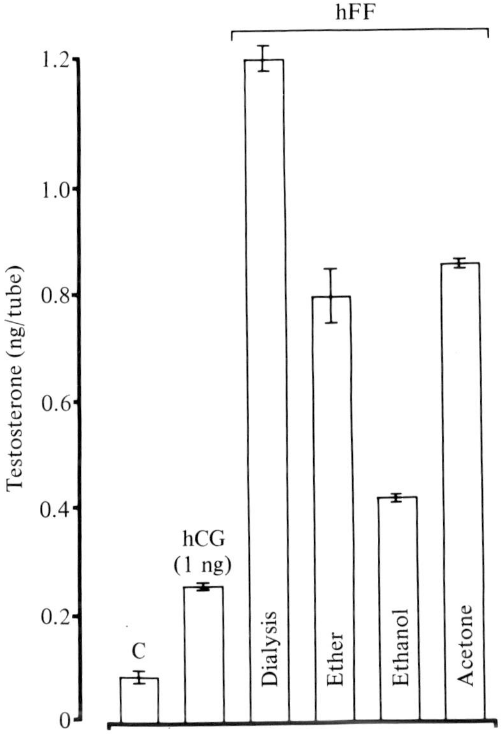

(b)

activity was associated with a high-molecular-weight protein and was not due to the steroid content of the follicular fluid.

To rule out the possibility that some components of hFF may directly influence the estimation of testosterone by radioimmunoassay (RIA), the samples (medium from culture of Leydig cells) were either heated at 100°C for 15 minutes to destroy proteins or the steroids were extracted with diethyl ether prior to RIA. There were no differences in the levels of testosterone in untreated and treated samples, suggesting that hFF did not directly influence the estimations of levels of testosterone (Khan *et al.*, 1988).

Having established the macromolecular nature of the stimulator, attempts were made to characterize the substance(s) by gel chromatography, chromatofocusing and SDS-PAGE.

The hFF proteins were subjected to chromatography on a column of AcA-54 (LKB Products AB, Bromma, Sweden) after precipitation with 80% ammonium sulfate and dialysis. The analysis of individual fractions showed that the interstitial-cell stimulatory activity eluted in a region that corres-

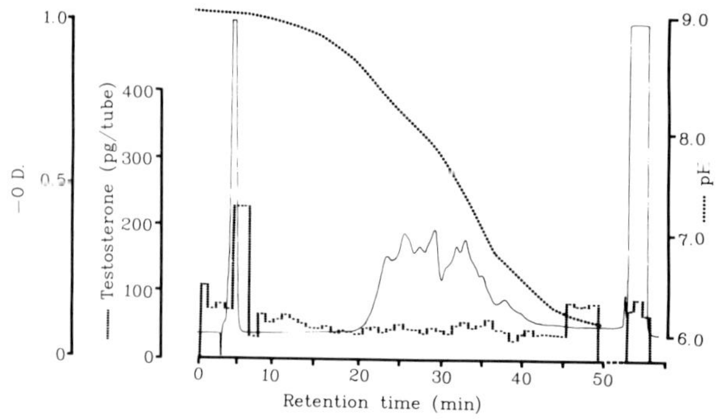

Fig. 3 A chromatofocusing profile, with a narrow pH range (8.0–9.5), of interstitial-cell stimulatory activity (Khan *et al.*, 1988).

ponded to molecular weights of between 30 kDa and 50 kDa. Pools of five fractions were also analyzed for hCG and LH immunoreactivity. These two hormones also eluted in the same region but their levels were very low compared to the bioactivity (Khan *et al.*, 1988).

The pooled fractions from gel chromatography containing ICSA were then further purified by chromatofocusing in the pH range 6.0–9.0 on a fast protein liquid chromatography (FPLC) system. The bioactivity was found in the void volume (above pH 9.0). These results indicated that the active substance was distinct from hCG which exhibits an acidic pI (below pH 6.0). The active fractions were further purified by chromatofocusing in a narrow pH range (8.0–9.5). As shown in Figure 3, the bioactivity was eluted as a single peak in the pH region between pH 8.8 and 9.5. As the pI value of the active substance was very close to the reported pI of human LH (Robertson and Diczfalusy, 1977), individual fractions were also analyzed for immunoreactive LH. However, no LH immunoreactivity was detected in these fractions. These studies indicated that the steroidogenic factor was distinct from both LH and hCG in terms of its physicochemical properties.

The purified fractions were analyzed by SDS-PAGE under reducing and non-reducing conditions. The results showed that the active fractions were not homogeneous. A protein band was present in the molecular-weight region between 20 kDa and 30 kDa and might represent the interstitial-cell stimulatory factor (Khan *et al.*, 1988).

Mechanism of action of ICSA

The above experiments suggested that the hFF factor stimulated production of testosterone in Leydig cells by a mechanism distinct from that associated with LH/hCG. Further experiments were performed to determine the site of action of this factor. The results of these experiments showed that the hFF

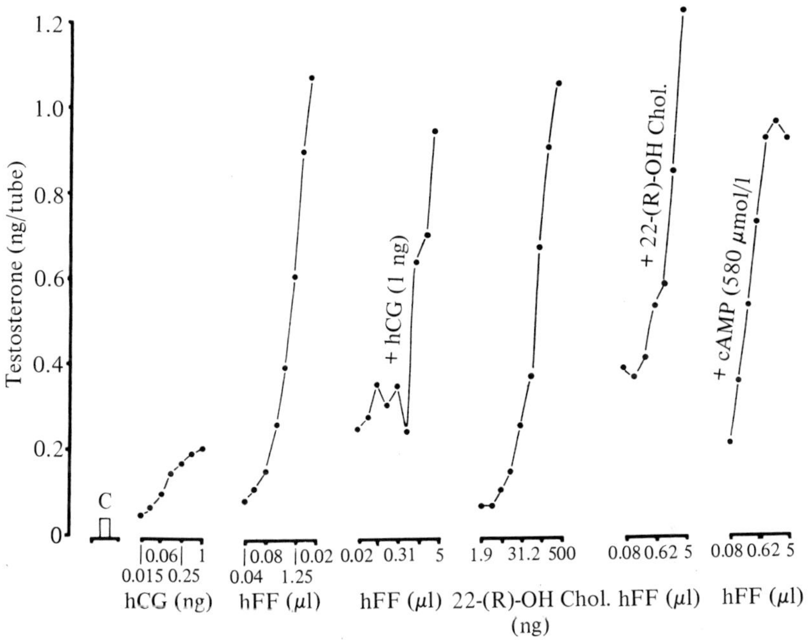

Fig. 4 Influence of hCG, hFF and 22-R-hydroxycholesterol (22-(R)-OH Chol.) on production of testosterone by rat interstitial cells *in vitro* and the influence of hFF on the interstitial cells incubated in the presence of maximal concentrations of hCG, cAMP and half-maximal concentrations of 22-R-hydroxycholesterol (Khan *et al.*, unpublished data).

factor further enhanced the production of testosterone in Leydig cells that had been stimulated maximally by cholera toxin or dibutyryl cyclic AMP, indicating that the effect of this factor was not mediated through stimulation of adenyl cyclase activity. The incubation of Leydig cells in the presence of 22-R-hydroxycholesterol resulted in enhanced synthesis of testosterone by these cells (Fig. 4). However, this stimulation bypasses the step of cholesterol side-chain cleavage in mitochondria which involves the mitochondrial cytochrome P450 (Rommerts *et al.*, 1986). The dose–response curves obtained with hFF and 22-R-hydroxycholesterol for rat Leydig cells were very similar and parallel to each other (Fig. 4). Moreover, when added in the presence of half maximal doses of 22-R-hydroxycholesterol, the effects of hFF on steroidogenesis were additive (Khan *et al.*, unpublished data). Thus, the hFF factor may act at the level of mitochondria to enhance the rate of synthesis of steroids in Leydig cells. Further experiments are needed to examine this hypothesis.

When the time course of the effects of hFF was studied by incubating Leydig cells for different time intervals, it was found that the hFF factor induced a significant increase in the production of testosterone after 30 minutes, while the effects of hCG were only evident after 1 hour under the experimental conditions and with the doses employed. These results again indicate that the hFF factor acts at an intermediate step in steroidogenesis, between stimulation by LH/hCG and the mitochondrial side-chain cleavage of cholesterol.

Concluding remarks

A macromolecular factor from human follicular fluid, which stimulates steroidogenesis of Leydig cells, has been partially characterized. The factor has a molecular weight between 30 kDa and 50 kDa and a pI value of 8.8 to 9.5. It appears to be distinct from human LH and hCG in terms of its physicochemical and immunological properties. Moreover, this factor affects steroidogenesis in Leydig cells by a mechanism that is distinct from that associated with LH/hCG and that does not involve the activation of adenyl cyclase for the stimulation of steroidogenesis.

The steroidogenic factor apparently originates in the ovary during follicular maturation and may enhance the action of pituitary LH in the stimulation of the ovarian production of steroids. Hence, it may play a role in the regulation of ovarian function.

Acknowledgements

We are grateful to Heike Westhoven and Bettina Schuhmann for expert technical assistance.

References

Bartlett, J.M.S. & Sharpe, R.M. (1987). Effect of local heating of the rat testis on the levels in interstitial fluid of a putative paracrine regulator of the Leydig cells and its relationship to changes in Sertoli cell secretory function. **Journal of Reproduction and Fertility** 80:279–287.

Cha, K.-Y., Barnes, R.B., Marrs, R.P. & Lobo, R.A. (1986). Correlation of the bioactivity of luteinizing hormone in follicular fluid with oocyte maturity in the spontaneous cycle. **Fertility and Sterility** 45:338–341.

di Zerega, G.S., Marrs, R.P., Roche, P.C., Campeau, J.D. & King, O.R. (1983). Identification of proteins in pooled human follicular fluid which suppress follicular response to gonadotropins. **Journal of Clinical Endocrinology and Metabolism** 56:35–41.

Hsueh, A.J.W. (1986). Paracrine mechanisms involved in granulosa cell differentiation. **Clinics in Endocrinology and Metabolism** 15:185–207.

Hunter, M.G., Sullivan, M.H.F., Dix, C.J., Aldred, L.F. & Cooke, B.A. (1982). Stimulation and inhibition by LHRH analogues of cultured rat Leydig cell function and lack of effect on mouse Leydig cells. **Molecular and Cellular Endocrinology** 27:31–44.

Khan, S.A., Hallin, P., Bartlett, J., De Geyter, C.H. & Nieschlag, E. (1988).

Characterization of a factor from human ovarian follicular fluid which stimulates Leydig cell testosterone production. **Acta Endocrinologica** 118:283–293.

Reichert, L.E. Jr & Abou-Issa, H. (1977). Studies on a low molecular weight testicular factor which inhibits binding of FSH to its receptor. **Biology of Reproduction** 17:614–621.

Risbridger, G.P., Averill, S. & de Kretser, D.M. (1987). Does bovine follicular fluid stimulate Leydig cell steroidogenesis? In: Spera, G. & de Kretser, D.M., eds. **Morphological Basis of Human Reproductive Function**, New York, Plenum Press, pp.63–64.

Robertson, D.M. & Diczfalusy, E. (1977). Biological and immunological characterization of human luteinizing hormone. II. A comparison of the immunological and biological activities of pituitary extracts after electrofocusing using different standard preparations. **Molecular and Cellular Endocrinology** 9:57–67.

Rommerts, F.F.G., Hoogerbrugge, J.W. & van der Molen, H.J. (1986). Stimulation of steroid production in isolated Leydig cells by unknown factors in testicular fluid differs from effects of luteinizing hormone. **Journal of Endocrinology** 109:111–117.

Sharpe, R.M. (1986). Paracrine control of the testis. **Clinics in Endocrinology and Metabolism** 15:185–207.

Sharpe, R.M. & Cooper, I. (1984). Intratesticular secretion of a factor(s) with major stimulatory effects on Leydig cell testosterone secretion *in vitro*. **Molecular and Cellular Endocrinology** 37:159–168.

Sluss, P.M., Schneyder, A.L., Franke, M.A. & Reichert, L.E. Jr (1987). Porcine follicular fluid contains both follicle-stimulating hormone agonist and antagonist activities. **Endocrinology** 120:1477–1481.

Syed, V., Khan, S.A. & Ritzen, E.M. (1985). Stage-specific inhibition of interstitial cell testosterone secretion by rat seminiferous tubules. **Molecular and Cellular Endocrinology** 40:257–264.

Tonetta, S.A. & di Zerega, G.S. (1986). Paracrine regulation of follicular maturation in primates. **Clinics in Endocrinology and Metabolism** 15:135–156.

Yang, K.-P., Samaan, N.A. & Ward, D.N. (1979). Effects of luteinizing hormone receptor-binding inhibitor on the *in vitro* steroidogenesis by rat ovary and testis. **Endocrinology** 104:552–558.

Intrafollicular roles of inhibin, interferon-α, and related peptides

J.K. FINDLAY, Z. ZHIWEN, L.A. HUTCHINSON, R.S. CARSON,
H.G. BURGER AND A.C. HERINGTON

Medical Research Centre, Prince Henry's Campus, Monash Medical Centre, Melbourne, Victoria 3004, Australia.

Keywords

Inhibin, activin, transforming growth factor-β, epidermal growth factor, insulin-like growth factor-1, interferon-α, granulosa cells, theca cells, follicular recruitment and development, local regulation.

Introduction

There is increasing evidence for the concept that regulation of ovarian function involves modulation of the actions of gonadotropins by intraovarian peptides which act as para- and/or autocrine regulators (Findlay and Risbridger, 1987). Paracrine regulators are those that are produced by one cell and act on neighboring cells, whereas autocrine regulators act on the same cells that produce them (Sporn and Todaro, 1980). There are several criteria for the classification of substances as local regulators (Franchimont, 1986), including evidence for local production under physiological regulation and local action. In this chapter we will consider whether or not the inhibin-related peptides, which include transforming growth factor-β (TGF-p2), and the interferon-α (IFN-α) family of lymphokines, control the functions of granulosa and theca cells, and thereby fulfil the criteria for intraovarian regulators.

Inhibin-related peptides

Members of the inhibin and TGF-β family include two forms of inhibin ($\alpha\beta_A$, $\alpha\beta_B$) with follicle-stimulating hormone (FSH)-suppressing activity, two forms of activin ($\beta_A\beta_A$, $\beta_A\beta_B$) with FSH-stimulating activity (see Burger *et al.*, 1987) and erythroid differentiating activity (Eto *et al.*, 1987), three forms of TGF-β (Massague, 1987), Mullerian inhibiting substance (MIS) (Cate *et al.*, 1986), a T-cell suppressing factor (Wrann *et al.*, 1987), the protein encoded by the Vgl mRNA of *Xenopus* (Weeks and Melton, 1987), and the putative peptide coded by the decapentaplegic-C gene complex of *Drosophila* (Padgett *et al.*, 1987). There are significant homologies between the nucleotide sequences of the β-genes of inhibin and the genes that encode these other activities. It should be noted that activin is formed by the association of two inhibin β-subunits, whereas inhibin consists of α- and β-subunits and has the opposite biological activity to activin with respect to the release of FSH by pituitary gonadotrophs (Vale *et al.*, 1986; Ling *et al.*, 1986) and erythroid differentiation (Yu *et al.*, 1987).

Interest in inhibin-related peptides as intragonadal regulators stems from two observations. Franchimont *et al.* (1979) showed that crude extracts that contained inhibin activity exerted a direct inhibitory effect on the synthesis of DNA by actively dividing spermatogonia. TGF-β, which has a close structural homology to inhibin, is well established as a local regulator in extragonadal tissues (see Sporn *et al.*, 1987).

Ovarian production of inhibin-related peptides

Inhibin

We and others have established that inhibin is produced locally within ovarian follicles by granulosa cells and by luteal cells (in rats and humans) and that its endogenous production is hormonally and locally regulated (see Burger *et al.*, 1988). FSH is the predominant endocrine regulator of the production of inhibin by granulosa cells, while luteinizing hormone (LH) at low doses is able to cause release of inhibin from granulosa cells after their exposure to FSH (Bicsak *et al.*, 1986; Zhiwen *et al.*, 1988a). Higher doses of LH/human chorionic gonadotropin (hCG) inhibit pregnant mare's serum gonadotropin (PMSG)/FSH-induced production of inhibin *in vitro* (Zhiwen *et al.*, 1988b) and *in vivo* (Lee, 1983). Stimulation of production of inhibin by 8-bromo cyclic AMP or prostaglandin E_2, is consistent with the hypothesis that FSH-stimulated production of inhibin is mediated through cyclic AMP (Zhiwen *et al.*, 1987a). Studies with rats *in vivo* have shown that the amount of mRNA that encodes the α- (Davis *et al.*, 1986) and β-subunits of inhibin (Davis *et al.*, 1988) was increased significantly after treatment with PMSG and that, in cycling rats, expression of both genes occurs primarily in the granulosa cells of healthy, maturing follicles (Woodruff *et al.*, 1988).

Several factors for which there is evidence of local ovarian production have been shown to influence the secretion of inhibin by granulosa cells *in vitro*. We and others have shown that somatomedin-C (IGF-1) is capable of stimulating production of inhibin *in vitro* (Bicsak *et al.*, 1986; Zhiwen *et al.*, 1987a) and that IGF-1 alone was effective over the physiological dose range of 3–100 ng/ml. Concomitant addition of FSH (100 ng/ml) and IGF-1 resulted in a significant increase in production of inhibin at all doses of IGF-1 (3–100 ng/ml). The dose-dependent effects of FSH and IGF-1 were time dependent, with a synergistic effect apparent after 48 hours of culture. There is now strong evidence for hormonally regulated production of IGF-1 by granulosa cells. Hammond *et al.* (1985) reported synthesis of immunoreactive IGF-1 by porcine granulosa cells and also reported that synthesis of immunoreactive IGF-1 was increased by gonadotropins, estradiol and growth hormone (Hsu

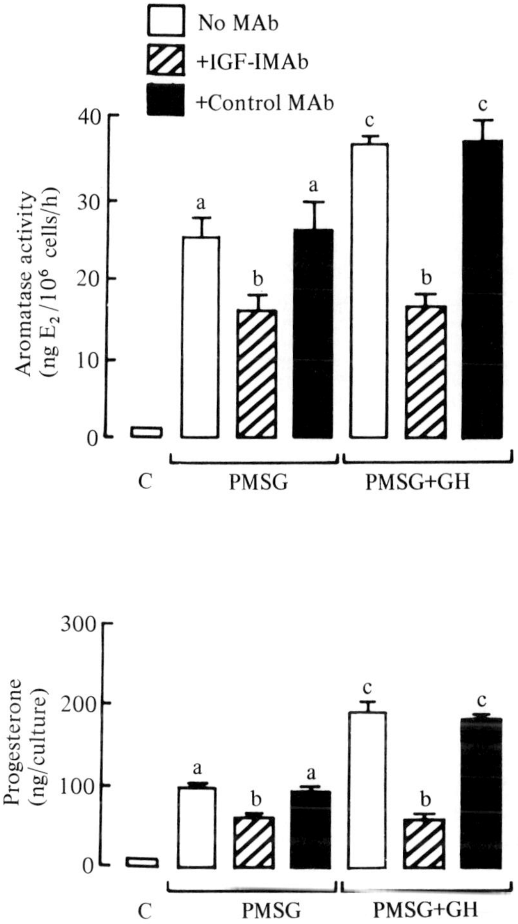

Fig. 1 Aromatase activity and production of progesterone by rat granulosa cells during a 3-day culture in the presence of both PMSG (100 mU/ml) and growth hormone (200 ng/ml), in the presence or absence of monoclonal antibody specific for IGF-1 or control monoclonal antibody (1:1000 dilution). a,b,c denote significant differences, *$p<0.01$ (Hutchinson *et al.*, 1987b).

and Hammond, 1987a, 1987b). Growth hormone (GH) *in vivo* increased levels of IGF-1 in rat ovaries (Davoren and Hsueh, 1986). We have shown (Fig. 1) that the stimulatory effects of FSH and of FSH plus GH on aromatase activity and the synthesis of progesterone by rat granulosa cells *in vitro* can be reduced by 40–60% by co-incubation with a monoclonal antibody against IGF-1 (Hutchinson *et al.*, 1987b). More recently, we have found evidence for expression of mRNA for IGF-1 in rat granulosa cells (Freed *et al.*, unpublished observations). In addition, FSH is known to increase type-1 IGF receptors on cultured rat granulosa cells (Adashi *et al.*, 1986). It would appear, then, that both production and action of IGF-1 are themselves under the control of FSH and GH. The time during normal recruitment and selection of the dominant follicle when IGF-1 may influence production of inhibin remains to be determined.

Epidermal growth factor (EGF) inhibits FSH-stimulated production of inhibin by rat granulosa cells *in vitro* (Franchimont *et al.*, 1986; Bicsak *et al.*, 1986; Zhiwen *et al.*, 1987a). In our study (Zhiwen *et al.*, 1987a) the inhibitory effect of EGF on basal secretion of inhibin was apparent after 2 days and was sustained over the subsequent 2 days. Maximal inhibition to 50% of control levels was observed at a dose of 100 ng EGF/ml on day 4. EGF also inhibited basal secretion of progesterone in a similar manner. There was a dose-dependent inhibition of FSH-stimulated secretion of inhibin with an IC50 of 0.5 ng/ml (0.08 nmol/l), about one-eighth of that in the absence of FSH. In addition, EGF inhibited the stimulation of production of inhibin by 8-bromo-cyclic AMP and prostaglandin E_2. The possibility that EGF might be toxic to granulosa cells was eliminated by an examination of several biochemical parameters related to cell growth. There is, therefore, a direct inhibitory effect of EGF both on basal and FSH-stimulated production of inhibin by granulosa cells, which suggests an important regulatory role for this growth factor in ovarian folliculogenesis. There is evidence that EGF or EGF-like material may be produced locally within the follicle. EGF-like activity in porcine follicular fluid has been demonstrated by radioreceptor assay (Hsu *et al.*, 1987) and mRNA for pre-proEGF has been detected in mouse ovaries (Rall *et al.*, 1985). The origin of the EGF-like activity in rats appears to be the ovarian theca/interstitial cells (Skinner *et al.*, 1987b). Medium conditioned by interstitial cells but not by granulosa cells was active in a radioreceptor assay for EGF and maintained the growth of an EGF-dependent line of cells. Fractionation of the activity revealed it to be different from authentic mouse EGF. In addition, EGF receptors have been found on membranes of bovine granulosa cells (Vlodavsky *et al.*, 1978), and granulosa cells of a number of species (but not of rats) proliferate in response to EGF *in vitro* (Gospodarowicz and Bialecki, 1979). In general, EGF has the ability to regulate the functions of granulosa cells by inhibiting differentiated functions (production of inhibin and steroid) and promoting proliferation. On a population basis, the major proliferative activity of granulosa cells occurs in the early antral phase (Hirschfield and Midgley, 1978). This observation does not preclude a role for EGF in proliferation and differentiation of individual granulosa cells at all stages of folliculogenesis.

There is now evidence that production of inhibin by granulosa cells can be regulated at a local level by activin and TGF-β, themselves members of the inhibin family of genes. Activin derived from a human leukemia cell line was shown to stimulate, in a dose-dependent manner (1–100 ng/ml), the basal production of inhibin by rat granulosa cells *in vitro* (Sugino *et al.*, 1988). There was an additive and not a synergistic effect of activin and FSH on the secretion of inhibin. TGF-β, which is structurally homologous to activin, caused a dose-dependent increase in both basal and FSH-stimulated production of inhibin by rat granulosa cells *in vitro* (Zhiwen *et al.*, 1988b). The effects of TGF-β and FSH appeared to be additive, and there was a suggestion of increased sensitivity of the production of inhibin by granulosa cells to FSH when cells were co-incubated with TGF-β. The stimulatory effect of TGF-β on basal and FSH-stimulated production of inhibin was evident on day 1 and maximal by day 4. In addition, TGF-β (1 ng/ml) significantly enhanced the inhibitory action of EGF on FSH-induced production of inhibin (IC50: EGF alone, 1.3 ng/ml; EGF plus TGF-β, ⟨0.1 ng/ml) (Zhiwen *et al.*, 1988b), an action probably involving enhancement of EGF receptors (Feng *et al.*, 1986). There is evidence for local production of both activin and TGF-β within the ovarian follicle (see below) underlining the interaction that occurs between members of the same family of genes to regulate the biosynthesis and action of their products.

Activin

Apart from the demonstration of the expression of the β inhibin genes in granulosa cells (Mason *et al.*, 1985; Woodruff *et al.*, 1988), and the isolation of activin from follicular fluid of the pig (Vale *et al.*, 1986; Ling *et al.*, 1986) and cow (McLachlan *et al.*, 1987), little is known about the production of activin and its regulation. The processes within the granulosa cell that control the association of a β-subunit with either an α-subunit to form inhibin, or with another β-subunit to form activin, remain to be elucidated. The lack of a specific assay for activin has also hampered progress in the study of its production. Inhibin and activin have functionally opposing effects in the pituitary cell (Vale *et al.*, 1986) and in erythroid differentiation assays (Yu *et al.*, 1987). Although radioimmunoassays (RIA) for inhibin show insignificant cross-reaction with activin (McLachlan *et al.*, 1987; Robertson *et al.*, 1988), a specific RIA for activin has not been reported. The major biological activity detected in follicular fluid directly in assays with cultures of pituitary cells and, indirectly, by the effect of ovariectomy on the secretion of gonadotropin *in vivo*, is inhibitory, suggesting a dominance of the production of inhibin over that of activin by the ovary. This suggestion is not inconsistent with the hypothesis that activin produced within the follicle acts locally in a paracrine/autocrine fashion to regulate folliculogenesis and not as a peripheral endocrine hormone that regulates pituitary secretion of gonadotropins.

Transforming growth factor-β

Stimulation by FSH of expression of the TGF-β gene(s) in the ovary was recently reported, but the cellular site of expression was not specified (Hernandez *et al.*, 1987). A study employing immunological and biological assays provided evidence that TGF-β activity was produced by cells derived from rat and bovine thecal tissue (Skinner *et al.*, 1987a). There was no evidence for production of TGF-β activity by granulosa cells. These results imply that FSH induction of the expression of TGF-β gene(s) involves a paracrine regulator of granulosa cell origin that acts on theca cells, because granulosa and not theca cells have receptors for FSH. It will be important to verify the cellular origin and timing of expression of TGF-β gene(s) in the follicle and the factors that control and modulate this expression.

Intraovarian actions of inhibin-related peptides

Differentiation and function of theca cells

Recent studies have shown opposing paracrine actions of inhibin and activin on the LH-induced secretion of androgen by theca cells (Hsueh *et al.*, 1987). While inhibin augmented the LH-stimulated production of androstenedione, activin suppressed the response to LH. Together, activin and inhibin antagonized each other's actions in the presence of LH. Neither substance affected the production of androstenedione in the absence of LH. Since the theca has not been demonstrated as a site of production of either inhibin or activin, this effect would represent a paracrine influence of granulosa cells on theca cells to regulate the supply of androgen substrate required by the granulosa cells to produce estrogen.

An autocrine action of TGF-β on the functions of theca cells has not been reported, although it is likely that TGF-β could have paracrine actions on granulosa cells (see below) and the oocyte (Feng *et al.*, 1988) to influence the growth and differentiation of the follicle and oocyte meiosis, respectively.

Differentiation and function of granulosa cells

Ying *et al.* (1986, 1987) reported an inhibitory effect of porcine inhibin ($\alpha\beta_A$ and $\alpha\beta_B$) on FSH-induced production of estrogen by cultured rat granulosa cells from diethyl stilbestrol (DES)-treated, immature, hypophysectomized rats. The extent of the inhibition was around 40% at doses of 10 ng/ml. This effect of inhibin could be reversed by co-culture with TGF-β or activin and there were no effects of inhibin on the basal secretion of estrogen.

In contrast, Hutchinson *et al.* (1987a) found no inhibitory effect of a pure, 31-kDa bovine inhibin ($\alpha\beta_A$) on FSH-induced aromatase activity or production of progesterone by granulosa cells from DES-treated, immature, intact rats. Sugino *et al.* (1988), using higher doses (>200 ng/ml) of a different preparation of pure bovine 32-kDa inhibin ($\alpha\beta_A$), showed only a slight suppressive effect on production of progesterone by rat granulosa cells *in vitro*. Such experiments are complicated by the endogenous production of inhibin (and probably activin) by the granulosa cells under these conditions (Zhiwen *et al.*, 1987a, 1987b, 1988a, 1988b), so the true effective dose of inhibin is difficult to determine. There were also methodological differences between the studies, e.g. hypophysectomized versus intact rats and different culture conditions. Resolution of this putative action of inhibin requires a demonstration of inhibin receptors on granulosa cells.

Activin has a stimulatory action on the FSH-induced production of estrogen by rat granulosa cells *in vitro* (Hutchinson *et al.*, 1987a; Ying *et al.*, 1987), an effect which is dose and time dependent. In contrast to its action on aromatase activity, we found that bovine activin caused a dose- and time-dependent decrease in FSH-induced production of progesterone by rat granulosa cells (Hutchinson *et al.*, 1987a). In contrast, Sugino *et al.* (1988), using human erythroid differentiating factor (EDF) as a source of activin, reported that it enhanced FSH-induced production of progesterone as well as binding sites for hCG in a time- and dose-dependent manner. EDF alone had no effects, similar to bovine activin (Hutchinson *et al.*, 1987a). Reasons for the different actions of EDF and bovine activin on FSH-induced production of progesterone are not known. The major differences under investigation are the source of activin and the serum-free culture conditions – Ham's F12/DMEM (Sugino *et al.*, 1988) versus McCoy's 5A with added insulin (Hutchinson *et al.*, 1987a).

TGF-β has an overall stimulatory action on the functions of granulosa cells. In addition to its effects on the production of inhibin (Zhiwen *et al.*, 1988b), summarized above, TGF-β enhances gonadotropin-induced production of estrogen (Ying *et al.*, 1986; Adashi *et al.*, 1986; Hutchinson *et al.*, 1987) and progesterone (Hutchinson *et al.*, 1987a; Knecht *et al.*, 1987; Dodson and Schomberg, 1987), and levels of hCG receptors (Knecht *et al.*, 1986; Dodson and Schomberg, 1987) and EGF receptors (Feng *et al.*, 1986). Knecht *et al.* (1987) reported that TGF-β enhanced the stimulatory and inhibitory effects of FSH on the accumulation of cAMP, whereas Dodson and Schomberg (1987) did not observe any significant action of TGF-β on FSH-stimulated production of cAMP by granulosa cells. It was thought that TGF-β does not exert a proliferative effect on rat granulosa cells. However, Dorrington *et al.* (1988) recently reported that, in the presence of FSH (10 ng/ml), TGF-β caused a dose- and time-dependent increase in incorporation of thymidine by granulosa cells of immature rats, irrespective of previous treatment with DES. The increase in incorporation of thymidine was paralleled by an increase in cell number. Of particular interest is the observation that the increase in incorporation of thymidine was an early, FSH-dependent event, with a maximum at 20–24 hours and lower values at 44–48 hours. Differentiation induced by FSH, as assessed by steroidogenesis, is low at 24 hours, with the major increase occurring between 24 and 48 hours. Dorrington *et al.* (1988) claim that the early stimulation of growth followed by differentiation *in vitro* is consistent with the sequence of events that occur *in vivo* and with the concept that there is an inverse relationship between growth and differentiation of rat granulosa cells (Epstein-Almog and Orly, 1985). The finding is also novel because TGF-β was thought to inhibit rather than stimulate epithelioid cells, such as granulosa cells (Sporn *et al.*, 1987).

TGF-β presumably acts via its own receptors (Massague, 1987), there being no apparent affinity of activin or inhibin for TGF-β receptors (Massague, 1987). If the actions of activin on FSH-induced production of progesterone are confirmed, they suggest a unique role for activin in the differentiation of granulosa cells. Activin could delay the onset of luteinization, while at the same time maintaining the estrogenic capacity of the follicle. These speculations also underline the importance of what determines the ratio of production of inhibin to that of activin by granulosa cells during differentiation.

Interferon-α peptides

Although the IFN-α peptides are known as antiviral and antiproliferative agents (Pestka *et al.*, 1987), there is evidence that IFN-α can modulate the responses of cells to other regulators and tropic hormones. Normal women treated with IFN-α had decreased circulating concentrations of estradiol and progesterone without significant alterations in plasma concentrations of FSH, LH, prolactin or thyroid-stimulating hormone (TSH) (Kauppila *et al.*, 1982), data which suggest a direct action of IFN-α on the ovary. Similarly, men treated with IFN-α had reduced levels of testosterone and normal levels of gonadotropins (Orava *et al.*, 1986). IFN-α inhibited, in a dose- and time-dependent manner, the LH-induced production of testosterone *in vitro* by immature porcine Leydig cells (Orava *et al.*, 1985) and the FSH-induced production of estrogen by rat Sertoli cells (Branca *et al.*, 1987). We have recently demonstrated a time- and dose-dependent inhibition by rat IFN-α of production of inhibin by rat granulosa cells (Fig. 2). The maximum inhibition was about 50% of control values at doses between 300 U/ml and 1000 U/ml, and the minimum effective dose was around 10–30 U/ml. IFN-α had a similar inhibitory effect on the production of progesterone in the same experiment (data not shown).

This evidence for a local action of IFN-α in the ovary supports the need for a thorough investigation of the production of IFN-α and its action on the production of peptides and steroids by follicular cells. In view of its inhibitory action on the eicosanoid pathways in monocytes and macrophages (Browning, 1987) and endometrial cells (Salamonsen *et al.*, 1988), IFN-α may influence fundamental aspects of regulation in follicular cells through control of eicosanoid metabolism. Granulosa cells produce a range of eicosanoid metabolites (Carson *et al.*, 1986), some of which are known to be important for the process of ovulation (Espey, 1974).

Future directions

The evidence for inhibin- and IFN-α-related peptides acting as local regulators within the ovary has depended largely on demonstrations *in vitro* of their actions on ovarian cells, coupled with, in the case of the inhibins, demonstrations of the cellular origins of the peptides by immunological and

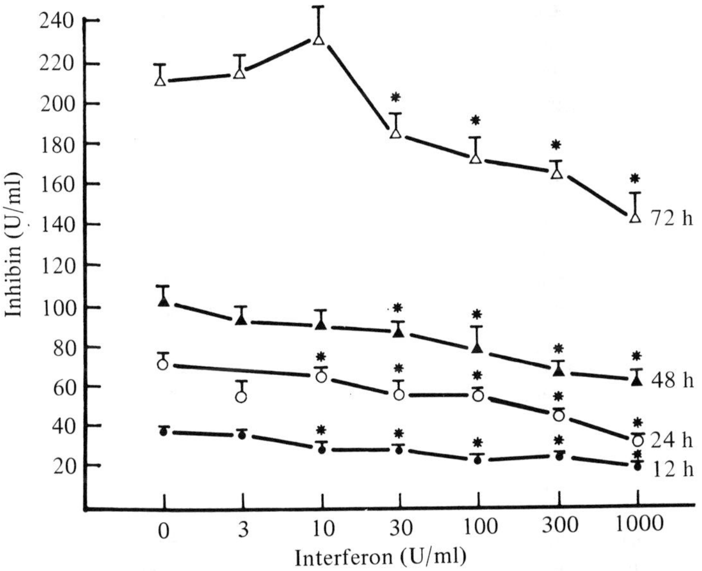

Fig. 2 The time- and dose-dependent inhibitory effects of rat interferon-α on FSH-induced production of inhibin *in vitro* by granulosa cells from DES-treated, immature rats. Rat-FSH-I6 was used at 1.0 ng/ml and inhibin was measured by specific RIA. Each point represents a mean ± S.E.M. of triplicate determinations. *p<0.05 vs. control within each time course.

biological methods, and more recently by analysis of mRNA transcribed from the inhibin genes. The task, now, is to apply these observations to a physiological setting to explain the recruitment, selection and dominance of ovarian follicles. We need to determine when, during the course of cellular growth and differentiation, these factors are produced, and when they are able to act on ovarian cells.

Work to date has concentrated on the 31-kDa inhibins, activins and TGF-β. However, it is known that both inhibin (Robertson *et al.*, 1986) and TGF-β (Sporn *et al.*, 1987) are processed from larger forms at the time of or after release by the cell. In the case of TGF-β, the hormone appears to be secreted in a latent form which can subsequently be activated in an acidic environment. This observation suggests that regulation of the local action of the inhibin-related peptides may involve not only secretion of the peptide and the responsiveness of its target-cell receptors, but also post-translational, post-secretory modifications of the molecule. For inhibin, such modifications involve cleavage of large N-terminal fragments of the α- and β-chains for which there are no known functions.

Studies *in vivo* to verify the physiological roles of putative intraovarian regulators present a particular challenge. Measurement of circulating concentrations of a particular peptide, if it can be detected, may not reflect intraovarian concentrations, so greater reliance will have to be placed on immunoneutralization models and demonstrations of expression of the genes in different physiological situations. Other experimental models could include genetic deletions of specific factors and transfection with antisense RNA. It may be that further clues about the importance of these peptides at the local level can be obtained from clinical syndromes, such as resistant ovary syndrome, polycystic ovarian disease, luteinized unruptured follicle, and unexplained infertility.

Acknowledgements

This work was supported financially by the National Health and Medical Research Council of Australia, Biotechnology Australia Pty. Ltd (Z.Z.), and the Australian Meat and Livestock Research and Development Corporation (L.A.H.). The authors are grateful to Faye Coates for editorial assistance and Michael Whitehead for artwork.

References

Adashi, E.Y. & Resnick, C.E. (1986). Antagonistic interactions of transforming growth factors in the regulation of granulosa cell differentiation. **Endocrinology** 119:1879–1881.

Adashi, E.Y., Resnick, C.E., Svoboda, M.E. & Van Vyk, J.J. (1986). Follicle-stimulating hormone enhances somatomedin-C binding to cultured rat granulosa cells. **Journal of Biological Chemistry** 261:3923–3926.

Bicsak, T.A., Tucker, E.N., Cappel, S., Vaughan, J., Rivier, J., Vale, W. & Hseuh, A.W. (1986). Hormonal regulation of granulosa cell inhibin biosynthesis. **Endocrinology** 119:2711–2719.

Branca, A.A., Franke, M.A., Sluss, P.M. & Reichert, L.E. Jr (1987). Interferon inhibits FSH-stimulated oestradiol production in rat Sertoli cell cultures. **Medical Science Research** 15:739.

Browning, J. (1987). Interferons and rheumatoid arthritis: insight into interferon biology? **Immunology Today** 8:372–374.

Burger, H.G., de Kretser, D.M., Findlay, J.K. & Igarashi, M., eds. (1987). Inhibin non-steroidal regulation of follicle-stimulating hormone secretion. **Serono Symposia**, Vol. 42, New York, Raven Press.

Burger, H.G., Zhiwen, Z., Davis, S., Lee, V., Carson, R.S., Herington, A., Findlay, J.K., Farnworth, P., Wang, Q.-F., Au, S., de Kretser, D.M. & Robertson, D.M. (1988). Inhibin-regulation and mechanism of action. In: Hodgen, G.D. & Rosenwacks, Z., eds. **First Conrad International Workshop on Non-Steroidal Gonadal Factors: Physiological Roles and Possibilities in Contraceptive Development**, Virginia, Jones Institute Press, pp.137–148.

Carson, R.S., Mitchell, M.D. & Trounson, A.O. (1986). Regulation of prostaglandin biosynthesis by human ovarian follicular fluid: a mechanism for ovulation? **Prostaglandins** 32:49–56.

Cate, R.L., Mattaliano, R.J., Hession, C., Tizard, R., Farber, N.N., Cheung, A., Ninfa, E.G., Fery, A.Z., Gash, D.J., Chow, E.P., Fisher, R.A., Bertonis, J.N., Torres, G., Wallner, G.P., Ramachandran, K.L., Ragin, R.C., Manganaro, T.F., MacLaughlin, D.T. & Donohoe, P.K. (1986). Isolation of bovine and human genes for Mullerian Inhibiting Substance and expression of the human gene in animal cells. **Cell** 45:685–698.

Davis, S.R., Burger, H.G., Robertson, D.M., Farnworth, P.G., Carson, R.S. & Krozowski, Z. (1988). PMSG stimulates inhibin gene expression in the immature rat ovary: dose–response characteristics and relationship to serum gonadotropins, inhibin and ovarian steroid content. **Endocrinology** 123:2399–2407.

Davis, S.R., Dench, R., Nikolaidis, I., Clements, J.A., Forage, R.G. & Burger, H.G. (1986). Inhibin A-subunit gene expression in the ovaries of immature female rats is stimulated by pregnant mare serum gonadotrophin. **Biochemical and Biophysical Research Communications** 138:1196–1202.

Davoren, J.B. & Hsueh, A.J.W. (1986). Growth hormone increases ovarian levels of immunoreactive somatomedin C/insulin-like growth factor-1 *in vivo*. **Endocrinology** 118:888–890.

Dodson, W.C. & Schomberg, D.W. (1987). The effect of transforming growth factor-β on follicle-stimulating hormone-induced differentiation of cultured rat granulosa cells. **Endocrinology** 120:512–516.

Dorrington, J., Chuma, A.V. & Bendell, J.J. (1988). Transforming growth factor-β and follicle-stimulating hormone promote rat granulosa cell proliferation. **Endocrinology** 123:353–359.

Epstein-Almog, R. & Orly, J. (1985). Inhibition of hormone-induced steroidogenesis during cell proliferation in serum-free cultures of rat granulosa cells. **Endocrinology** 116:2103–2112

Espey, L.L. (1974). Ovarian proteolytic enzymes and ovulation. **Biology of Reproduction** 10:216–235.

Eto, Y., Tsuji, T., Takezava, M., Takano, S., Yokogava, Y. & Shibai, H. (1987). Purification and characterization of erythroid differentiation factor (EDF) isolated from human leukemia cell line THP-1. **Biochemical and Biophysical Research Communications** 142:1095–1103.

Feng, P., Catt, K.J. & Knecht, M. (1986). Transforming growth factor-β regulates the inhibitory actions of epidermal growth factor during granulosa cell differentiation. **Journal of Biological Chemistry** 261:14167–14170.

Feng, P., Catt, K.J. & Knecht, M. (1988) Transforming growth factor-β stimulates meiotic maturation of the rat oocyte. **Endocrinology** 122:181–186.

Findlay, J.K. & Risbridger, G.P. (1987). Intragonadal control mechanisms. In: Burger, H.G., ed. **Bailliere's Clinical Endocrinology and Metabolism**, London, Bailliere Tindall, pp.223–243.

Franchimont, P., ed. (1986). **Paracrine Control: Clinics in Endocrinology and Metabolism**, London, W.B. Saunders, pp.IX–Xlll.

Franchimont, P., Hazee-Hagelstein, M.T., Charlet-Renard, Ch. & Jaspar, J.N. (1986). The effect of mouse epidermal growth factor on DNA and protein synthesis, progesterone and inhibin production by bovine granulosa cells in culture. **Acta Endocrinologica** lll:122–127.

Franchimont, P., Verstraelen-Proyard, J., Hazee-Hagelstein, M.T., Renard, Ch., Demoulin, A., Bourguignon, J.P. & Hutsin, J. (1979). Inhibin from concept to reality. **Vitamins and Hormones** 37:243–302.

Gospodarowicz, D. & Bialecki, H. (1979). Fibroblast and epidermal growth factors are mitogenic agents for cultured granulosa cells of rodent, porcine and human origin. **Endocrinology** 104:757–764.

Hammond, J.M., Lino, J., Barano, L.S., Skaleris, D., Knight, A.B., Romanus, J.A. & Rechler, M.M. (1985). Production of insulin-like growth factors by ovarian cells. **Endocrinology** 117.2553–2555.

Hernandez, E.R., Twardzik, D.R., Purchio, A. & Adashi, E.Y. (1987). Gonadotropin dependent ovarian transforming growth factor-β gene expression. **Proceedings of the Society for the Study of Reproduction** 20th Annual Meeting, Illinois, USA, Abstract 35.

Hirschfield, A.N. & Midgley, A.R. Jr (1978). Morphometric analysis of follicular development in the rat. **Biology of Reproduction** 19:597–605.

Hsu, C.-J. & Hammond, J.M. (1987a). Gonadotropins and estradiol stimulate the secretion of insulin-like growth factor-1 by porcine granulosa cells in culture. **Endocrinology** 120:198–207.

Hsu, C.-J. & Hammond, J.M. (1987b). Concomitant effect of growth hormone on secretion of insulin-like growth factor-1 and progesterone by cultured porcine granulosa cells. **Endocrinology** 121:1343–1348.

Hsu, C.-J., Holmes, S.D. & Hammond, J.M. (1987). Ovarian growth factor-like activity. Concentrations in porcine follicular fluid during follicular enlargement. **Biochemical and Biophysical Research Communications** 147:242.

Hsueh, A.W., Dahl, K.D., Vaughan, J., Tucker, E., Rivier, J., Bardin, C.W. & Vale, W. (1987). Heterodimers and homodimers of inhibin subunits have different paracrine action in the modulation of luteinizing hormone-stimulated androgen biosynthesis. **Proceedings of the National Academy of Sciences, USA** 84:5082–5086.

Hutchinson, L.A., Findlay, J.K., de Vos, F.L. & Robertson, D.M. (1987a). Effects of bovine inhibin, transforming growth factor-β and bovine activin-α on granulosa cell differentiation. **Biochemical and Biophysical Research Communications** 146:1405–1412.

Hutchinson, L.A., Herington, A.C. & Findlay, J.K. (1987b). IGF-1 mediates growth hormone- and FSH-stimulated steroidogenesis in cultured rat granulosa cells. **Proceedings of the Sixty-Ninth Annual Meeting of the Endocrine Society, USA** Abstract No.833.

Kauppila, A., Cantell, K., Janne, O., Kokko, E. & Vihko, R. (1982). Serum sex steroid and peptide hormone concentrations, and endometrial estrogen and progestin receptor levels during administration of human leukocyte interferon. **International Journal of Cancer** 29:291–294.

Knecht, M., Feng, P. & Catt, K.J. (1986). Transforming growth factor-β regulates the expression of luteinizing hormone receptors in ovarian granulosa cells. **Biochemical and Biophysical Research Communications** 139:800–807.

Knecht, M., Feng, P. & Catt, K.J. (1987). Bifunctional role of transforming growth factor-β during granulosa cell development. **Endocrinology** 120:1243–1249.

Lee, V.K. (1983). PMSG-treated immature female rat – a model system for studying control of inhibin secretion. In: Greewald, G.S. & Terranova, P.F., eds. **Factors Regulating Ovarian Function**, Raven Press, New York, pp.157–161.

Ling, N., Ying, S.-Y., Ueno, N., Shimasaki, S., Esch, F., Hotta, N. & Guillemin, R. (1986). Pituitary FSH is released by a heterodimer of the β-subunits from the two forms of inhibin. **Nature** 321:779–782.

Mason, A.J., Hayflick, J.S., Ling, N., Esch, F., Ueno, N., Ying, S.-Y., Guillemin, R., Niall, H. & Seeburg, P.H. (1985). Complementary DNA sequences of ovarian follicular fluid inhibin show precursor structure and homology with transforming growth factor-β. **Nature** 318:659–663.

Massague, J. (1987). The TGF-β family of growth and differentiation factors. **Cell** 49:437–438.

McLachlan, R.I., Robertson, D.M., Healy, D.L., Burger, H.G. & de Kretser, D.M. (1987). Circulating immunoreactive inhibin levels during the normal human menstrual cycle. **Journal of Clinical Endocrinology and Metabolism** 65:954–961.

Orava, M., Cantell, K. & Vihko, R. (1985). Human leukocyte interferon inhibits human chorionic gonadotropin-stimulated testosterone production by porcine Leydig cells in culture. **Biochemical and Biophysical Research Commmunications** 127:809–815.

Orava, M., Cantell, K. & Vihko, R. (1986). Treatment with preparations of human leukocyte interferon decreases serum testosterone concentrations in men. **International Journal of Cancer** 38:295–296.

Padgett, R.W., St Johnston, R.D. & Gelbart, W.M. (1987). A transcript from a *Drosophila* pattern gene predicts a protein homologous to the transforming growth factor-β family. **Nature** 325:81–84.

Pestka, S., Langr, R.J., Zoon, K.C. & Samuel, C.E. (1987). Interferons and their actions. **Annual Review of Biochemistry** 56:727–777.

Rall, L.B., Scott, J., Bell, G.I., Crawford, R.J., Penschow, J.D., Niall, H.D. & Coghlan, J.P. (1985). Mouse prepro-epidermal growth factor synthesis by the kidney and other tissues. **Nature** 313:228–231.

Robertson, D.M., de Vos, F.L., Foulds, L.M., McLachlan, R.I., Burger, H.G., Morgan, F.J., Hearn, M.T.W. & de Kretser, D.M. (1986). Isolation of 31-kd form of inhibin from bovine follicular fluid. **Molecular and Cellular Endocrinology** 44:271–277.

Robertson, D.M., Tsonis, C.G., McLachlan, R.I., Handelsman, D.J., Leask, R., Baird, D.T., McNeilly, A.S., Hayward, S., Healy, D.L., Findlay, J.K., Burger, H.G. & de Kretser, D.M. (1988). Comparison of inhibin immunological and *in vitro* biological activities in human serum. **Journal of Clinical Endocrinology and Metabolism** 67:438–443.

Salamonsen, L.A., Stuchbery, S.J., Godkin, J.D. & Findlay, J.K. (1988). Interferon-α mimics effects of ovine trophoblast protein 1 on prostaglandin and protein secretion by ovine endometrial cells *in vitro*. **Journal of Endocrinology** 117:Rl–R4.

Skinner, M.K., Keski-Oja, J., Osteen, K.G. & Moses, H.L. (1987a). Ovarian thecal cells produce transforming growth factor-β which can regulate granulosa cell growth. **Endocrinology** 121:786–792.

Skinner, M.K., Lobb, D. & Dorrington, J.H. (1987b). Ovarian thecal/interstitial cells produce an epidermal growth factor-like substance. **Endocrinology** 121:1892–1899.

Sporn, M.B., Roberts, A.B., Wakefield, L.M. & de Crombrugghe, B. (1987). Some recent advances in the chemistry and biology of transforming growth factor-β. **Journal of Cell Biology** 105:1039–1045.

Sporn, M.B. & Todaro, G.J. (1980). Autocrine secretion and malignant transformation of cells. **New England Journal of Medicine** 303:878–880.

Sugino, H., Nakamura, T., Hasegawa, Y., Miyamoto, K., Abe, Y., Igarashi, M., Eto, Y., Shiba, H. & Titani, K. (1988). Erythroid differentiation factor can modulate follicular granulosa cell functions. **Biochemical and Biophysical Research Communications** 153:281–288.

Vale, W., Rivier, J., Vaughan, J., McClintock, R., Corrigan, A., Woo, W., Karr, D. & Spiess, J. (1986). Purification and characterization of an FSH-releasing protein from porcine ovarian follicular fluid. **Nature** 321:776–779.

Vlodavsky, I., Brown, K.D. & Gospodarowicz, D. (1978). Comparison of the binding of epidermal growth factor to cultured granulosa and luteal cells. **Journal of Biological Chemistry** 253:3744–3755.

Weeks, D.L. & Melton, D.A. (1987). A maternal mRNA localized to the vegetal hemisphere of *Xenopus* eggs codes for a growth factor related to TGF-β. **Cell** 51:861–867.

Woodruff, T.K., d'Agostino, J.B., Schartz, N.B. & Mayo, K.E. (1988). Dynamic changes in inhibin messenger RNAs in rat ovarian follicles during the reproductive cycle. **Science** 239:1296–1299.

Wrann, M., Bodmer, S., deMartin, R., Siepl, C., Hofer-Warbinek, R., Frei, K., Hofer, E. & Fontana, A. (1987). T Cell suppressor factor from human glioblastoma cells is a 12.5-kDa protein closely related to transforming growth factor-β. **EMBO Journal** 6:1633–1636.

Ying, S.-Y., Becker, A., Ling, N., Ueno, N. & Guillemin, R. (1986). Inhibin and β-type transforming growth factor (TGF-β) have opposite modulating effects on follicle stimulating hormone (FSH)-induced aromatase activity of cultured rat granulosa cells. **Biochemical and Biophysical Research Communications** 136:969–975.

Ying, S.-Y., Becker, A., Svanson, G.. Tan, P., Vadleigh, D., Czvik, J., Ling, N., Ueno, N., Esch, F., Chiang, T.-C., Hu, R., Dong, M.-H., Sato, K., Munegumi, T. & Guillemin, R. (1987). Reciprocal relationship between the secretion of follicle stimulating hormones (FSH) and production of inhibin in the rat. In: Burger, H.G., de Kretser, D.M., Findlay, J.K. & Igarashi, M., eds. **Inhibin-Non-Steroidal Regulation of Follicle Stimulating Hormone Secretion**, Vol. 42, New York, Raven Press, pp.135–148.

Yu, J., Shao, L., Lemas, V., Yu, A.L., Vaughan, J., Rivier, J. & Vale, W. (1987). Importance of FSH-releasing protein and inhibin in erythrodifferentiation. **Nature** 330:765–767.

Zhiwen, Z., Carson, R.S. & Burger, H.G. (1988a). Selective control of rat granulosa cell inhibin production by FSH and LH *in vitro*. **Molecular and Cellular Endocrinology** 56:35–40.

Zhiwen, Z., Carson, R.S., Herington, A.C., Lee, V.W.K. & Burger, H.G. (1987a). Follicle-stimulating hormone and somatomedin C stimulate inhibin production by rat granulosa cells *in vitro*. **Endocrinology** 120:1633–1638.

Zhiwen, Z.W., Findlay, J.K., Carson, R.S., Herington, A.C. & Burger, H.G. (1988b). Transforming growth factor-β enhances basal and FSH-stimulated inhibin production by rat granulosa cells *in vitro*. **Molecular and Cellular Endocrinology** 58:161–166.

Zhiwen, Z., Herington, A.C., Carson, R.S., Findlay, J.K. & Burger, H.G. (1987b). Direct inhibition of rat granulosa cell inhibin production by epidermal growth factor *in vitro*. **Molecular and Cellular Endocrinology** 54:213–220.

The inhibin/activin family and pro-opiomelanocortin-derived peptides as intratesticular regulators of cellular function

P.L. MORRIS, C.-L.C. CHEN, Z.M. FENG, J. VAUGHAN, W.W. VALE AND C.W. BARDIN

The Population Council and The Clayton Foundation Laboratories for Peptide Biology, The Salk Institute for Biological Studies, La Jolla, CA 92037, USA.

Keywords

Inhibin, activin, pro-opiomelanocortin, α-MSH, β-endorphin, ACTH, Leydig cells, Sertoli cells, short-loop feedback.

Introduction

In-vitro studies indicate that the Sertoli and Leydig cell peptides, inhibin and activin, respectively, exert negative and positive feedback control of pituitary secretion of follicle-stimulating hormone (FSH) (Ying, 1988; Vale *et al.*, 1988). FSH, in turn, can potentially close this long-loop feedback system through its stimulation of inhibin secretion (Bicsak *et al.*, 1987; Ying *et al.*, 1987; Morris *et al.*, 1988). Recent studies indicate that inhibin and activin also regulate the production of testosterone by Leydig cells (Hsueh *et al.*, 1987). These actions of inhibin and activin are believed to represent part of a regulatory system that operates between cellular compartments within the testis.

The peptides derived from pro-opiomelanocortin (POMC), including α-melanocyte-stimulating hormone (MSH), adrenocorticotropic hormone (ACTH), and β-endorphin, form another group of intratesticular messengers. These latter hormones are synthesized in Leydig cells and are secreted into the testicular interstitial fluid (TIF) of rats at concentrations several-fold higher than in the peripheral blood. These observations are strengthened by the demonstration of immunostainable POMC and POMC mRNA in Leydig cells (Chen *et al.*, 1984; Bardin *et al.*, 1987a). Both the synthesis and secretion of the POMC-derived peptides by Leydig cells appear to be regulated by gonadotropins rather than glucocorticosteroids, which are potent modulators of these gonadotropins in the anterior pituitary (Valenca and Negro-Vilar, 1986; Chen and Madigan, 1987). Studies on the function of POMC-derived peptides in the testis suggest that β-endorphin inhibits Sertoli cell division (Orth, 1986) and protein secretion (Morris and Bardin, 1987), while ACTH and α-MSH stimulate production of Sertoli cell proteins (Bardin *et al.*, 1984; Boitani *et al.*, 1985, 1986; Bardin *et al.*, 1987a). Although the testis is known to synthesize other opiate precursors, their role as intratesticular regulators is not established (Bardin *et al.*, 1987a).

In the present chapter, we review the evidence for inhibin and POMC gene expression and peptide secretion by testicular cells. We will also outline the evidence in support of the postulate that these hormones exert autocrine and/or paracrine effects on Sertoli and Leydig cells.

Evidence that inhibin and activin are produced by the testis

Isolation of inhibin from rete testis fluid

Inhibin and activin were first isolated from ovarian follicular fluid (Robertson *et al.*, 1985; Miyamoto *et al.*, 1985; Ling *et al.*, 1985; Rivier *et al.*, 1985). The first purification and partial characterization of male inhibin was from ovine rete testis fluid. Using an in-vitro bioassay, two preparations of inhibin were purified approximately 500-fold, with an overall recovery of approximately 8% (Bardin *et al.*, 1987b). Both inhibin forms are heterodimers consisting of one 18.0-kDa and one 16.5-kDa subunit. These subunits were sequenced separately using automated Edman degradation with a gas-phase sequencer. The α-subunit of one inhibin preparation was truncated at the N-terminus, which corresponded to residues 16–30 of the α-subunit of the larger inhibin. The N-terminal 26 residues of ovine inhibin α differ from porcine inhibin only at residues 3 and 26, where we observed Pro rather than Ala and Ala rather than Val, respectively. The N-terminal sequence of the β-chain of the hydrophobic peak of purified material was identical to that of the β-chain of the hydrophilic inhibin. The N-terminus of the 16.5-kDa ovine subunit deviates from the porcine inhibin βA-subunit by a single change at position 17 (Tyr for Phe). It is notable that porcine and human βA-chains are identical to one another. No inhibin containing the βB-subunit or activin was isolated from rete testis fluid.

Cloning inhibin cDNA from testicular libraries

Inhibin α-subunit cDNAs that contain the complete coding sequence for the precursor protein, the entire 3'-untranslated region, and part of 5'-untranslated region were isolated using human testicular libraries. The predicted amino acid sequence for the human testicular inhibin α-subunit precursor protein is identical to that of the α-subunit from human placenta, rather than that from human ovary. Positions -13 and -15 of the signal peptide are Val and Ser in human ovarian α-inhibin (Mason *et al.*, 1986; Keinan *et al.*, 1989), and His and Cys in the human placental (Mayo *et al.*, 1986) and testicular (Keinan *et al.*, 1988) inhibins. It is of note that the predicted amino acid sequences of the mature inhibin α-subunit are the same as those in human testis, ovary, and placenta (Chen *et al.*, 1988; Keinan *et al.*, 1989).

Seven clones containing cDNA inserts of the inhibin βB-subunit were isolated and three were sequenced (Feng and Chen, unpublished). The results indicate that the predicted amino acid sequence is the same as for the mature human ovarian inhibin βB-subunit. No cDNAs corresponding to the βA-subunit were identified in the phage plaques from which the βB-subunit cDNAs were isolated. These observations suggest that the amount of βB-subunit mRNA is much larger than that of the βA-subunit mRNA in human testes. It follows that inhibin in the human male will differ from that in the ram by having predominantly βB- rather than βA-subunits.

Localization of inhibin and activin in testicular cells

Immunostainable inhibin α-subunit was demonstrated in the seminiferous tubular epithelium (Bardin *et al.*, 1987b). There was light staining at the basal portions of the epithelium in a pattern consistent with localization in Sertoli cells. The most intense staining, however, was localized in the portion of the epithelium adjacent to the lumen of the tubule. In addition, Sertoli cell-enriched cultures secrete immunoactive and bioactive inhibin in response to FSH. This gonadotropin also regulates inhibin α-subunit mRNA in these cultures. These observations are consistent with the production of inhibin by Sertoli cells. The absence of activin in rete testis fluid suggested that this hormone was either not produced by the testis or that it was produced in cells different from those that synthesize inhibin. Recent studies indicate that this activin is produced by Leydig cells (Lee *et al.*, 1988). In these experiments, immunoactive and bioactive activin were secreted by cultured Leydig cells and a Leydig cell line contained inhibin β-subunit but not α-subunit mRNA. These observations suggest that, in the testis, inhibin is synthesized predominantly in Sertoli cells while activin is predominantly synthesized in Leydig cells.

Regulation of inhibin gene expression and inhibin protein secretion

Regulation of inhibin mRNA

The existence of inhibin α-subunit mRNA in the testis was determined by Northern blot hybridization analysis (Keinan *et al.*, 1989). A single hybridizable mRNA was observed in samples of human testicular RNA. The α-subunit mRNA was also identified in the testis of various other species, including monkey, ram, rat, and mouse. All the inhibin α-subunit mRNA detected in the testes of primates and rodents showed a single band of about 1.5 kb by Northern blot analysis, as did mRNA from porcine ovary (Keinan *et al.*, 1989).

The expression of the inhibin α-subunit gene in rat testis was studied by Northern blot analysis using a human inhibin α-subunit cDNA as a hybridization probe. The results of this study suggested that the inhibin α-subunit gene is developmentally regulated. The concentration of rat testicular inhibin α-subunit mRNA peaked between 20 and 25 days of age and slowly declined with increasing age in a pattern similar to that of other Sertoli cell mRNAs (Keinan *et al.*, 1989; Meunier *et al.*, 1988). Inhibin βA- and βB-subunit mRNA concentrations also rose and declined in a similar pattern but the relative levels were 10% or less of α-subunit mRNA (Meunier *et al.*, 1988; Feng and Chen, unpublished).

Hypophysectomy decreased testicular inhibin α-subunit mRNA levels in rats. Administration of FSH to hypophysectomized animals restored the level of α-subunit mRNA in the testis (Keinan *et al.*, 1989). By contrast, the concentration of inhibin βB-subunit mRNA increased in hypophysectomized rats (Feng and Chen, unpublished).

The regulation of levels of inhibin mRNAs in Sertoli cell-enriched primary cultures was also investigated. There was detectable inhibin α-subunit mRNAs in Sertoli cells cultured for 4 days without gonadotropin. FSH markedly increased the inhibin α-subunit mRNA (Keinan *et al.*, 1989) but had no effect on levels of mRNA for the βB-subunit (Feng and Chen, unpublished). These results suggest that FSH is one of the factors that maintain the differential regulation of α-subunit mRNA in Sertoli cells. The expression of higher levels of the α- than of the β-subunit in the cell is a mechanism by which the synthesis of inhibin rather than activin may be favored by these cells. Testosterone was without effect on inhibin subunit mRNA levels.

Regulation of inhibin secretion by Sertoli cell-enriched cultures

Basal conditions

During the first day in culture, concentrations of inhibin in media increased; over the next 2 days, inhibin levels remained relatively constant and then rose again between 3 and 4 days. The absolute concentrations of inhibin measured in media from cultures maintained under basal conditions (insulin, transferrin, epidermal growth factor (EGF), bacitracin) ranged from 92.4 to 113.5 fmol/ml after 4 days of culture. When these results were normalized to 10^6 cells, basal accumulation was 189 ± 11 fmol/ml (Morris *et al.*, 1988).

Effects of FSH

During the first 24 hours there was no effect of FSH on inhibin accumulation. After 48 hours, there was a significant increase ($p<0.01$) in levels of inhibin at a dose of 300 ng/ml of FSH. By 3 days in culture, there was a dose-dependent increase in inhibin levels at all doses of FSH between 10 ng/ml and 1000 ng/ml; the maximal effective dose was achieved at 100 ng/ml. After 4.5 days in culture, there was a similar, dose-dependent response of levels of inhibin to FSH. Since FSH stimulates adenylyl cyclase in Sertoli cells, it was important to determine whether the increase in inhibin secretion is related to accumulation of cAMP. That this is actually the case was suggested by a study showing that forskolin stimulates inhibin accumulation. We conclude, therefore, that FSH is a major regulator of inhibin secretion via a cAMP-dependent mechanism (Bicsak *et al.*, 1987; Morris *et al.*, 1988).

Effects of testosterone

Using bioassays, several investigators suggested that testosterone is also a major regulator of inhibin secretion (Au *et al.*, 1983, 1986; Verhoeven and Franchimont, 1983). Using the immunoassay, only a small decrease in inhibin accumulation resulted from treatment with testosterone and this decrease occurred only at the highest dose of testosterone examined (10^{-6} mol/l). These effects of testosterone on levels of inhibin were modest compared to those of FSH and would not have been detected by bioassay or even by immunoassay without studies at various times and doses (Morris *et al.*, 1988). This possibly explains why Bicsak *et al.* (1987) did not observe an effect of testosterone. Possible hormone interactions were investigated using multiple doses of testosterone and FSH but none was detected (Morris *et al.*, 1988).

Effects of EGF

Treatment with EGF had no effect on the number of immature Sertoli cells maintained in serum-free medium. Treatment with EGF produced an increase in levels of inhibin. In the presence of a maximal dose of FSH (300 ng/ml), EGF had an additive effect on inhibin accumulation. The pattern of the response to FSH was the same with and without EGF, except that the dose of 1 ng/ml of FSH had a significant effect on the production of inhibin in the absence of EGF ($p < 0.002$), as compared to production in basal cultures maintained with EGF. It is of note that this low dose of FSH only has an effect on inhibin accumulation in the absence of EGF (Morris *et al.*, 1988).

Effects of androstenedione

Multiple doses of androstenedione (but not testosterone) produced a dose-dependent decrease in accumulation of inhibin after 3 days of culture. Androstenedione also suppressed FSH-induced inhibin secretion. This steroid suppressed inhibin accumulation stimulated by all doses of FSH. Inhibin secretion was reduced in a uniform manner by androstenedione and, therefore, the hormone had no effect on the overall pattern of the FSH response. Since the effects of androstenedione were clearly different from those of testosterone and dihydrotestosterone (Bicsak *et al.*, 1987), it was possible that the action of the former steroid was related to its conversion to estrogen. However, after 4 days of treatment with estradiol there was no change in inhibin accumulation after exposure to doses from $2x10^{-13}$ to $2x10^{-5}$ mol/l. In addition, estradiol had no effect on the dose-dependent stimulation of the accumulation of inhibin by FSH. From these observations, it appears that the action of androstenedione is not mediated through its conversion to estrogen or to a more potent androgen. The mechanism of action remains to be established since neither the androgen nor the estrogen receptors are implicated by the present results. We conclude that, since androstenedione is a

Table 1. *Tissue-specific formation of POMC mRNAs of various sizes*

Authentic	Large	Small
Pituitary	Pituitary (2)	Brain
Hypothalamus	Hypothalamus (2)	Testis (1) (2)
Testis	Ectopic tumor	Epididymis
		Ovary
		Uterus
		Placenta
		Adrenal (1)

In a few instances the reason for the large or the small POMC mRNA is known. These reasons include: (1) different transcription start sites; (2) altered splicing of RNA; (3) different lengths of poly(A) added to the gene transcript.

major secretory product of Leydig cells of the prepubertal testis, this steroid may be a regulator of Sertoli cell function at this time.

Regulation of POMC gene expression and secretion of POMC-derived peptides

Presence of POMC-derived peptides and mRNA in testis

Following the demonstration of POMC-derived peptides in Leydig cells by a variety of immunological and chemical procedures (for review, see Bardin *et al.*, 1987a), we sought to identify mRNA for POMC in testis. A POMC cDNA probe hybridized with mRNA from pituitary, testis, brain and epididymis, but not from liver (Chen *et al.*, 1984). In our initial reports, the mRNA in testis, epididymis, ovary and other reproductive tissues was termed 'POMC-like' since its size is approximately 150–200 bases shorter than that in pituitary and hypothalamus (Chen *et al.*, 1984; Chen and Madigan, 1987). Both large and small heterogeneous POMC-like mRNAs have now been demonstrated in several extrapituitary tissues. Since there is only one POMC gene in the rat and most other species, heterogeneous-sized POMC mRNA could arise for a variety of reasons, including: different transcription initiation sites; variations in the splicing of precursor RNA; multiple sites for polyadenylation; and poly(A) tails could be of different lengths. Table 1 shows the distribution of heterogeneous mRNA in several tissues and the reason for the heterogeneity where it is known. In testis, different sites of initiation of transcription and poly(A) tails of different lengths are both responsible for the shorter mRNA (Lacaze-Masmonteil *et al.*, 1987; Jeanotte *et al.*, 1987; Kilpatrick *et al.*, 1987).

Histochemical evidence suggests that POMC-like mRNA in the testis

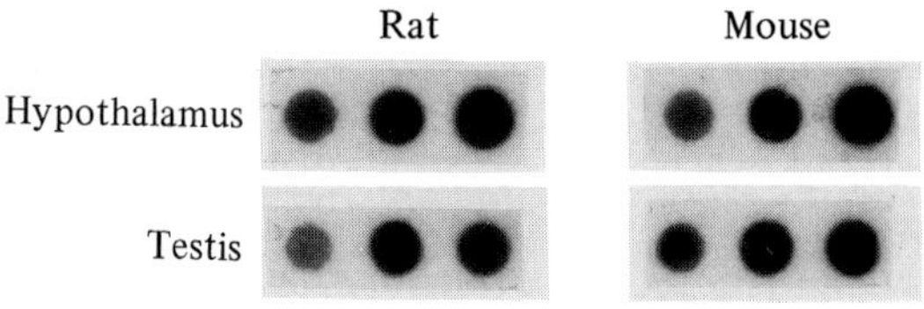

Fig. 1 Comparison of POMC mRNA concentrations by dot-blot analysis. Poly-(A)$^+$ RNA (1, 2 and 4 μg) isolated from hypothalamus or testis of rat and mouse were spotted on nitrocellulose filters, and the concentrations of POMC mRNA were determined by hybridization with a ^{32}P-labeled cDNA probe. The concentrations of POMC mRNA were the same in both hypothalamus and pituitary.

should be localized in the Leydig cells. Several lines of evidence support this possibility. POMC-like mRNA was found in a mouse Leydig cell line (TM_3) but not in extracts from a mouse Sertoli cell line (TM_4) (Chen *et al.*, 1984); in a transplantable murine Leydig cell tumor (Melner and Puett, 1984); and in rat testes by in-situ cDNA hybridization (Krieger *et al.*, 1984). In several studies, the ^{3}H-labeled cDNA was localized in the cytoplasm of most Leydig cells (Pintar *et al.*, 1984; Gizang-Ginsberg and Wolgemuth, 1985). The finding of POMC-like mRNA in Leydig cells supports the postulate that POMC-derived peptides are synthesized in this portion of the testis. The initial immunocytochemical studies did not show dramatic immunostaining in germ cells relative to that in Leydig cells (Tsong *et al.*, 1982a, 1982b; Shaha *et al.*, 1984), except in studies with an antibody raised against α-N-acetyl-endorphin (Cheng *et al.*, 1984). In the first experiments using in-situ hybridization there were a few grains over the cells in the seminiferous tubule so that localization in the germ cells could not be excluded. Subsequent studies have shown that POMC mRNA can be detected in germ cells by Northern blotting (Gizang-Ginsberg and Wolgemuth, 1987; Boitani *et al.*, 1988). Interestingly, in spermatids, both different transcription start sites and poly(A) tails of different lengths are responsible for the shorter POMC mRNA relative to that in the pituitary (Kilpatrick *et al.*, 1987). In other germ cells and Leydig cells, only different transcription start sites are believed to contribute to the shorter mRNA (Chen and Boitani, unpublished).

The initial measurements of POMC mRNA indicated that its concentration in testis was the same as in hypothalamus (Chen *et al.*, 1984; Fig. 1), even though the concentration of POMC-derived peptides was 500- to 1000-fold higher in the hypothalamus (Bardin *et al.*, 1987a). Insight into a possible reason for this marked discrepancy between the concentrations of peptide in these tissues was suggested by the demonstration that the shorter mRNA in testis results from the use of an alternate initiation site in exon 3 of the gene (Fig. 2). Since this start site is located in the sequence that corresponds to gamma-MSH peptide, there is some question as to whether such an mRNA

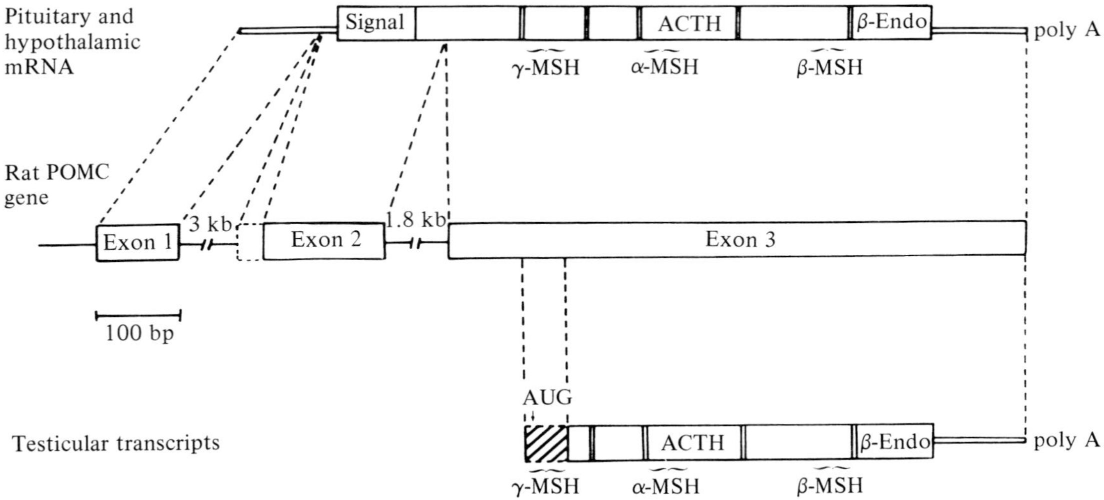

Fig. 2 The origin of authentic, large, and small POMC mRNA from the POMC gene. The structure of the rat POMC gene is schematically represented together with the structure of cytoplasmic POMC transcripts in the pituitary and hypothalamus, as well as in the testis (Jeanotte *et al.*, 1987). POMC exons are indicated as open boxes. The box shown by the dashed line at exon 2 is the alternative splicing site in the pituitary (Oates and Herbert, 1984). The positions of the POMC-derived peptides are shown in the transcripts of the POMC transcripts and the pairs of basic residues cleaved during POMC processing are indicated as double lines. The shaded area indicates the position of the multiple sites of initiation of testicular and adrenal transcripts (Jingami *et al.*, 1984; Jeanotte *et al.*, 1987; Lacaze-Masmonteil *et al.*, 1987).

can be translated at all. If translation could occur, it is unlikely that the resulting peptide could be secreted because of the absence of a signal sequence at the N-terminus of the authentic POMC precursor. The difficulties posed by the shortened POMC mRNA in testis must be rationalized to take into account the unequivocal evidence for the secretion of POMC-derived peptides by Leydig cells both *in vivo* and *in vitro* (Valenca and Negro-Vilar, 1986; Fabbri *et al.*, 1988). One explanation is that the shorter mRNA is translated and the truncated precursor uses an internal signal sequence to allow secretion of small quantities of peptide. Alternatively, the testis could produce a small amount of authentic sized POMC mRNA which is not usually detected on Northern blots because its level represents as little as 1/1000 of that of the shorter form. Preliminary studies favor the latter explanation. These results suggest that the concentration of the major class of POMC mRNA in the testis and other reproductive organs may not relate directly to the measured concentrations of POMC-derived peptides.

Regulation of POMC-like mRNA and POMC-derived peptides

The fact that immunostainable β-endorphin and other POMC-derived peptides in Leydig cells appeared to increase during periods of testosterone synthesis in fetal life and again at puberty suggests that the expression of these peptides may be dependent upon gonadotropin secretion. Consistent with this possibility was the demonstration that there was an increase in the number of cells that display immunostainable material in neonatal mice after 5 days of treatment with human chorionic gonadotropin (hCG) (Shaha *et al.*, 1984). In this latter experiment, treatment with hCG was initiated in groups of mice at 5, 10, and 15 days of age and this treatment resulted in a marked increase in the number of stainable Leydig cells in each treated group.

That POMC in adult Leydig cells is under the control of the pituitary gland was also suggested by the observation that testicular levels of β-endorphin, α-endorphin, and ACTH declined after hypophysectomy (Tsong *et al.*, 1982a). The levels of immunoreactive β-endorphin and ACTH present in the interstitial fluid which surrounds the Leydig cells also declined after hypophysectomy and increased after treatment with hCG. Interestingly, short and long-term treatments with a superactive agonist of luteinizing hormone-releasing hormone (LHRH) stimulated and suppressed, respectively, the concentration of β-endorphin in interstitial fluid in parallel with changes in levels of testosterone (Valenca and Negro-Vilar, 1986). Such findings are consistent with the hypothesis that POMC-derived peptides are secreted by Leydig cells in the interstitium of the testis under the control of hormones that are known to stimulate and suppress these cells. These observations, together with in-vitro studies that demonstrate secretion of β-endorphin by Leydig cells (Fabbri *et al.*, 1988), provide the strongest evidence that POMC-derived peptides are not only secreted but that their secretion is appropriately regulated (Bardin *et al.*, 1984, 1987a).

Since the levels of immunoassayable POMC-derived peptides in testis decreased after hypophysectomy in parallel with decreases in testicular weight (Tsong *et al.*, 1982a), we sought to determine whether the accumulation of POMC mRNA in testicular cells is also regulated by gonadotropins. To address this question, testicular poly(A) RNAs were isolated from rats which had been hypophysectomized for different periods of time. The total amount of poly(A) RNA isolated from each pair of testes decreased in parallel with decreases in testicular weight, as did the total content of POMC mRNA per pair of testes. Treatment with hCG resulted in an increase in the content of POMC mRNA in the testis (Chen and Madigan, 1987). The transcript whose level decreased and increased with these treatments was about 200 bp shorter than the POMC mRNA found in the pituitary.

Several studies suggest that the seminiferous tubules also regulate the quantity of POMC mRNA in Leydig cells. Experiments using in-situ hybridization localized POMC-like mRNA primarily to Leydig cells in interstitial regions surrounded completely or in part by tubules at stages IX to XII of the cycle of the seminiferous epithelium (Gizang-Ginsberg and Wolgemuth, 1985). In addition, in mutant mice with germ cells arrested in early spermatogenesis, the abundance of POMC transcripts was normal. By contrast, transcripts were virtually undetectable in testes of mutant mice devoid of germ cells (Gizang-Ginsberg and Wolgemuth, 1987). These observations suggest that the level of the short POMC mRNA in Leydig cells is regulated by several humoral factors but, as noted above, it is not certain whether this mRNA is translated into secreted peptides. It is appropriate to state at present that neither the function nor the regulation of the POMC mRNA in germ cells is understood.

The effects of inhibin/activin and POMC-derived peptides on testicular cells

In 1980, 2 years before Tsong *et al.* (1982a) reported the presence of immunostainable POMC-derived peptides in Leydig cells, impure extracts of ACTH were shown to increase the growth rate of a cell line derived from Sertoli cells, namely, TM_4 (Brinkman *et al.*, 1980). Similar results were obtained with synthetic ACTH-(1–24) (Mather *et al.*, 1985). Synthetic ACTH, β-MSH, α-MSH, and desacetyl α-MSH also stimulated the synthesis and accumulation of cAMP in Sertoli cells (Bardin *et al.*, 1984; Mather *et al.*, 1984, 1985; Boitani *et al.*, 1986). The action of these POMC-derived peptides, like those of FSH and isoproterenol, was potentiated by forskolin and the phosphodiesterase inhibitor, methylisobutyl xanthine (MIX).

The activities of α-MSH and desacetyl α-MSH were compared (Boitani *et al.*, 1985, 1986, 1989) since the latter peptide was identified in testicular extracts (Margioris *et al.*, 1983). Both α-MSH and desacetyl α-MSH stimulated the accumulation of cAMP in media of primary Sertoli cell-

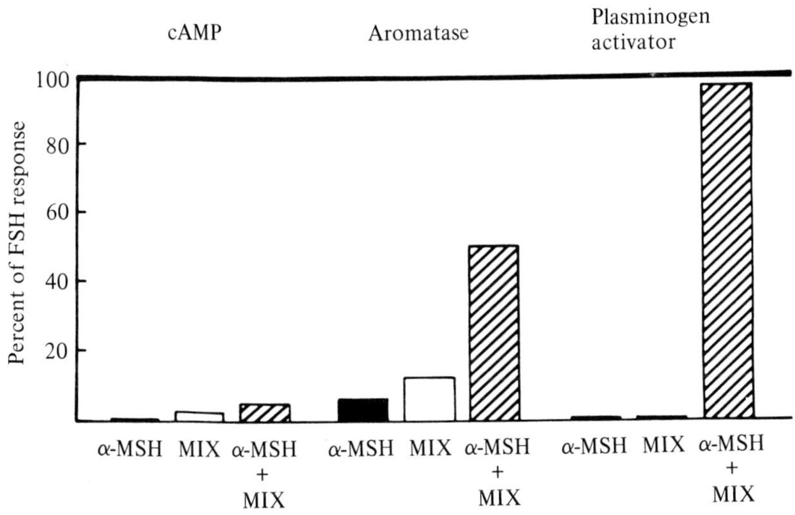

Fig. 3 The relative responses of cAMP accumulation, aromatase activity and plasminogen activator activity (urokinase) to various agents, expressed as a percentage of the FSH response in Sertoli cell-enriched cultures.

enriched cultures when these cells were incubated in the presence of MIX, FSH or forskolin. Both peptides shifted the dose–response curve for FSH to the left, making the cells more sensitive to this gonadotropin. When either cAMP accumulation or aromatase activity was used as a parameter, the apparent potencies of the effects of α-MSH, its desacetyl derivative, and ACTH on Sertoli cells were similar. By contrast, the comparative effects of α-MSH on three different Sertoli cell products – cAMP, aromatase, and plasminogen activator (urokinase) – (as shown in Fig. 3) are diverse both with respect to the action of peptide with and without MIX and relative to the action of FSH. For example, neither α-MSH nor MIX had appreciable effect on urokinase activity in 10-day-old Sertoli cell-enriched cultures, but α-MSH plus MIX suppressed the activity of this enzyme as effectively as FSH (Boitani *et al.*, 1989). From the results of these and other studies, we conclude that the ACTH/MSH peptides make up one of a group of modulators that regulate Sertoli cell function via the cAMP system. Even though these modulators do not appear to exert uniform effects on all Sertoli cell proteins, a single endpoint appears equally responsive to ACTH, α-MSH, and desacetyl α-MSH. These effects on Sertoli cells are unlike those on the adrenal cortex and melanocytes which can distinguish between these individual peptides (Table 2). In view of this, we conclude that ACTH, α-MSH, and related peptides (ACTH/MSH) are a group of peptides that have similar action on Sertoli cells.

In contrast to the stimulatory effects of ACTH/MSH, β-endorphin inhibits

Table 2. *The relative differential responses of cells to POMC-derived peptides*

Cell type	Peptide	
	α-MSH	ACTH
Adrenal cortical cell	+	++++
Melanocyte	++++	+
Sertoli cell[a]	++++	++++

[a]Sertoli cells respond similarly to α-MSH, desacetyl α-MSH, β-MSH, and ACTH but less well to gamma-MSH.

Sertoli cell division, adenylate cyclase activity, and protein secretion. The inhibitory action of β-endorphin on the testis was first shown in experiments using the opiate antagonists, nalmefene and naloxone, which were injected intratesticularly in neonatal rats that were killed 5 days later (Fig. 4; Gerendai *et al.*, 1983, 1986). Both opiate antagonists increased the secretion of the Sertoli product, androgen-binding protein (ABP), and the compensatory hypertrophy that follows unilateral castration, which is dependent upon the Sertoli cell division. Naloxone also increased the rate of Sertoli cell division in explant cultures of neonatal testes (Orth, 1986). Since the hypertrophy that follows unilateral orchidectomy of neonatal rats is believed to be due to the increase in serum levels of FSH, the opiate antagonists appear to block the action of an endogenous opiate that inhibits FSH. The increases in testicular size and rABP secretion following antagonist administration are consistent with the hypothesis that β-endorphin and/or other testicular opioids inhibit Sertoli cell growth and secretion during early development and that these compounds are, at this time, antagonistic to FSH which stimulates Sertoli cells (Vogel *et al.*, 1983; Gunsalus *et al.*, 1984). The demonstration of opiate receptors on Sertoli cells and the inhibition of FSH-induced secretion of rABP *in vitro* by an opiate antagonist are consistent with this hypothesis (Fabbri *et al.*, 1985).

In view of the observations outlined above, it seemed pertinent to study the effects of POMC-derived peptides on inhibin secretion. Treatment with β-endorphin, ACTH, α-MSH, met-enkephalin, or dynorphin B had no effect on basal accumulation of inhibin. By contrast, treatment with β-endorphin reduced the inhibin response to FSH stimulation (Morris *et al.*, 1987a). None of the other POMC-derived peptides, met-enkephalin, or dynorphin B (1–9) had a similar effect. Since the response to FSH is mediated by cyclic AMP, the effect of directly elevating intracellular cAMP levels by treatment with

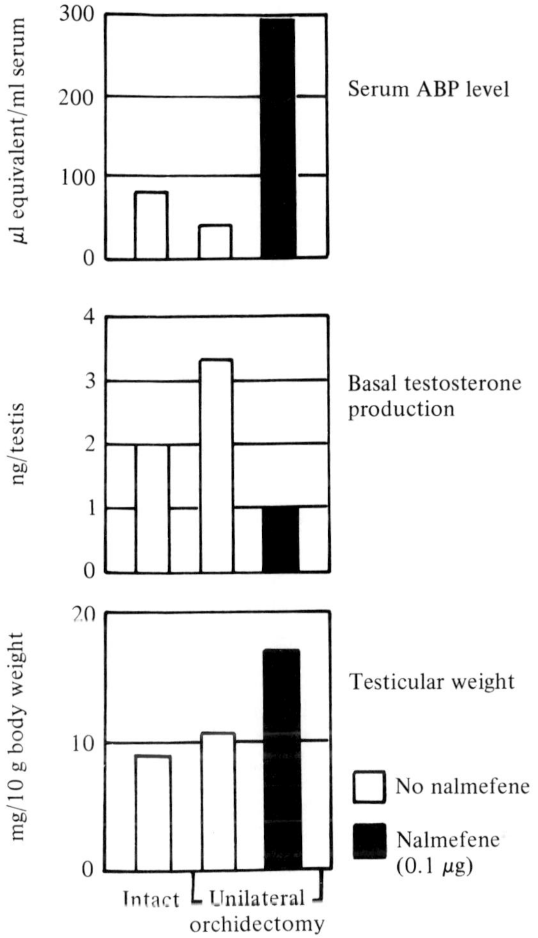

Fig. 4 Effects of nalmefene in hemicastrate rats. Five-day-old rats were injected intratesticularly (in the right testis) with nalmefene, and the left testis was removed. Animals were killed at 11 days of age. The black bars indicate a difference from the hemicastrate, vehicle-treated (no nalmefene) control rats.

forskolin was studied. This agent increased the accumulation of inhibin in Sertoli-enriched cultures from 130 ± 2.3 to 175 ± 3.6 fmol/ml. Treatment with β-endorphin had no effect on the forskolin-stimulated accumulation of inhibin, whereas the effects of FSH and forskolin were additive. Taken together, these results suggest that the inhibitory effect of β-endorphin on the inhibin response to FSH may be due to effects on the FSH receptor or on the coupling of the FSH receptor to the adenylyl cyclase (AC) system. To

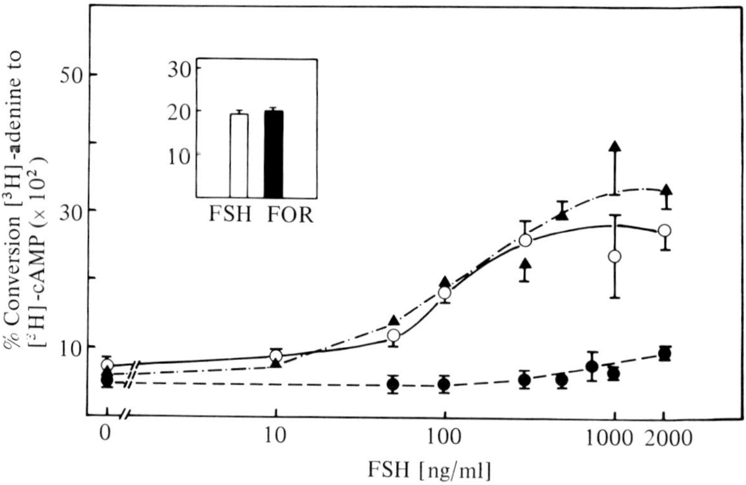

Fig. 5 Acute stimulation of adenylyl cyclase (AC) activity by FSH in the presence and absence of opiates. Sertoli cell-enriched cultures were maintained in serum-free medium alone (open circles) or with 1 μmol/l methionine-enkephalin (solid triangles) or 0.3 μmol/l β-endorphin (solid circles). After 4 days, the effect of FSH on conversion of [^{3}H]-adenine to [^{3}H]-cAMP was measured in intact cells (Morris *et al.*, 1987b). Assays were performed at a density of 2.2±0.5 (S.D.)x10^6 cells per 2 ml per 35-mm dish. Insert: acute cyclase stimulation by 5 μmol/l forskolin and 100 ng/ml FSH (Morris *et al.*, 1987b).

investigate this latter possibility, the ability of opiates to modify the action of FSH on AC activity was investigated (Morris *et al.*, 1987a).

There was no difference in basal AC activity (without FSH) in Sertoli cells maintained with or without met-enkephalin or β-endorphin. In agreement with previous studies, FSH stimulated AC activity in a dose-dependent manner. The acute effects of all doses of FSH were significantly ($p<0.001$) reduced when the cells were treated for 4 days with β-endorphin (Morris *et al.*, 1987a). By contrast, met-enkephalin was without effect on the FSH response (Fig. 5). No inhibitory effect of β-endorphin was observed on the activation of AC by a suboptimal (5 μmol/l) dose of forskolin. These observations suggest that the inhibitory effects of β-endorphin on Sertoli cell function are mediated via an antagonism of the action of FSH. Moreover, it appears that this effect is on the FSH receptor or its coupling to AC.

The results in Figure 4 are also consistent with the hypothesis that an intratesticular opiate facilitates the secretion of androgen. It is not clear how this effect of the antagonist is mediated over such an extended period of time (i.e. in rats from 5 to 11 days of age). Nonetheless, a stimulatory effect of β-endorphin on androgen secretion by Leydig cells was confirmed with in-vitro studies (Bardin *et al.*, 1987a; Morris and Bardin, 1987). These findings suggest that POMC-derived peptides have autocrine effects on Leydig cells.

The effects of inhibin and activin on Leydig cells

Since a variety of Sertoli cell factors have been shown to regulate Leydig function, the effects of inhibin on the production of androgen *in vitro* were examined. Suspensions of testicular cells were prepared from testes removed from neonatal or adult hypophysectomized rats. A preparation of inhibin isolated from ram rete testis fluid by immunoaffinity chromatography had no effect on the basal rate of testosterone secretion. When administered with luteinizing hormone (LH), inhibin shifted the dose–response curve for LH to the left and activin shifted the curve to the right. Thus, inhibin increased and activin decreased the sensitivity of testicular cells to LH (Hsueh *et al.*, 1987).

In another study, the effects of activin and inhibin on androstenedione secretion were studied in primary Leydig cell-enriched cultures established from the testes of 20-day-old rats (Morris, unpublished). Levels of androstenedione were measured since it is the primary androgen secreted by Leydig cells from rats of this age. Although there was no effect of inhibin on basal androstenedione secretion over the initial 24 hours, after 3 days there was a modest but significant stimulatory effect on basal secretion of this hormone. Inhibin enhanced the androstenedione response (1.6- to 1.9-fold) to a submaximal dose of hCG over a 3-day culture period. By contrast, the same dose of inhibin suppressed the androgen response to a maximal dose of hCG over a 3-day period. These results suggest that the period of exposure of Leydig cells, as well as the amount of gonadotropin present, affects the response of the cell to inhibin. Activin, regardless of dose or time in culture, had no effect on basal androstenedione secretion. Activin did suppress by one-third the androstenedione response to all doses of hCG at 24 hours of culture. After 3 days, the effects of activin were no longer significant. These studies on immature Leydig cells led us to conclude that inhibin has a biphasic effect on the production of androgen, which is dependent on the dose of hCG, and that the opposing actions of inhibin and activin are evident in different time frames.

Discussion and conclusion

In the immature rat, recent evidence shows that the interstitial fluid compartment contains POMC-derived peptides (Valenca and Negro-Vilar, 1986) and larger uncharacterized proteins secreted by Leydig cells and other interstitial cells (Morris *et al.*, 1987a). Numerous studies suggest that the ACTH/MSH family of peptides may be stimulators of Sertoli cell function and that β-endorphin is an inhibitory paracrine regulator. By contrast, β-endorphin may be an autocrine stimulator of Leydig cells (Morris and Bardin, 1987). The present findings support this hypothesis. Moreover, modulation of FSH-stimulated inhibin secretion by β-endorphin but not α-MSH, ACTH, methionine-enkephalin, or dynorphin B (1–9), is in agreement with earlier studies suggesting that the peptides derived from different portions of the POMC molecule have differential effects on Sertoli cells (Boitani *et al.*, 1985, 1986; Bardin *et al.*, 1984, 1987a). The results to date support the hypothesis that β-endorphin antagonizes the actions of FSH on the Sertoli cell. The inhibitory effect of β-endorphin on Sertoli cells appears to occur at the level of the receptor for FSH or its coupling to AC since no impairment of basal inhibin secretion or forskolin-activated AC activity by β-endorphin has been observed.

Recent studies show that inhibin regulates Leydig cell function by facilitating testosterone secretion from crude preparations of interstitial cells in response to LH (Bicsak *et al.*, 1987; Hsueh *et al.*, 1987). Since β-endorphin, an opiate produced by Leydig cells, inhibits Sertoli cell function (Bardin *et al.*, 1987a; Morris *et al.*, 1987b), these results suggest that β-endorphin and inhibin are components of an intratesticular short-loop system that modulates the functions of Sertoli and Leydig cells.

Acknowledgements

This work was supported by the Clayton Foundation; by NIH grants HD-16149, HD-13527, DK-34449, HD-13541, HD-12357, DK-26741; and by USAID grant pha-G116 and Cooperative Agreement DPE-3005-A-00-3003-00.

References

Au, C.L., Robertson, D.M. & de Kretser, D.M. (1983). *In vitro* bioassay of inhibin in testes of normal and cryptorchid rats. **Endocrinology** 112:239–244.

Au, C.L., Robertson, D.M. & de Kretser, D.M. (1986). Measurement of inhibin and an index of inhibin production by rat testes during postnatal development. **Biology of Reproduction** 35:37–43.

Bardin, C.W., Chen, C.-L.C., Morris, P.L., Gerendai, I., Boitani, C., Liotta, A.S., Margioris, A. & Krieger, D.T. (1987a). Pro-opiomelanocortin-derived peptides in testis, ovary and tissues of reproduction. **Recent Progress in Hormone Research** 43:1–28.

Bardin, C.W., Morris, P.L., Chen, C.-L.C., Shaha, C., Voglmayr, J., Rivier, J., Spiess, J. & Vale, W.W. (1987b). Testicular inhibin: structure and regulation by FSH, androgens and EGF. In: Burger, H.G., de Kretser, D.M., Findlay, J.K. & Igarashi, M., eds. **Inhibin: Non-Steroidal Regulation of Follicle-Stimulating Hormone Secretion**, Serono Symposia, Vol. 42, New York, Raven Press, pp.179–190.

Bardin, C.W., Shaha, C., Mather, J., Salomon, Y., Margioris, A.N., Liotta, A.S., Gerendai, I., Chen, C.-L. & Krieger, D.T. (1984). Identification and possible function of pro-opiomelanocortin-derived peptides in the testis. **Annals of the New York Academy of Sciences** 438:346–364.

Bicsak, T.A., Vale, W., Vaughan, J., Tucker, E.M., Cappel, S. & Hsueh, A.J.W. (1987). Hormonal regulation of inhibin production by cultured Sertoli cells. **Molecular and Cellular Endocrinology** 49:211–217.

Boitani, C., Chen, C.-L.C., Canipari, R. & Bardin, C.W. (1988). Expression of pro-opiomelanocortin (POMC) gene in male rat germ cells and response of Sertoli cells to POMC-derived peptides. In: Cooke, B.A., ed. **5th European Testes Workshop Proceedings**, Italy, Serono Symposia Series, Abstract G2.

Boitani, C., Chen, C.-L.C., Margioris, A.N., Morris, P.L. & Bardin, C.W. (1985). Pro-opiomelanocortin-derived peptides in the testis: evidence for a possible role in Leydig and Sertoli cell function. **Medical Biology** 63:251–258.

Boitani, C., Farini, D., Canipari, R. & Bardin, C.W.(1989). Estradiol and plasminogen activator secretion by cultured rat Sertoli cells in response to melanocyte-stimulating hormones. **Journal of Andrology** 10:202–209.

Boitani, C., Mather, J.P. & Bardin, C.W. (1986). Stimulation of cAMP production in rat Sertoli cells by α-MSH and desacetyl α-MSH. **Endocrinology** 118: 1513–1518.

Brinkman, A.O., Leemborg, F.G., Roodnat, E.M., De Jong, F.H. & van der Molen, H.J. (1980). A specific action of estradiol on enzymes involved in testicular steroidogenesis. **Biology of Reproduction** 23:801–809.

Chen, C.-L.C. & Madigan, M. (1987). Regulation of testicular proopiomelanocortin-like gene expression. **Endocrinology** 121:590–596.

Chen, C.-L.C., Mather, J.P., Morris, P.L. & Bardin, C.W. (1984). Expression of pro-opiomelanocortin-like gene in the testis and epididymis. **Proceedings of the National Academy of Sciences, USA** 81:5672–5675.

Chen, C.-L.C., Morris, P.L., Keinan, D., Feng, Z.M., Shaha, C., Vale, W.W. & Bardin, C.W. (1988). Proopiomelanocortin and inhibin gene expression regulate a short-loop system between testicular Leydig and Sertoli cells. **Cell-to-Cell Communication in Endocrinology**, New York, Raven Press, pp.139–153.

Cheng, M.C., Clements, J.A., Smith, A.I., Lolait, S.J. & Funder, J.W. (1984). N-Acetyl endorphin in rat spermatogonia and primary spermatocytes. **Journal of Clinical Investigation** 75:832–835.

Fabbri, A., Knox, G., Buczko, E. & Dufau, M.L. (1988). β-Endorphin production by the fetal Leydig cell: regulation and implications for paracrine control of Sertoli cell function. **Endocrinology** 122:749–756.

Fabbri, A., Tsai-Morris, C.H., Luna, S., Fraioli, F. & Dufau, M.L. (1985). Opiate receptors are present in the rat testis. Identification and localization in Sertoli cells. **Endocrinology** 117:2544–2546.

Gerendai, I., Nemeskeri, A. & Csernus, A. (1983). Naloxone has a local effect on the testis of immature rats. **Andrologia** 15:398–403.

Gerendai, I., Shaha, C., Gunsalus, G.L. & Bardin, C.W. (1986). The effects of opioid receptor antagonists suggest that testicular opiates regulate Sertoli and Leydig cell function in the neonatal rat. **Endocrinology** 118:2039–2044.

Gizang-Ginsberg, E. & Wolgemuth, D.J. (1985). Localization of mRNA in mouse testes by in-situ hybridization: distribution of alpha-tubulin and development stage specificity of pro-opiomelanocortin transcripts. **Developmental Biology** 111:293–305.

Gizang-Ginsberg, E. & Wolgemuth, D.J. (1987). Expression of the proopiomelanocortin gene is developmentally regulated and affected by germ cells in the male mouse reproductive system. **Proceedings of the National Academy of Sciences, USA** 84:1600–1604.

Gunsalus, G.L., Carreau, S., Vogel, D.L., Musto, N.A. & Bardin, C.W. (1984). Use of androgen-binding protein to monitor development of the seminiferous epithelium.

In: Serio, M., Motta, M., Zanisi, M. & Martini, L., eds. **Sexual Differentiation: Basic and Clinical Aspects**, New York, Raven Press, pp.53–64.

Hsueh, A.J.W., Dahl, K.D., Vaughan, J., Tucker, E., Rivier, J., Bardin, C.W. & Vale, W. (1987). Hetero- and homodimers of inhibin subunits have different paracrine action in the modulation of LH-stimulated androgen biosynthesis. **Proceedings of the National Academy of Sciences, USA** 84:5082–5086.

Jeanotte, L., Burbach, J.P.H. & Drouin, J. (1987). Unusual proopiomelanocortin ribonucleic acids in extrapituitary tissues: intronless transcripts in testes and long poly(A) tails in hypothalamus. **Molecular Endocrinology** 1:749–757.

Jingami, H., Nakanishi, S., Immura, H. & Numa, S. (1984). Tissue distribution of messenger RNAs coding for opioid peptide precursors and related RNA. **European Journal of Biochemistry** 142:441–447.

Keinan, D., Madigan, M.B., Bardin, C.W. & Chen, C.-L.C. (1989). Expression and regulation of testicular α-subunit inhibin gene *in vivo* and *in vitro*. **Molecular Endocrinology** 3:29–35.

Kilpatrick, D.L., Borland, K. & Jin, D.F. (1987). Differential expression of opioid peptide genes by testicular germ cells and somatic cells. **Proceedings of the National Academy of Sciences, USA** 84:5695–5699.

Krieger, D.T., Margioris, A.N., Liotta, A.S., Shaha, C., Gerendai, I., Pintar, J. & Bardin, C.W. (1984). Pro-opiomelanocortin (POMC)-derived peptides in the rodent male reproductive tract. In: Delitala, G., Motta, M. & Serio, M., eds. **Opioid Modulation of Endocrine Function**, New York, Raven Press, pp.223–235.

Lagaze-Masmonteil, T., Dekeyzer, Y., Luton, J.-P., Kahn, A. & Bertagna, X. (1987). Characterization of proopiomelanocortin transcripts in human non-pituitary tissues. **Proceedings of the National Academy of Sciences, USA** 84:7261–7265.

Lee, W., Schwall, R., Mason, A.J. & Mather, J.P. (1988). Interstitial cell cultures secrete an activity with characteristics of the inhibin β-β homodimer, activin. In: Cooke, B.A., ed., **5th European Testes Workshop Proceedings**, Italy, Serono Symposia Series, Abstract A1.

Ling, N., Ying, S.-Y., Ueno, N., Esch, F., Denoroy, L. & Guillemin, R. (1985). Isolation and partial characterization of a M_r 32,000 protein with inhibin activity from porcine follicular fluid. **Proceedings of the National Academy of Sciences, USA** 82:7217–7221.

Margioris, A., Liotta, A.S., Vaudry, H., Bardin, C.W. & Krieger, D.T. (1983). Characterization of immunoreactive pro-opiomelanocortin-related peptides in rat testes. **Endocrinology** 112:663–671.

Mason, A.J., Niall, H.D. & Seeburg, P.H. (1986). Structure of two human ovarian inhibins. **Biochemical and Biophysical Research Communications** 135:957–964.

Mather, J., Bardin, C.W., Byer, A. & Salomon, Y. (1985). Modulation of adenylate cyclase activity in Sertoli cells *in vitro*. In Saez, J.M., Forest, M.G., Dazord, A. & Bertrand, J., eds. **Recent Progress in Cellular Endocrinology of the Testis**, Vol. 122, Paris, INSERM, pp.183–186.

Mather, J.P., Morris, P.L., Perez-Infante, V., Salomon, Y.A., Nakhla, A., Gunsalus, G.L. & Bardin, C.W. (1984). Hormonal control of Sertoli cell function. In: Labrie, F. & Proulx, L., eds. **Endocrinology: Proceedings of the 7th International Congress of Endocrinology**, Amsterdam, Elsevier, pp.615–618.

Mayo, K.E., Cerelli, G.M., Spiess, J., Rivier, J., Rosenfeld, M.G., Evans, R.M. & Vale, W. (1986). Inhibin A-subunit cDNAs from porcine ovary and human placenta.

Proceedings of the National Academy of Sciences, USA 83:5849–5853.

Melner, M.H. & Puett, D. (1984). Evidence for the synthesis of multiple proopiomelancortin-like precursors in murine Leydig tumor cells. **Archives of Biochemistry and Biophysics** 232:197–199.

Meunier, H., Rivier, C., Evans, R. & Vale, W. (1988). Gonadal and extra-gonadal expression of inhibin α, βA and βB subunits in various tissues predicts diverse functions. **Proceedings of the National Academy of Sciences, USA** 85:247–251.

Miyamoto, K., Hasegawa, Y., Fukada, M., Nomura, M., Igarashi, M., Kangawa, K. & Matsuo, H. (1985). Isolation of porcine follicular fluid inhibin of 32K daltons. **Biochemical and Biophysical Research Communications** 129:396–403.

Morris, P.L. & Bardin, C.W. (1987). Intratesticular opiates as regulators of Leydig cell function. **Annals of the New York Academy of Sciences** 513:380–382.

Morris, P.L., Cheng, C.Y. & Bardin, C.W. (1987a). Identification of prolactin-responsive proteins in Leydig cell-enriched culture media. **Annals of the New York Academy of Sciences** 513:390–392.

Morris, P.L., Vale, W.W. & Bardin, C.W. (1987b). β-Endorphin regulates the FSH stimulation of inhibin by Sertoli cells. **Biochemical and Biophysical Research Communications** 148:1513–1519.

Morris, P.L., Vale, W.W., Cappel, S. & Bardin, C.W. (1988). Inhibin production by primary Sertoli cell-enriched cultures: regulation by FSH, androgens and EGF. **Endocrinology** 122:717–725.

Oates, E. & Herbert, E. (1984). 5' Sequences of porcine and rat proopiomelancortin mRNA. **Journal of Biological Chemistry** 259:7421–7425.

Orth, J.M. (1986). FSH-induced Sertoli cell proliferation in the developing rat is modified by β-endorphin. **Endocrinology** 119:1876–1878.

Pintar, J.E., Schachter, B.S., Herman, A.B., Durgerian, S. & Krieger, D.T. (1984). Characterization and localization of proopiomelanocortin in mRNA in the adult rat. **Science** 225:632–634.

Rivier, J., Spiess, J., McClintock, R., Vaughan, J. & Vale, W. (1985). Purification and partial characterization of inhibin from porcine follicular fluid. **Biochemical and Biophysical Research Communications** 133:120–127.

Robertson, D.M., Foulds, L.M., Leversha, L., Morgan, F.H., Hearn, M.T.W., Burger, H.G., Wettenhall, R.E.H. & de Kretser, D.M. (1985). Isolation of inhibin from bovine follicular fluid. **Biochemical and Biophysical Research Communications** 126:220–226.

Shaha, C., Liotta, A.S., Krieger, D.T. & Bardin, C.W. (1984). The ontogeny of immunoreactive β-endorphin in the fetal, neonatal, and pubertal testes from mouse and hamster. **Endocrinology** 114:1584–1591.

Tsong, S.-D., Phillips, D.M., Bardin, C.W., Halmi, N., Liotta, A.J., Margioris, A. & Krieger, D.T. (1982a). ACTH and β-endorphin related peptides are present in multiple sites in the reproductive tract of the rat. **Endocrinology** 110:2204–2206.

Tsong, S.D., Phillips, D.M., Halmi, N., Krieger, D.T. & Bardin, C.W. (1982b). β-Endorphin is present in the male reproductive tract of five species. **Biology of Reproduction** 27:755–764.

Vale, W., Rivier, C., Hsueh, A., Campen, C., Meunier, H., Bicsak, T., Vaughan, J., Corrigan, A., Bardin, W., Sawchenko, P., Petraglia, F., Yu, J., Plotsky, P., Spiess, J. & Rivier, J. (1988). Chemical and biological characterization of the inhibin family protein hormones. **Recent Progress in Hormone Research** 44:1–34.

Valenca, M.M. & Negro-Vilar, A. (1986). Pro-opiomelanocortin-derived peptides in testicular interstitial fluid: Characterization and changes in secretion after human chorionic gonadotropin or luteinizing hormone-releasing hormone analog treatment. **Endocrinology** 118:32–37.

Verhoeven, G. & Franchimont, P. (1983). Regulation of inhibin secretion by Sertoli cell-enriched cultures. **Acta Endocrinologica** 102:136–143.

Vogel, D.L., Gunsalus, G.L., Bercu, B.B., Musto, N.A. & Bardin, C.W. (1983). Sertoli cell maturation is impaired by neonatal passive immunization with antiserum to luteinizing hormone-releasing hormone. **Endocrinology** 112:1115–1121.

Ying, S.-Y. (1988). Inhibins, activins, and follistatins: gonadal proteins modulating the secretion of follicle-stimulating hormone. **Endocrine Reviews** 9:267–293.

Ying, S.-Y., Czvik, J., Becker, A., Ling, N., Ueno, N. & Guillemin, R. (1987). Secretion of follicle-stimulating hormone and production of inhibin are reciprocally related. **Proceedings of the National Academy of Sciences, USA** 84:4631–4635.

Modulation of FSH by low-molecular-weight synthetic fragments of human seminal inhibin

A.R. SHETH, K.S. HURKADLI, S.D. MAHALE AND K.S.N. IYER

Institute for Research in Reproduction (ICMR), Indian Council of Medical Research, Parel, Bombay 400 012, India.

Keywords

Inhibin-like proteins, human seminal plasma, prostate, synthetic peptides, FSH-suppressing activity.

Introduction

A family of inhibin-like proteins has been isolated from human testis, human placenta, and from bovine, porcine and human follicular fluid (de Jong, 1988). A distinctly different inhibin-like protein has been isolated from human seminal plasma that originates from prostatic epithelial cells (Beksac *et al.*, 1984; Sheth *et al.*, 1984; Sathe *et al.*, 1987). This protein, now referred to as prostatic inhibin peptide (PIP), consists of 94 amino acid residues (Fig. 1). In adult male rats, PIP specifically suppresses levels of follicle-stimulating hormone (FSH) without affecting levels of luteinizing hormone (LH) (Fig. 2).

Recently, we synthesized two synthetic fragments of PIP which modulate the levels of FSH (Fig. 3). A synthetic carboxyl-terminal nonapeptide representing residues 86–94 of PIP caused a twofold increase in levels of circulating FSH in adult male rats (Fig. 4) without significantly altering levels of LH and prolactin (PRL) except at higher doses (Table 1; Iyer *et al.*, 1987). The peptide exerted its action directly at the pituitary level since in picogram doses it significantly increased the release of FSH from isolated rat pituitary glands into the medium (Fig. 5; Hurkadli *et al.*, 1989). Our recent studies have shown that, *in vitro*, the peptide exhibits similar effects on human, monkey and cattle pituitaries (Hurkadli, unpublished). This nonapeptide will be of particular value when a specific increase in levels of FSH is desired, e.g. in cases of polycystic ovarian syndrome or for the induction of superovulation for in vitro fertilization and embryo transfer programs.

Addition of a tyrosine residue at the NH_2-terminal of the nonapeptide and blocking of the SH group of the cysteine residue at position 87 completely alter the activity of the peptide such that elevation of levels of FSH is replaced by suppression of levels of FSH in rats both *in vivo* (Fig. 6; Iyer *et al.*, 1989) and *in vitro* (Fig. 7). This decapeptide is also active *in vitro* when applied to human, monkey and sheep pituitaries. To our knowledge, ours is the smallest inhibin peptide that is effective in many species both *in vivo* and *in vitro*. Because of its small size, the decapeptide will be easier and less expensive to prepare than

Complete Sequence of Human beta–Inhibin

```
      1                   5                   10                  15
NH2. Ser Cys Tyr Phe Ile Pro Asn Glu Gly Val Pro Gly Asp Ser Thr
                         20                  25                  30
     Arg Lys Cys Met Asp Leu Lys Gly Asn Lys His Pro Ile Asn Ser
                         35                  40                  45
     Glu Trp Gln Thr Asp Asn Cys Glu Thr Cys Thr Cys Tyr Glu Thr
                         50                  55                  60
     Glu Ile Ser Cys Cys Thr Leu Val Ser Thr Pro Val Gly Tyr Asp
                         65                  70                  75
     Lys Asp Asn Cys Gln [Arg] Ile Phe Lys Lys Glu Asp Cys Lys Tyr
                         80                  85                  90
     Ile Val Val Glu Lys Lys Asp Pro Lys Lys Thr Cys Ser Val Ser
                     94
     Glu Trp Gly Ile .COOH
```

Fig. 1 Amino acid sequence of a prostatic inhibin peptide (PIP).

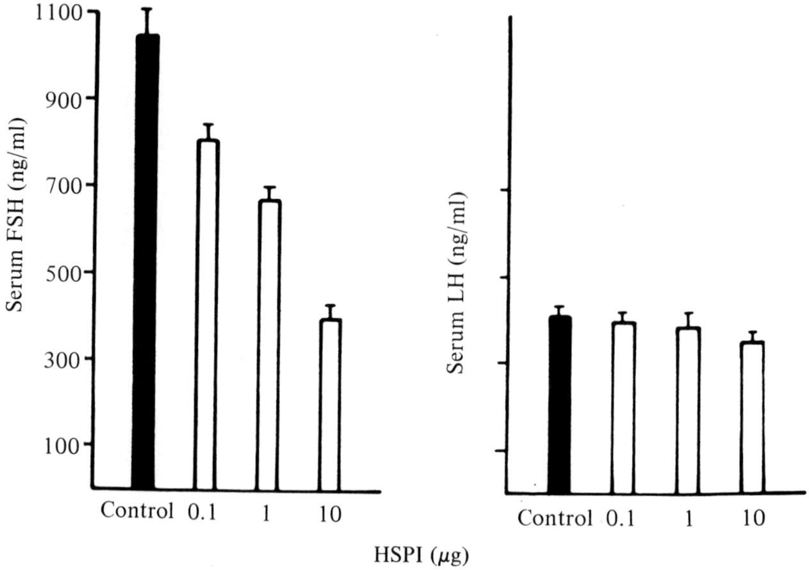

Fig. 2 Effect of PIP on levels of LH and FSH in adult male rats.

Nonapeptide

86 94

Thr-Cys-Ser-Val-Ser-Glu-Trp-Gly-Ile-COOH

Decapeptide

85 94

Thy-Thr- Cys -Ser-Val-Ser-Glu-Trp-Gly-Ile-COOH

Acm

Fig. 3 Amino acid sequence of synthetic fragments of PIP. The nonapeptide increases secretion of FSH whereas the decapeptide decreases the secretion of FSH.

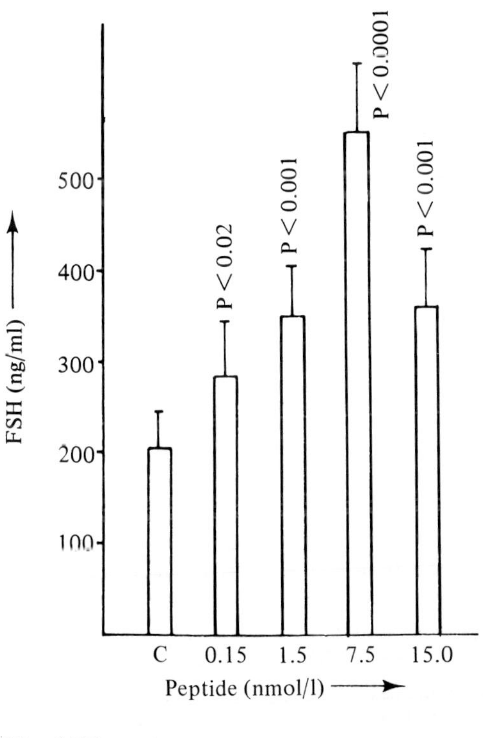

Fig. 4 Effect of the nonapeptide on levels of FSH in adult male rats.

Table 1. *Levels of circulating LH and PRL (ng/ml) after administration of the nonapeptide (values are means ± S.D. of results from 5–6 rats in each group)*

		Nonapeptide (nmol/l)			
Hormone	Saline control (ng/ml)	0.15	1.5	7.5	15.0
LH	1.17±0.83	1.49 ± 0.69	1.25 ± 0.37	2.27[a] ± 0.63[a]	+ 0.43 ± 0.43
PRL	38.67±9.16	52.01 ±17.22	51.15 ±18.93	51.76 ±21.15[a]	61.71[b] ±10.56

[a]$p<0.04$.
[b]$p<0.003$.

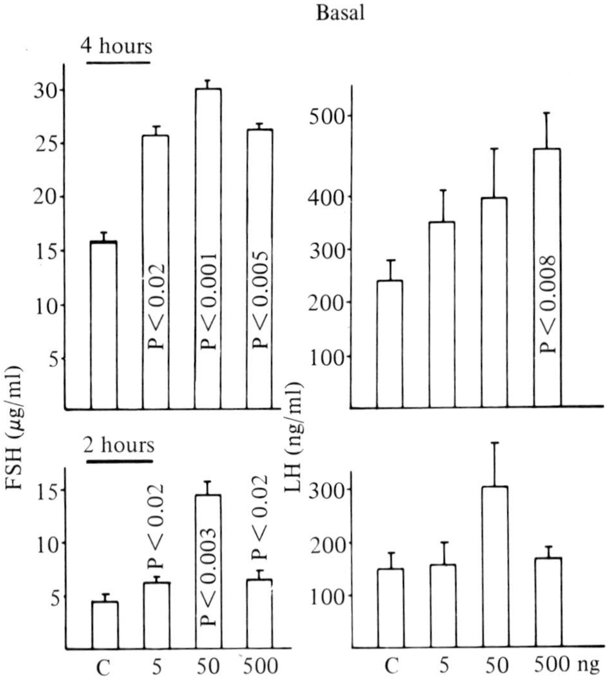

Fig. 5 Incubation of the nonapeptide with rat pituitaries *in vitro*. Increases in levels of FSH and LH after 2 hours and 4 hours are apparent.

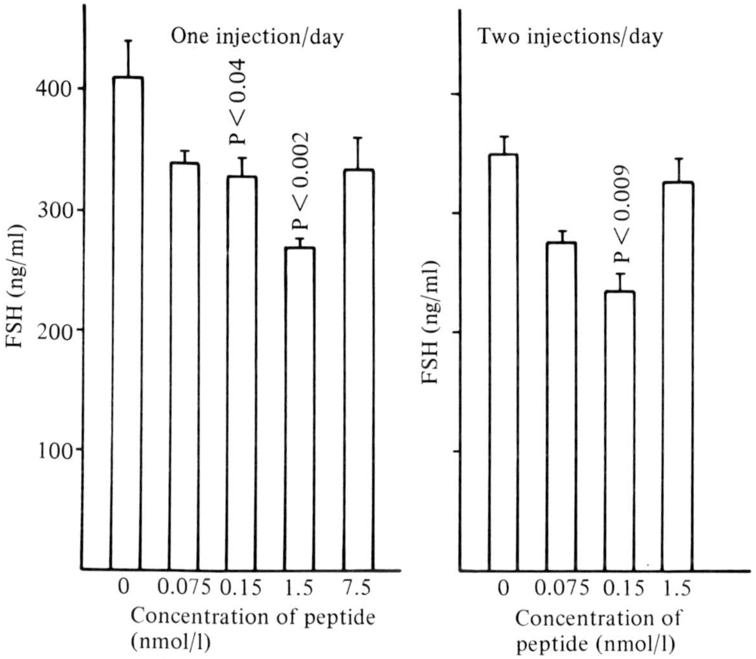

Fig. 6 Effect of the decapeptide on levels of FSH when administered (once or twice a day) to adult male rats.

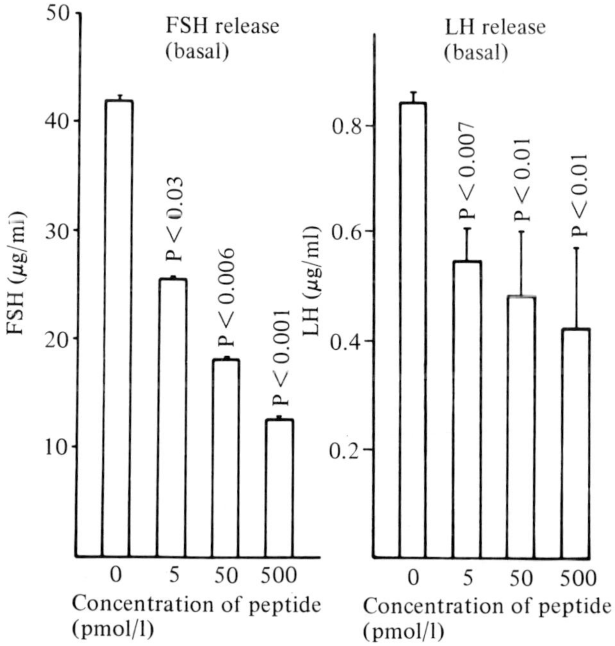

Fig. 7 Effects of the decapeptide on release of FSH and LH from rat pituitaries at 4 hours *in vitro*.

larger proteins and may not cause formation of antibodies even after long-term usage.

The design and synthesis of analogs of the decapeptide, with a view to increasing the potency of the FSH-suppressing activity, are in progress.

References

Beksac, M.S., Khan, S.A., Elissaon, R., Skakkabaek, N.E., Sheth, A.R. & Diczfalusy, E. (1984). Evidence for the prostatic origin of immunoreactive inhibin-like material in human seminal plasma. **International Journal of Andrology** 7:389–392.

de Jong, F.H. (1988). Inhibin. **Physiological Review** 168(2):555–600.

Hurkadli, K.S., Mahale, S.D., Iyer, K.S.N. & Sheth, A.R. (1989). Enhancement of *in vitro* release of FSH from rat pituitaries by a synthetic nonapeptide fragment of human seminal plasma inhibin. **Life Sciences** 45:1357–1363.

Iyer, K.S.N., Mahale, S.D., Hurkadli, K.S. & Sheth, A.R. (1987). Preferential elevation of the levels of follitropin by a synthetic carboxy-terminal nonapeptide 86–94 of human seminal plasma inhibin. **Indian Journal of Experimental Biology** 25:742–744.

Iyer, K.S.N., Mahale, S.D., Hurkadli, K.S. & Sheth, A.R. (1989). A synthetic decapeptide analogue of human seminal plasma inhibin exhibiting specific suppression of follicle-stimulating hormone release in rats. **Indian Journal of Experimental Biology** 27:10–13.

Sathe, V.S., Sheth, N.A., Sheth, A.R. & Phadke, M.A. (1987) Biosynthesis and localization of inhibin in human prostate. **The Prostate** 10:33–40.

Sheth, A.R., Vanage, G.R., Hurkadli, K.S. & Sheth, N.A. (1984). Role of the prostate in the regulation of pituitary secretion of follicle-stimulating hormone. **Medical Hypotheses** 15:141–148.

Transforming growth factor beta and related peptides: a role in testicular intercellular communication

M. BENAHMED, C. SORDOILLET, D.J. HARTMANN,[1] G. ESPOSITO, C. COCHET,[2] E. TABONE,[3] E. DE PERETTI, M.A. CHAUVIN AND A.M. MORERA

Groupe de Recherches sur les Communications Cellulaires, Laboratoire de Biochimie, l'Hopital Sainte Eugenie, Centre Hospitalier, Lyon-Sud 69310, Pierre-Bénite, France. [1]*Centre de Radioanalyse, Institut Pasteur, Lyon, France.* [2]*INSERM U.244 CENG, Grenoble, France.* [3]*Centre Léon Berard, Lyon, France.*

Keywords

Transforming growth factor-β, TGF-β-related peptides, gonadal maturation, differentiation, Sertoli cells, Leydig cells, peritubular myoid cells, para-autocrine regulation, steroid hormones, lactate, extracellular matrix components.

Introduction

Fertility in the male is dependent upon the daily production of a vast number of competent spermatozoa via the complex process of spermatogenesis. It has been known for decades that spermatogenesis depends upon a functional neuroendocrine system. Neurons of the extrahypothalamic central nervous system influence the hypothalamic secretion of gonadotropin-releasing hormone (GnRH) which modulates the secretion of luteinizing hormone (LH) and follicle-stimulating hormone (FSH) from the pituitary. There is general agreement that, in mammalian testes, the neuroendocrine control of spermatogenesis appears to be mediated via the action of hormones on gonadal somatic cells without any direct action on germ cells (Fritz, 1978, 1985; Fritz and Tung, 1986); LH acts directly only on Leydig cells, while FSH acts directly only on Sertoli cells, as evaluated by the capacity of these gonadotropins to bind to specific receptors on the membranes of their respective target cells (Catt *et al.*, 1980; Payne *et al.*, 1982). Testosterone (produced by Leydig cells after stimulation by LH), which is essential for spermatogenesis and fertility (Steinberger *et al.*, 1973), acts directly on peritubular myoid cells (Skinner and Fritz, 1984) and probably to a lesser extent on Sertoli cells, but it does not bind specifically to germ cells (Fritz and Tung, 1986). Although the exact mechanisms by which the (hormonally regulated) gonadal somatic cells influence spermatogenesis remain to be elucidated, it is likely that multiple intercellular interactions are required to create a unique cytoarchitectural and physicochemical microenvironment within mammalian seminiferous tubules.

Testicular intercellular communication

Gonadal intercellular interactions may occur both between somatic cells and between somatic and germ cells. Intercellular interactions between somatic cells involve mainly: (1) Sertoli cells that form the seminiferous tubule which provides the cytoarchitectural support for germ cells; (2) peritubular myoid cells, which are positioned between Sertoli and Leydig cells and surround the seminiferous tubules; and (3) Leydig cells which are present in the vascular interstitial tissue. Intercellular interactions between somatic and germ cells involve mainly Sertoli cells and germ cells within the seminiferous tubule.

Intercellular interactions can occur in a number of different ways (Fig. 1), as follows.

1. The formation of components of the extracellular matrix (ECM). The ECM is composed of four main classes of compounds: elastin and collagen molecules, other glycoproteins (e.g. fibronectin, laminin) and proteoglycans (Kleinman *et al.*, 1981). The essential importance of the ECM in cellular functions has been recognized only recently (Buck and Horwitz, 1987). In the testis, peritubular myoid and Sertoli cells cooperate in the formation and deposition of components of the ECM present in the basal lamina. Primary or secondary cultures of peritubular myoid cells synthesize and secrete fibronectin, collagen I and IV, and chondroitin sulfate, while primary cultures of Sertoli cells produce laminin, collagen IV and heparin sulfate but not fibronectin and collagen I (Tung and Fritz, 1980; Skinner and Fritz, 1984) However, although peritubular myoid and Sertoli cells are the main cells that produce components of the ECM, other types of testicular cell, such as Leydig cells, also produce these components (Tabone *et al.*, 1989). The list of components of the ECM identified in the testis is growing but the mechanisms of action of such components in cellular interactions remain to be elucidated.
2. The formation and secretion of diffusible nutritional factors for the survival of neighboring cells. In the testis, Sertoli and germ cells are involved in such interactions. The nutritional role of Sertoli cells has been postulated since the first description of these cells (Sertoli, 1865). Sertoli cells have been shown to produce and secrete: (a) the bioenergetic metabolites, e.g. pyruvate and lactate (Robinson and Fritz, 1981), that are used by germ cells (Jutte *et al.*, 1981); and (b) the proteins involved in transport of iron and copper to germ cells, namely, transferrin and ceruloplasmin (Skinner, 1987).
3. The formation and secretion of diffusible regulatory factors that induce a cellular response linked to cell differentiation and/or growth. Several types of molecule involved in these interactions have been identified: (a) steroid hormones, namely, estradiol (Van der Molen and Rommerts, 1981) and testosterone (Adashi and Hsueh, 1981); (b)

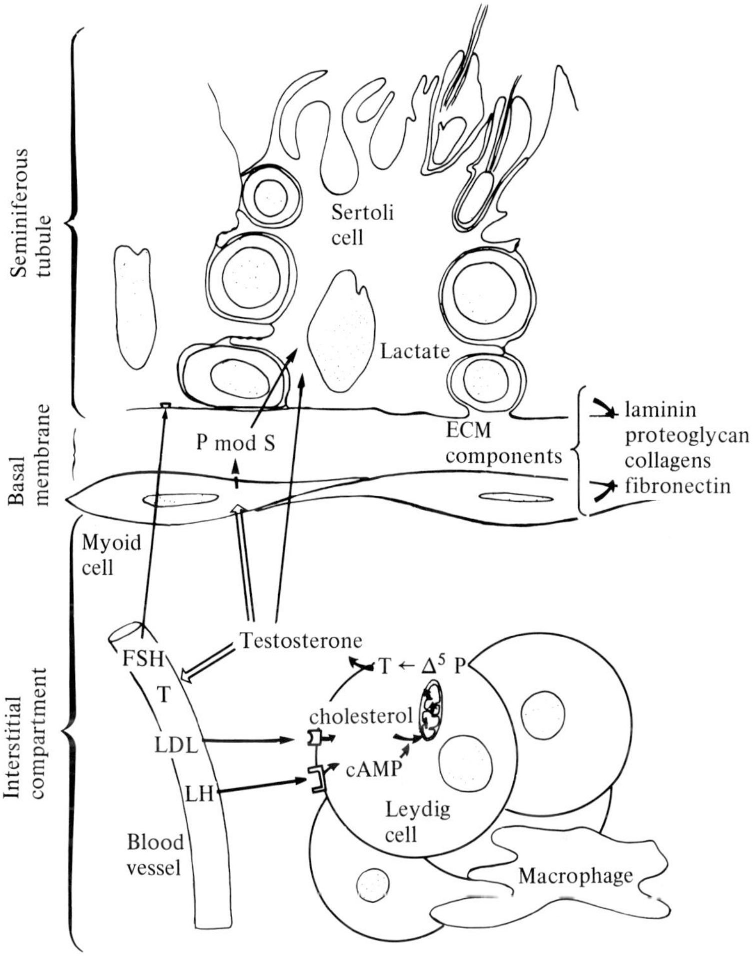

Fig. 1 Summary of the local control of testicular somatic functions by different factors. For details, see the text.

polypeptide growth factors, such as insulin-like growth factors (IGFs) (Ritzen, 1983; Lin *et al.*, 1986; Benahmed *et al.*, 1987a; Morera *et al.*, 1987b; Smith *et al.*, 1987), fibroblast growth factor (FGF) (Ueno *et al.*, 1987; Sordoillet *et al.*, 1988), epidermal growth factor (EGF)-like activity (Ascoli, 1981; Hsueh *et al.*, 1981; Elson *et al.*, 1984; Verhoeven and Cailleau, 1986), Sertoli cell growth factor (Bellvé and Feig, 1984); (c) different peptides, such as β-endorphin (Tsong *et al.*, 1982; Fabbri and Dufau, 1988) angiotensin II (Khanum and Dufau, 1988) and arginine–vasopressin (Kasson *et al.*, 1986; Tahri-Joutei and Pointis, 1988); and (d) uncharacterized factors

(Grotjan and Heindel, 1982; Bergh, 1983; Sharpe, 1984, 1986; Syed *et al.*, 1985; Janecki *et al.*, 1985; Verhoeven and Cailleau, 1985; Rommerts *et al.*, 1986; Benahmed *et al.*, 1985, 1987b; Khan *et al.*, 1988; Carreau *et al.*, 1988; Jegou *et al.*, 1989).

The recently available methods for the separation of cells (Meistrich *et al.*, 1981; Mather and Phillips, 1984; Rommerts *et al.*, 1985) have led to the preparation of highly purified populations of cells from the testis. A high degree of purity in populations of cultured cells is required for the study of the site of synthesis and the site of action of the components involved in the different types of intercellular interaction.

In this chapter, using as a model porcine immature (3-week-old) somatic testicular cells (Leydig, peritubular myoid, and Sertoli cells), cultured in a defined medium (Benahmed *et al.*, 1985, 1986), we show that transforming growth factor-β (TGF-β) (and its gonadal related peptides) represent a family of polypeptides that is involved in the different types of intercellular communication within the testis.

TGF-β and related peptides

The biology and structure of TGF-β and its related peptides have been discussed recently in several reviews (Lawrence *et al.*, 1985; Goustin *et al.*, 1986; Sporn *et al.*, 1986, 1987; Massague *et al.*, 1987; Massague, 1987; Roberts *et al.*, 1988) and, consequently, we shall only summarize the information that seems most relevant to our current discussion. TGF-β has been shown to have widespread effects on growth, differentiation, embryogenesis, and tissue repair.

TGF-β influences the rate of proliferation of many types of cell, acting as an inhibitor of the growth of most types of cell and, in particular, of epithelial cells. Indeed, although TGF-β was originally assayed by its ability to stimulate proliferation of normal rat kidney (NRK) fibroblasts in soft agar, it was shown to be virtually identical to a growth inhibitor identified in medium conditioned by monkey kidney cells (Holley *et al.*, 1980). Subsequently, inhibitory effects of TGF-β on growth of numerous lines of neoplastic and non-neoplastic cells, both in monolayer and in soft agar (Sporn *et al.*, 1987), have been described.

In cells of mesenchymal origin, TGF-β stimulates or inhibits proliferation, depending on the presence of other growth factors operant in these cells, e.g. platelet-derived growth factor (PDGF), FGF and EGF. Although the mechanisms underlying the antiproliferative action of TGF-β remain unknown, this factor can block the mitogenic action of PDGF, EGF, FGF and interleukin-1 on specific types of cell (Sporn *et al.*, 1986).

In addition to its action on their growth, TGF-β may affect the differentiation of cells both in an inhibitory and a stimulatory manner; TGF-β has an inhibitory action on the adipogenic differentiation of 3T3 fibroblasts and influences the function of immune cells, the differentiation of epithelial cells, myogenesis, osteogenesis, and chondrogenesis (Deuel, 1987). TGF-β is also a potent regulator of steroidogenesis in corticoadrenal cells (Hotta and Baird, 1986; Feige *et al.*, 1987) and ovarian granulosa cells (Adashi and Resnick, 1986; Dodson and Schomberg, 1987; Knecht *et al.*, 1987). Furthermore, TGF-β stimulates the transport of both glucose (Inman and Colowick, 1985) and amino acids, and glycolysis (Boerner *et al.*, 1985) in fibroblasts.

One major finding relevant to the importance of TGF-β is its effect on the formation of extracellular matrix; TGF-β has recently been found to be a potent regulator of the expression of certain components of the ECM, including fibronectin, type I collagen, various forms of chondroitin/dermatan sulfate proteoglycan, as well as of the expression of the cell adhesion proteins (integrins) (Ignotz and Massague, 1986). Another action of TGF-β related to enhanced formation of the ECM is its ability to inhibit the proteolytic degradation of matrix proteins. The action of TGF-β on components of the ECM is of major importance with respect to the role of these components in embryonic development and tumorigenesis.

TGF-β is the prototype of a large family of structurally related, multifunctional, dimeric proteins. Within this family, there is a group of variants of TGF-β which are disulfide-linked dimers of 25 kDa. TGF-β1 and TGF-β2 are produced as precursors of 391 and 414 amino acids, respectively. The existence of a precursor polypeptide of 391 amino acids was predicted from cDNA cloning of the human gene for TGF-β, transcribed as a 2.5-kb mRNA (Derynck *et al.*, 1985). The homodimers of the C-terminal 112 residues of TGF-β1 and TGF-β2 represent the biologically active forms of these proteins, and coexpression of the TGF-β1 and TGF-β2 polypeptide chains in the same cell can give rise to the heterodimer TGF-β1,2 which has been found, to date, only in porcine platelets. Recently, TGF-β3, another member of the family of TGF-β2, has been identified both in human tissue (Ten Dijke *et al.*, 1988) and in chick embryos (Jakowlew *et al.*, 1988). The similarities among the members of the TGF-β family reside in the C-terminal, cysteine-rich portion of the precursor proteins and all family members have an identical carboxy-terminus, namely, cys-X-cys-X-COOH. TGF-β1 represents the form of TGF-β that was originally isolated from human platelets. TGF-β2, present in porcine but not in human platelets, is less abundant and represents 15–20% of the total TGF-β. TGF is secreted by virtually all types of cell in a biologically inactive form (Lawrence *et al.*, 1984; Pircher *et al.*, 1984). The latent form may be activated by various treatments that involve acidic, alkaline or chaotropic agents (Lawrence *et al.*, 1985) and by plasmin and cathepsin D (Lyons *et al.*, 1988). The activation of the latent form of TGF-β may represent a crucial step in the action of this peptide (Lawrence *et al.*, 1985; Pircher *et al.*, 1986).

TGF-β1 and TGF-β2 bind with high affinity (with values of Ka in the picomolar range) to three distinct components on the surface of target cells

(Massague *et al.*, 1987). Type I receptors for TGF-β are identified as an affinity-labeled complex of 65 kDa; type II receptors yield an affinity-labeled complex of 85, 95, or 110 kDa, depending upon the species; and type III receptors are dimers, the monomers of which have apparent molecular weights of 250–350 kDa (Cheifetz *et al.*, 1987). The type III receptor appears to be a proteoglycan since it contains chains of heparin sulfate and chondroitin sulfate (Segarini and Seyedin, 1988). Type I and type II receptors have higher affinity for TGF-β1 than for TGF-β2, whereas type III receptors have similar high affinity for TGF-β1 and TGF-β2 (Cheifetz *et al.*, 1987; Massague *et al.*, 1987). Whether the three different types of receptor for TGF-β are involved in mediation of the individual actions of the various forms of TGF-βs still remains an unresolved question.

The TGF-β family has been extended to include certain gonadal factors, such as inhibins, activins (Mason *et al.*, 1985; Vale *et al.*, 1986; Ling *et al.*, 1986) and anti-Mullerian hormone/Mullerian inhibiting substance (AMH/MIS) (Cate *et al.*, 1986; Picard *et al.*, 1986). Several recent reviews have been devoted to the biology and structure of inhibins (Rivier *et al.*, 1987; Franchimont, 1987; Ying, 1988; McLachlan *et al.*, 1988). Inhibins were purified from ovarian follicular fluid of several species and their structures have been deduced by molecular cloning techniques. Although inhibins from follicular fluid have been estimated to have different high molecular weights, the 32-kDa form is probably the biologically active form and the final product of proteolytic cleavage of the precursor to the α-subunit, as postulated by McLachlan *et al.* (1988).

Inhibins A and B are heterodimers with identical α-subunits (18 kDa) linked to different β-subunits (βA, βB, 14 kDa). Activins A and AB are dimers resulting from the association of two βA-subunits (Vale *et al.*, 1986) or the association of βA- and βB-subunits (Ling *et al.*, 1986).

The mature α- and β-subunits are structurally related to each other; the mature subunit of inhibin possesses seven cysteine residues whereas the β-subunits have nine cysteine residues, seven of which can be aligned with those of the α-subunit. In addition to a 70% similarity in primary sequence between βA- and βB-subunits, the pattern of distribution of the nine cysteine residues in the inhibin β-subunit is similar to that in TGF-β; this positional conservation of the cysteine residues is also apparent in the carboxy-terminal portion of AMH/MIS (Cate *et al.*, 1986; Picard *et al.*, 1986).

The male gonad as a site of production of TGF-β

Production of TGF-β by Sertoli cells was indicated by the detection of TGF-β activity in conditioned media from these cells and by the presence of mRNA specific for TGF-β in Sertoli cells. TGF-β activity in medium conditioned by Sertoli cells was characterized mainly by two criteria: (1) stimulation of anchorage-independent growth of two lines of mesenchymal cells (normal rat kidney cells and rat fibroblasts); and (2) displacement of TGF-β from its receptor (Benahmed *et al.*, 1988). The competition for TGF-β receptors is highly specific for TGF-β, as shown by the inability of several growth factors, including EGF, FGF, PDGF, IGF-1, and related gonadal peptides (activins, inhibins) (Massague *et al.*, 1987), to displace TGF-β from its receptors.

The production of TGF-β by Sertoli cells was further confirmed by the expression of the TGF-β gene in these cells. We have detected a 2.5-kb transcript of the TGF-β gene in the population of poly(A)$^+$ RNA from immature porcine Sertoli cells using the method of RNA transfer-blot hybridization (unpublished data).

Taking advantage of the radioreceptor assay, we have studied the regulation of secretion of TGF-β from Sertoli cells. After 48 hours of treatment with FSH, the secretion of receptor-reactive TGF-β (rrTGF-β) by cultured Sertoli cells was decreased in a dose-dependent manner. The maximal (>80% decrease) and half-maximal inhibitory effects on the secretion of rrTGF-β were observed with 10 ng/ml and 4.2 ng/ml FSH, respectively. A similar suppressive effect observed with 8-bromo-cyclic AMP (10^{-3} mol/l) on the secretion of rrTGF-β suggests that this effect of FSH might be exerted via the cAMP pathway (Benahmed *et al.*, 1988).

In contrast with the above results, 2 days of treatment of porcine Sertoli cells with estradiol (10^{-7} mol/l), dexamethasone (10^{-7} mol/l) or thyroxine (10^{-7} mol/l) resulted in an increase in the release of rrTGF-β. However, the suppressive action of FSH on the release of rrTGF-β seems to be predominant since the stimulatory effects of estradiol, dexamethasone and thyroxin were not observed in the presence of FSH. The findings suggest that cultures of Sertoli cells may prove a system suitable for investigating: (1) the hormonal regulation of secretion of TGF-β as well as transcription of its mRNA; and (2) the activation of the latent form of TGF-β. Indeed, although the rrTGF-β was measured after acidification, preliminary data indicate the presence of bioactive TGF-β in non-acidified conditioned medium from Sertoli cells, suggesting, therefore, the possible activation *in situ* of latent TGF-β.

TGF-β appears to be produced by the other somatic testicular cells. We have detected a 2.5-kb transcript of the TGF-β gene in poly(A)$^+$ RNA from porcine Leydig and myoid peritubular cells (unpublished data).

The male gonad as a site of action of TGF-β (and related peptides)

Let us now consider the actions of TGF-β and related peptides on the three different classes of somatic testicular cells, i.e. the Leydig, Sertoli, and peritubular myoid cells.

The role of TGF-β on the morphology and proliferation of Leydig cells

After treatment with TGF-β (1 ng/ml for 48 hours), Leydig cells lost their rounded shape and became more elongated, with a 'fibroblastic' appearance

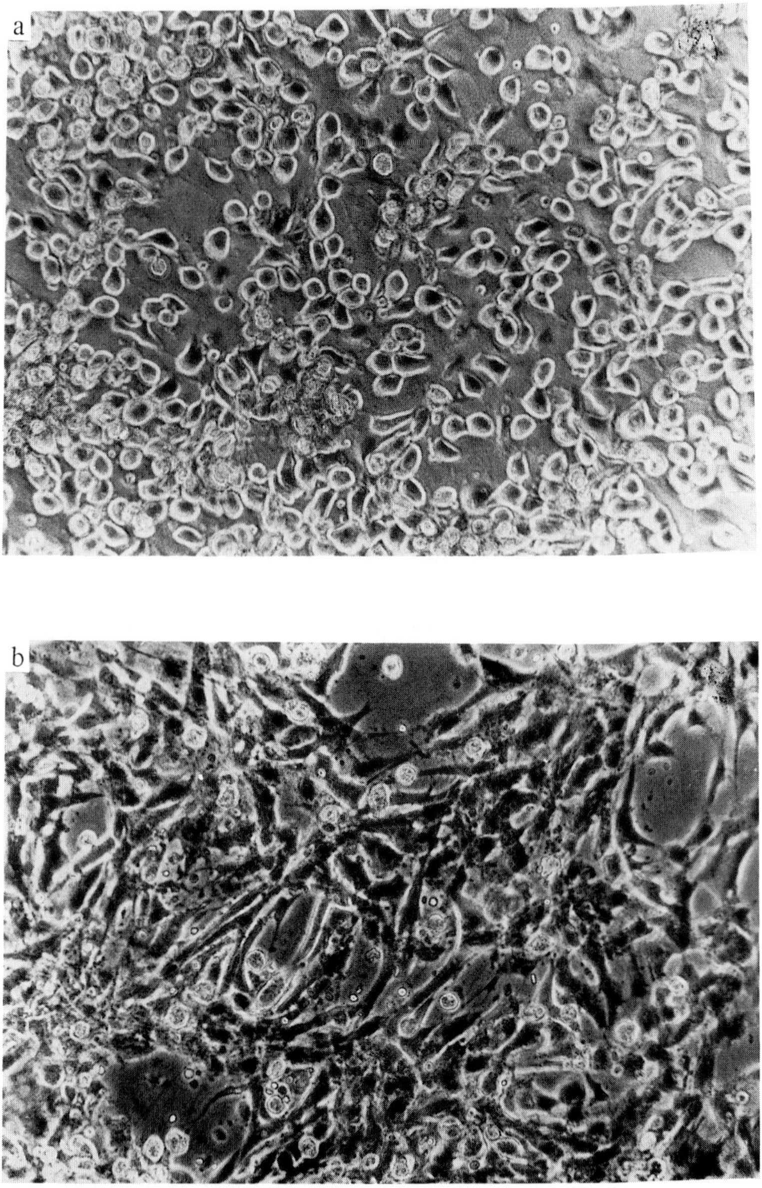

Fig. 2 Effects of TGF-β on the morphology of Leydig cells. Leydig cells were cultured for 48 hours in the absence (a) or presence (b) of TGF-β (1 ng/ml).

(Fig. 2). The proliferation of Leydig cells cultured in a chemically (serum-free) defined medium was not affected by TGF-β under any of the different sets of conditions presented here.

The role of TGF-β in the differentiation of Leydig cells

In the testis, Leydig cells are the principal source of androgens. The steroidogenic activity of Leydig cells depends on the stimulatory effect of LH. This gonadotropin controls steroidogenesis in Leydig cells via interactions with specific membrane receptors which initiate a sequence of interrelated events at the membrane and within the cell. Stimulation of the androgen pathway involves binding of LH to its specific plasma-membrane receptors, LH-induced binding of guanyl nucleotides, phosphorylation of membrane proteins, and activation of adenylate cyclase with formation of cAMP. Subsequently, cAMP-dependent protein kinase probably causes phosphorylation of some key proteins of the steroidogenic pathway and a consequent increase in the production of testosterone (Catt *et al.*, 1980; Dufau *et al.*, 1987).

In this regard, to appreciate the action of TGF-β on the differentiation of Leydig cells, the effects of TGF-β on several key biochemical steps, including binding of LH to receptors, formation of cAMP, and secretion of testosterone, have been studied.

Effects of TGF-β on binding of LH/hCG

TGF-β (0–10 ng/ml, 76 hours) inhibited binding of LH/human chorionic gonadotropin (hCG) with an ID_{50} of 0.2 ng/ml (Morera *et al.*, 1987b, 1988). The decrease in binding of LH/hCG was related to a decrease in the number of receptors for LH rather than to a decrease in the binding affinity (not shown). This inhibition was observed after 24 hours and was maximal after 48 hours of treatment with TGF-β (1 ng/ml) (Morera *et al.*, 1987a, 1988), a result that, therefore, excludes any direct interaction between TGF-β and LH at the level of gonadotropin receptor. Furthermore, although binding of LH/hCG was enhanced by IGF-1 (or insulin) (Lin *et al.*, 1986; Benahmed *et al.*, 1987a; Morera *et al.*, 1987b) and PDGF, the inhibitory action of TGF-β remained predominant in the presence of these factors (Fig. 3). The mechanisms underlying the decrease in the number of receptors for LH/hCG after treatment with TGF-β are, as yet, unknown.

The effect of TGF-β on adenylate cyclase activity

Both in rat (Lin *et al.*, 1987) and porcine cultured Leydig cells, TGF-β inhibited the hCG-stimulated formation of cAMP (not shown). Additional studies will be required to determine whether TGF-β influences the stimulatory or the inhibitory regulatory proteins in the membrane or the catalytic unit of adenylate cyclase, or combinations thereof and/or cAMP phosphodiesterase activity.

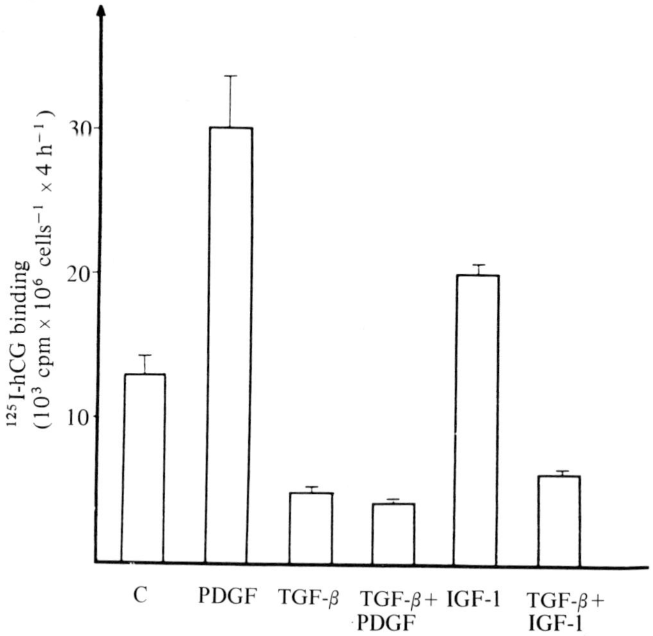

Fig. 3 The inhibitory effect of TGF-β on binding of LH/hCG. Leydig cells were cultured in the presence or absence of TGF-β (1 ng/ml, for 48 hours) alone or in combination with human platelet-derived growth factor (PDGF; 5 ng/ml) or insulin-like growth factor 1 (IGF-1; 100 ng/ml). The cells were then washed, and binding of LH/hCG was evaluated by incubating cells for 4 hours in the presence of saturating concentrations of ^{125}I-hCG. After several washings, Leydig cells were solubilized with NaOH-deoxycholate.

The effect of TGF-β on the secretion of steroid hormones

The biosynthesis from pregnenolone of testosterone, the major biologically important steroid produced by Leydig cells, occurs via several Δ5 intermediates (involving pregnenolone, 17α-hydroxypregnenolone, dehydroepiandrosterone and Δ5 androstene-3β-17β-diol) as well as several Δ4 intermediates (progesterone, 17α-hydroxyprogesterone, 4-androstene 3,17-dione) (Van der Molen and Rommerts, 1981). The testicular rate of conversion of pregnenolone through the Δ5 and Δ4 pathway depends upon the species. In contrast to the case in the rat, in both the human and the porcine testes, the Δ5 pathway appears to be the most significant, i.e. testosterone is synthesized via pregnenolone, dehydroepiandrosterone (DHEA) and Δ4 androstene-3, 17-dione.

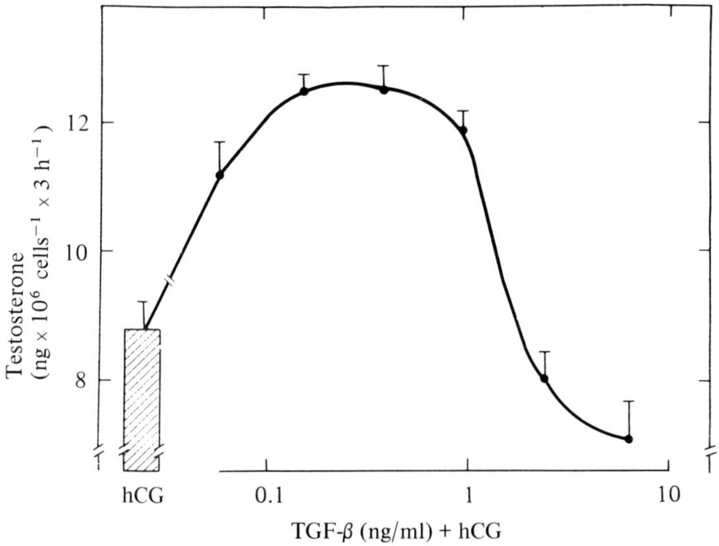

Fig. 4 The effect of TGF-β on the hCG-stimulated secretion of testosterone. Leydig cells were incubated with increasing concentrations of TGF-β (0–6.25 ng/ml) for 48 hours. The cells were then washed and incubated for 3 hours in the presence of hCG (1 ng/ml); production of testosterone was measured in the medium by a specific radioimmunoassay (Forest *et al.*, 1973).

The action of TGF-β was studied at both the level of DHEA and testosterone. Treatment of cultured porcine Leydig cells with increasing concentrations of TGF-β (0–2.5 ng/ml, for 48 hours) results in an inhibitory effect on secretion of DHEA in the medium, with a maximal decrease of 77% and an ID_{50} of 0.2 ng/ml TGF-β (Morera *et al.*, 1988). This inhibitory effect of TGF-β was observed in the case of both basal and stimulated secretion of DHEA with all concentrations of hCG tested. In contrast, the same treatment led to a biphasic effect on levels of stimulated secretion of testosterone. The effect was both stimulatory and inhibitory and depended on the concentration of TGF-β, as shown in Figure 4; treatment of Leydig cells with the maximally efficient concentration of hCG (1 ng/ml) and TGF-β in a range of low concentrations (0.06–0.4 ng/ml) resulted in an increase in the action of hCG with a maximal stimulatory effect of 43 ±2.4% observed with 0.16 ng/ml TGF-β. However, at high concentrations of TGF-β (1–6 ng/ml) this enhancement of the action of hCG disappeared and was completely suppressed by TGF-β at a concentration of 2.5 ng/ml. Conversely, in Leydig cells, TGF-β (1 ng/ml, for 48 hours) had an inhibitory effect on the secretion of testosterone stimulated by low concentrations of hCG (0.01–0.1 ng/ml), while

TGF-β had a stimulatory effect on the secretion of testosterone in the presence of high concentrations of hCG (0.3–5 ng/ml).

Both the potent inhibitory effect of TGF-β on the secretion of DHEA and its biphasic effect on the secretion of testosterone were observed when Leydig cells were stimulated with 8-bromo-cAMP (10^{-3} mol/l) instead of hCG and also when they were cultured in the presence of cholesterol that was bound to low-density lipoproteins (LDL). Indeed, although LDL cholesterol at saturating concentrations (100 μg protein/ml, for 24 hours) remained effective in terms of its ability to increase by two- to threefold the synthesis of DHEA and testosterone both in the presence and absence of TGF-β (1 ng/ml, for 48 hours), the lipoprotein cholesterol was unable to prevent the inhibitory effect of TGF-β on secretion of DHEA as well as its biphasic effect on the secretion of testosterone. Taken together, these findings suggest that the steroidogenic action of TGF-β is effected at a level distal to cyclic AMP and is unlikely to involve an inhibition of the metabolism of cholesterol (LDL).

The potent inhibitory action of TGF-β on basal and hCG-stimulated secretion of DHEA, coupled to the biphasic action of this factor on hCG-stimulated secretion of testosterone, led us to hypothesize that TGF-β may exert a dual control on levels of DHEA: it decreases the formation of DHEA and increases the breakdown of DHEA into testosterone.

In order to study whether TGF-β decreases the rate of formation of DHEA, use was made of a compound, WIN 24540, capable of rapid inhibition of the catabolism of DHEA into testosterone, via blockage of 3β-hydroxysteroid dehydrogenase/isomerase activity (Neumann *et al.*, 1970). Leydig cells cultured in the presence of TGF-β (1 ng/ml, for 48 hours) and WIN 24540 at a concentration of 10^{-5} mol/l (which completely blocks the production of testosterone) exhibit a decrease in both basal and hCG-stimulated secretion of DHEA and pregnenolone, while the conversion of pregnenolone into DHEA was not affected. These findings indicate that the decrease in the rates of secretion of DHEA (and other Δ5 steroids) after treatment with TGF-β was related to a decrease in the rate of formation of pregnenolone.

In contrast to the results just described, the transformation of Δ5 steroid hormones (e.g. pregnenolone) but not of Δ4 steroid hormones (e.g. progesterone) into testosterone was increased in Leydig cells treated with TGF-β (1 ng/ml, for 48 hours). These findings support the concept that TGF-β is a potent stimulator of 3β-hydroxysteroid dehydrogenase/isomerase activity. The increase in the activity of the enzyme was further confirmed by the increase in the rate of conversion of DHEA and Δ5 androstenediol but not of Δ4 androstenedione into testosterone (Fig. 5). TGF-β increased, in a dose-dependent manner, the activity of 3β-hydroxysteroid dehydrogenase/isomerase (reflected by the conversion of DHEA into Δ4 androstenedione) and the maximum effect was obtained with 0.16 ng/ml of TGF-β (Benahmed *et al.*, 1989).

Taken together, these findings indicate that TGF-β affects the production of testosterone in Leydig cells predominantly at two levels.

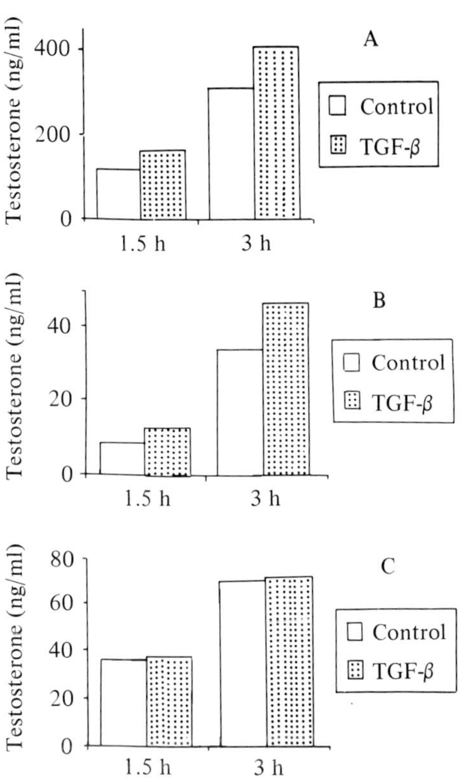

Fig. 5 The effect of TGF-β on the conversion of various steroid hormones into testosterone. Leydig cells were cultured for 48 hours in the absence (open squares) or in the presence (stippled squares) of TGF-β (1 ng/ml). The cells were then washed and incubated for 1.5 and 3 hours in the presence of Δ5 androstenediol (Δ5 diol) (A), DHEA (B) or Δ4 androstenedione (Δ4 dione) (C) and the conversion of these steroids into testosterone was measured by radioimmunoassay of testosterone in the culture medium.

1. TGF-β enhances the activity of 3β-hydroxysteroid dehydrogenase/isomerase activity, a key enzyme in the maturation of Leydig cells. Whether TGF-β controls the expression of the enzyme at the level of transcription or at post-transcriptional levels remains to be elucidated.
2. TGF-β decreases the formation of pregnenolone and the ability of 25-OH cholesterol, but not of LDL cholesterol, to reverse the inhibitory effect of TGF-β, a result that suggests that TGF-β acts before the association between cholesterol and cholesterol side-chain cleavage cytochrome P450 in the mitochondria.

Finally, in Leydig cells treated with TGF-β and LH/hCG, the accumulation of testosterone is the result of, at least, three different effects: (1) the increase in formation of pregnenolone following short-term treatment (3 hours) with hCG; (2) the decrease in formation of pregnenolone following treatment with high concentrations of TGF-β; and (3) the increase in 3β-hydroxysteroid dehydrogenase/isomerase activity that follows all treatment with all concentrations of TGF-β tested. We know that these effects of TGF-β are exerted directly on Leydig cells since we have shown (Morera *et al.*, 1988) that Leydig cells, affinity-labeled with ^{125}I-TGF-β, exhibit a major band of approximately 280 kDa which has the properties of a type III receptor for TGF-β, as defined by Cheifetz *et al.* (1987).

Interactions between TGF-β and other testicular factors in the control of steroidogenesis

The action of TGF-β on the differentiation of Leydig cells is modulated by several factors which include not only growth factors, as reported for effects of TGF-β on cell growth, but also extracellular matrix components. While the inhibitory effect of TGF-β on steroidogenesis in Leydig cells was not affected by FGF, such an effect was not observed in the presence of EGF. However, fibronectin alone, or in combination with collagen IV, amplifies the inhibitory action of TGF-β by decreasing the ID_{50} for secretion of steroid hormones (in preparation). Because these factors are secreted in the testis, these findings imply that the study of the local action of TGF-β must take into account both the secretion and the regulation of synthesis of other growth factors as well as components of the ECM.

Effects of TGF-β and a factor secreted by Sertoli cells (SCAIF) on the activity of Leydig cells

In the same gel-filtration fraction (mol. wt 20–30 kDa) from dialyzed and concentrated medium that had been conditioned by growth of Sertoli cells in which we found the receptor-reactive TGF-β, we have also found a potent inhibitor of the differentiated functions of Leydig cells, i.e. binding of LH/hCG and hCG-stimulated secretion of steroid hormones (Benahmed *et al.*, 1986). These findings raised the question of whether this factor, called SCAIF (for Sertoli cell androgenic inhibiting factor), and TGF-β are similar or closely related. Although a pure fraction of SCAIF is not yet available, we have compared the effects of pure porcine TGF-β and of a gel-filtration fraction of SCAIF, on Leydig cells. Our results indicated that SCAIF was more efficient in inhibiting binding of LH/hCG (Fig. 6) and on secretion of DHEA (data not shown) than was TGF-β. The maximal decrease in binding of LH/hCG was 75% and 40% in the presence of SCAIF and TGF-β, respectively (Fig. 6). SCAIF and TGF-β are probably closely related or very similar; the difference in the potencies of their inhibitory actions may be due to the fact that we

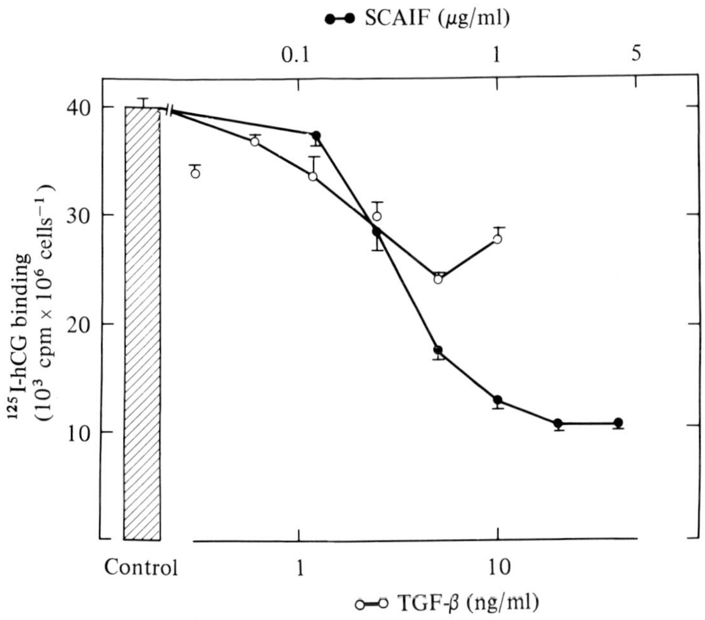

Fig. 6 Effect of SCAIF (Sertoli cell androgenic inhibiting factor) and TGF-β on binding of LH/hCG to Leydig cells. Leydig cells were incubated with various concentrations, up to 0.5 μg/ml, of SCAIF (closed circles) or increasing concentrations of TGF-β, 0–10 ng/ml (open circles) for 48 hours. The cells were then washed, and binding of LH/hCG was evaluated as described in the legend to Figure 2.

compared the effects of a partially purified preparation of SCAIF with that of pure TGF-β. Since TGF-β can act in opposite ways depending on the presence of other factors, it is tempting to speculate that the preparation of SCAIF contains, in addition to TGF-β, another factor(s) that can amplify the inhibitory effects. Furthermore, the likelihood that SCAIF and TGF-β are similar or closely related is strengthened by our previous demonstration that secretion of both SCAIF (Benahmed *et al.*, 1986) and TGF-β (Benahmed *et al.*, 1988) by Sertoli cells is similarly suppressed by FSH. However, further experiments are needed to determine the nature of SCAIF before we can conclude definitively that SCAIF is identical to TGF-β or that it is a separate factor.

The role of TGF-β in Sertoli cells

In immature cultured porcine Sertoli cells, lactate is produced in amounts similar to those reported in the case of rat Sertoli cells and the production is similarly regulated by FSH and insulin (Mita *et al.*, 1982; Grootegoed *et al.*, 1987).

Addition of TGF-β to cultured porcine Sertoli cells had a biphasic effect on the secretion of lactate. After a brief treatment (0–24 hours) with TGF-β, secretion of lactate was stimulated, whereas after long-term pretreatment (24–72 hours) with TGF-β, secretion of lactate was inhibited. The stimulatory action of FSH on the production of lactate was modified by TGF-β. Short-term treatment with TGF-β slightly increased (but in a non-additive manner) the action of the gonadotropin on the secretion of lactate. However, after a long-term treatment of the cells with TGF-β, the effect of FSH on the production of lactate was dramatically decreased at all concentrations of FSH tested (12.5–3000 ng/ml) (Esposito *et al.*, 1990).

The biochemical mechanisms involved in both the stimulatory and inhibitory effects of TGF-β remain unknown. However, the short-term stimulatory effect could be related to that of insulin (or IGF-1). Indeed, treatment with TGF-β or with insulin (or IGF-1) results in an increase in the secretion, again in a non-additive manner, of comparable amounts of lactate by cultured immature Sertoli cells.

The long-term inhibitory effect of TGF-β on the action of FSH on the production of lactate coupled with the suppression of secretion of rrTGF-β by Sertoli cells after treatment with FSH suggests that the stimulatory effect of gonadotropin on the secretion of lactate may involve the suppression of secretion of TGF-β by Sertoli cells.

The mechanisms underlying both the stimulatory and inhibitory actions of TGF-β on the basal and FSH-stimulated rates of secretion of lactate remain to be elucidated.

The role of TGF-β in peritubular myoid cells

Since peritubular myoid cells are one of the major sources of fibronectin in the testis, we have studied the effects of TGF-β on the secretion of this component of the ECM. TGF-β stimulates the synthesis of fibronectin by cultured porcine peritubular myoid cells (not shown) as reported in other models.

Gonadal peptides related to TGF-β

The recent report of Hsueh *et al.* (1987), indicating that inhibins stimulate the secretion of testosterone in cultured rat Leydig cells, suggests that this factor may well represent an intratesticular regulator of steroidogenesis.

To date, no data related to the effect of AMH/MIS on testicular cells have been reported.

Conclusions

Although the gonadotropins LH and FSH are the major regulators of testicular functions, it is important and necessary that local regulation of their actions be exerted on different types of testicular cell (Sharpe, 1986). However, both the nature and the mechanisms of action of the factors involved in such local regulation remain to be identified. The identification of an activity, such as that of TGF-β, the secretion and effects of which appear to be highly dependent upon systemic hormones, namely FSH and LH, illustrates this concept.

The secretion of the factor by Sertoli cells is modulated negatively by FSH or positively by steroid or thyroid hormones. Moreover, the effects of TGF-β on different types of testicular cell appear to be strongly modulated by hormones such as LH/hCG, with respect to steroidogenesis in Leydig cells, and FSH and IGF-1 (or insulin) with respect to secretion of lactate by Sertoli cells.

At this point, it is worthwhile to underline the close relationships that exist between TGF-β and FSH; such relationships may well play a key role in the maturation of the testis. Indeed, although FSH interacts specifically only with Sertoli cells (in terms of binding to specific receptors), this hormone is not only involved, as expected, in the maturation and functions of Sertoli cells, but also in those of Leydig cells (Payne *et al.*, 1982), of peritubular myoid cells (as evidenced by a decrease in secretion of fibronectin by co-cultures of peritubular myoid and Sertoli cells, after treatment with FSH) (Skinner *et al.*, 1985), and of germ cells (Parvinen, 1982). Although these effects of the gonadotropin clearly suggest that FSH modulates the activities of the different types of cell via factors secreted by Sertoli cells, such factors remain to be characterized. From the data presented here, it is tempting to propose that TGF-β (or a closely related if not identical activity) might be one of these factors. Furthermore, the possibility that the (negative) effects of FSH might be related to a 'panregulin' such as TGF-β (Sporn *et al.*, 1986) is consistent with the varied and widespread effects of the gonadotropin on different types of testicular cell. However, FSH may also exert its different activities via other (positive) factors, such as the inhibins, as recently suggested (Hsueh *et al.*, 1987).

The fact that factors such as TGF-β appear to be involved in the intragonadal control of different functions renders the concept of local control more complex than was initially anticipated. Indeed, this factor: (1) is secreted not only in the gonad but also in other organs; (2) is secreted in the male gonad by different types of somatic cell, including Leydig, Sertoli and peritubular myoid cells, so that its accumulation within the testis could be simultaneously dependent upon different controls related to each type of cell; (3) is secreted in an inactive form (latent TGF-β) (Lawrence *et al.*, 1984), and the biochemical events leading to the active form of the peptide might provide an important site for regulation by hormones involved in the control of testicular function. Furthermore, (4) the regulatory actions of TGF-β on growth and differentiation are modulated to a great extent by the presence of other factors which are potentially present in the testis and which include EGF, FGF, PDGF and components of the ECM; and (5) TGF-β is not only involved in intercellular

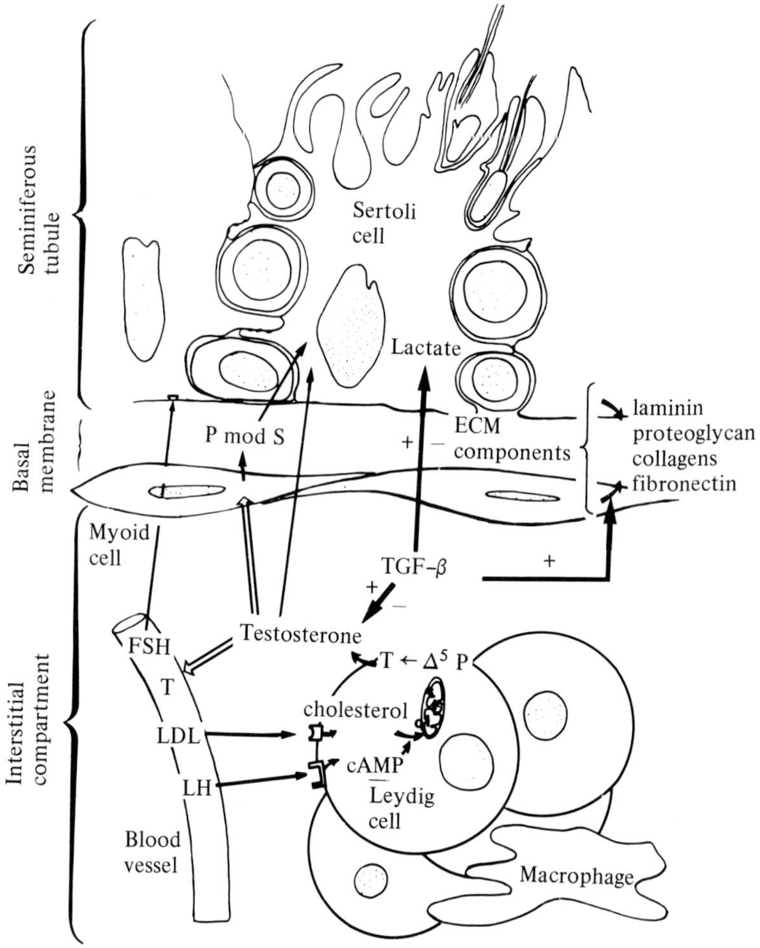

Fig. 7 Summary of the different effects of TGF-β on the functions of testicular somatic cells. Locally produced TGF-β exerts a bifunctional effect on the biosynthesis of steroid hormones (Leydig cells), the production of lactate (Sertoli cells), and a stimulatory effect on the production of extracellular matrix components by tubular somatic cells.

communications as a regulatory factor but it is also involved in other types of intercellular interaction since it is able to modulate both the formation of components of the ECM (e.g. fibronectin and collagen I) and the secretion of nutritional factors (e.g. lactate) (Fig. 7).

Although it is quite conceivable that deficiencies or aberrations in local control mechanisms can perhaps account for what is termed 'idiopathic oligospermia', the approaches to both the evaluation *in vivo* and the correction of such abnormalities will require considerable effort and ingenuity.

In the context of fertility control, although the manipulation of factors such as TGF-β, which are involved in the local control of the gonad, appears to be far from easy, the recent observations indicating that gonadal (Sertoli cell) peptides related to TGF-β, such as inhibins, may be involved in the local control of gonadal activity, appear to offer interesting opportunities in this field.

Acknowledgements

We thank Dr E.M. Chambaz for helpful suggestions and Dr D.A. Lawrence for a critical review of the manuscript. This work was supported by the Institut National de la Santé et de la Recherche Médicale (INSERM CRE 874001), Association pour la Recherche sur le Cancer (ARC) and Fondation pour la Recherche Médicale (FRM).

References

Adashi, E.Y. & Hsueh, A.J.W. (1981). Autoregulation of androgen production in a primary culture of rat testicular cells. **Nature** 293:737–739.

Adashi, E.Y. & Resnick, C.E. (1986). Antagonistic interactions of transforming growth factors in the regulation of granulosa cell differentiation. **Endocrinology** 119:1879–1881.

Ascoli, M. (1981). Regulation of gonadotropin receptors and gonadotropin responses in a clonal strain tumor cells by epidermal growth factor. **Journal of Biolological Chemistry** 256:179–183.

Bellvé, A.R. & Feig, L.R. (1984). Cell proliferation in the mammalian testis. Biology of the seminiferous growth factor (SGF). **Recent Progress in Hormone Research** 40:531–567.

Benahmed, M., Cochet, C., Keramidas, M., Chauvin, M.A. & Morera, A.M. (1988). Evidence for an FSH-dependent secretion of a receptor-reactive transforming growth factor β-like material by immature Sertoli cells in primary culture. **Biochemical and Biophysical Research Communications** 154:1222–1231.

Benahmed, M., Grenot, C., Tabone, E., Sanchez, P. & Morera, A.M. (1985). FSH regulates cultured Leydig cell function via Sertoli cell proteins: an *in vitro* study. **Biochemical and Biophysical Research Communications** 132:729–734.

Benahmed, M., Morera, A.M. & Chauvin, M.A. (1986a). Evidence for a Sertoli cell, FSH-suppressible inhibiting factor(s) of testicular steroidogenic activity. **Biochemical and Biophysical Research Communications** 135:169–178.

Benahmed, M., Morera, A.M., Chauvin, M.A. & de Peretti, E. (1987a). Somatomedin C/insulin-like growth factor 1 as a possible intratesticular regulator of Leydig cell activity. **Molecular and Cellular Endocrinology** 50:69–77.

Benahmed, M., Morera, A.M., Chauvin, M.A., de Peretti, E. & Revol, A. (1987b). FSH regulates testicular steroidogenesis through Sertoli cell factors: effects and preliminary characterization. In: Orgebin-Crist, M.C. & Danzo, B.J., eds. Cell Biology of the Testis and Epididymis. **Annals of the New York Academy of Sciences** 513:470–471.

Benahmed, M., Sordoillet, C., Chauvin, M.A., de Peretti, E. & Morera, A.M. (1989). On the mechanisms involved in the inhibitory and stimulating actions of TAFβ on porcine testicular steroidogenesis: an in-vitro study. **Molecular and Cellular Endocrinology** 67:155–164.

Benahmed, M., Tabone, E., Grenot, C., Sanchez, P., Chauvin, M.A. & Morera, A.M. (1986b). Paracrine control of Leydig cell activity by FSH-dependent proteins from Sertoli cells: *in vitro* study. **Journal of Steroid Biochemistry** 24:311–314.

Bergh, A. (1983). Paracrine regulation of Leydig cells by the seminiferous tubule. **International Journal of Andrology** 6:57–65.

Boerner, P., Resnick, R.J. & Racker, E. (1985). Stimulation of glycolysis and amino acid uptake in NRK-49F cells by transforming growth factor and epidermal growth factor. **Proceedings of the National Academy of Sciences, USA** 82:1350–1353.

Buck, C.A. & Horwitz, A.F. (1987). Cell surface receptors for extracellular matrix molecules. **Annual Review of Cellular Biology** 3:179–205.

Carreau, S., Papadopoulos, V. & Drosdowsky, M.A. (1988). Stimulation of adult rat Leydig cell aromatase activity by a Sertoli cell factor. **Endocrinology** 122:1103–1109.

Cate, R.L., Mattaliano, R.J., Hession, C., Tizard, R., Farber, N.M., Cheung, A., Ninfa, E.G., Frey, A.Z., Hash, D.J., Chow, E.P., Fisher, R.A., Bertonis, J.M., Torres, G., Wallner, B.P., Ramachandran, K.L., Ragin, R.C., Manganaro, T.F., MacLaughin, D.T. & Donahoe, P.K. (1986). Isolation of the bovine and human genes for Mullerian inhibiting substance and expression of the human gene in animal cells. **Cell** 45:685–698.

Catt, K.J., Harwood, R.N., Clayton, R.N., Davies, T.F., Chan, V., Katikineni, M., Nozu & Dufau, M.L. (1980). Regulation of peptide hormone receptors and gonadal steroidogenesis. **Recent Progress in Hormone Research** 36:557–622.

Cheifetz, S., Weatherbee, J.A., Tang, M.L.-S., Anderson, J.L., Mole, J.E., Lucas, R. & Massague, J. (1987). The transforming growth factor β system, a complex pattern of cross-reactive ligands and receptors. **Cell** 48:409–415.

Derynck, R., Jarret, J.A., Chen, E.Y., Eaton, D.H. & Bell, J.R. (1985). Human transforming growth factor β DNA sequence and expression in tumour cell lines. **Nature** 316:701–705.

Deuel, T.F. (1987). Polypeptide growth factors: roles in normal and abnormal cell growth. **Annual Review of Cellular Biology** 3:443–492.

Dodson, W.C. & Schomberg, D.W. (1987). The effect of TGF-β on follicle stimulating hormone-induced differentiation of cultured rat granulosa cells. Endocrinology 120:512–516.

Dufau, M.L., Khanum, A., Winters, C.A. & Tsai-Morris, C.H. (1987). Multistep regulation of Leydig cell function. **Journal of Steroid Biochemistry** 27:343–350.

Elson, S.D., Christopher, A.B. & Thorburn, G.D. (1984). Identification of epidermal growth factor-like activity in human male reproductive tissue and fluids. **Journal of Clinical Endocrinology and Metabolism** 58:589–594.

Esposito, G., Keramidas, M., Mauduit, C., Feige, J.J., Morera, A.M. & Benahmed, M. (1990). Direct regulating effects of TGFβ on lactate production in cultured porcine Sertoli cells. **Endocrinology**, in press.

Fabbri, A. & Dufau, M.L. (1988). Hormonal regulation of β endorphin in the testis. **Journal of Steroid Biochemistry** 30:347–352.

Feige, J., Cochet, C., Rainey, W.E., Madani, C. & Chambaz, E. (1987). Type beta transforming growth factor affects adrenocortical cell differentiated functions. **Journal of Biological Chemistry** 262:13491–13495.

Forest, M.G., Cathiard, A.M. & Bertrand, J. (1973). Total and unbound testosterone levels in newborns and in normal hypogonadal children: use of a sensitive radioimmunoassay for testosterone. **Journal of Clinical Endocrinology and Metabolism** 36:1132–1143.

Franchimont, P. (1987). L'inhibine. **Annales d'Endocrinologie** 48:441–454.

Fritz, I.B. (1978). Sites of action of androgens and follicle-stimulating hormone on cells of the seminiferous tubule. In: Litwack, G., ed. **Biochemical Actions of Hormones**, Vol. V, New York, Academic Press, pp.249–281.

Fritz, I.B. (1985). Past, present and future of molecular and cellular endocrinology of the testis. In: Saez, J.M., Forest, M.G., Dazord, A. & Bertrand, J., eds. **Recent Progress in Cellular Endocrinology of the Testis**, Vol. 123, Paris, Editions INSERM, pp.15–54.

Fritz, I.B. & Tung, P.S. (1986). Testicular peritubular cell–Sertoli cell interactions. In: Stefanini, M. *et al.*, eds. **Molecular and Cellular Endocrinology of the Testis**, Amsterdam, Elsevier, pp.27–36.

Goustin, A.S., Leof, E.B., Shipley, G.D. & Moses, H.L. (1986). Perspectives in cancer research: growth factors and cancer. **Cancer Research** 46:1015–1029.

Grootegoed, J.A., Mackenbach, P. & Oonk, R.B. (1987). Sertoli cell–germ cell interactions in the regulation of spermatogenesis. In: Parvinen, M., Huhtaniemi, I. & Pelliniemi, L.J., eds. **Development and Function of the Reproductive Organs**, Vol. II, **Serono Symposia Review** 14:91–101.

Grotjan, H.E. & Heindel, J.J. (1982). Effect of spent media from Sertoli cell cultures on *in vitro* testosterone production. **Annals of the New York Academy of Sciences** 383:456–457.

Holley, R.W., Bohlen, P., Fava, R., Baldwin, J.H. & Kleenan, G. (1980). Purification of kidney epithelial cell growth inhibitor. **Proceedings of the National Academy of Sciences, USA** 77:5989–5992.

Hotta, M. & Baird, A. (1986). Differential effects of transforming growth factor type beta on the growth and function of adrenocortical cells *in vitro*. **Proceedings of the National Academy of Sciences, USA** 83:7795–7799.

Hsueh, A.J.W., Dahl, K.D., Vaughan, J., Tucker, E., Rivier, J., Bardin, C.W. & Vale, W. (1987). Heterodimers and homodimers of inhibin subunits have different paracrine action in the modulation of luteinizing hormone-stimulated androgen biosynthesis. **Proceedings of the National Academy of Sciences, USA** 84:5082–5086.

Hsueh, A.J.W., Welsh, T.H. & Jones, P.B.C. (1981). Inhibition of ovarian and testicular steroidogenesis by epidermal growth factor. **Endocrinology** 108:2002–2004.

Ignotz, R.A. & Massague, J. (1986). Transforming growth factor β stimulates the expression of fibronectin and collagen and their incorporation into the extracellular matrix. **Journal of Biological Chemistry** 261:4337–4345.

Inman, W.H. & Colowick, S.P. (1985). Stimulation of glucose uptake by transforming growth factor β. Evidence for the requirement of epidermal growth factor receptor activation. **Proceedings of the National Academy of Sciences, USA** 82:1346–1349.

Jakowlen, S., Dillard, P.J., Kondaiah, P., Sporn, M.B. & Roberts, A.B. (1988). Complementary deoxyribonucleic acid cloning of a novel transforming growth factor-β messenger ribonucleic acid from chick embryo chondrocytes. **Molecular Endocrinology** 28:747–755.

Janecki, A.J., Jakubowiak, A. & Lukaszyk, A. (1985). Stimulatory effect of Sertoli cell secretory products on testosterone secretion by purified Leydig cells in primary culture. **Molecular and Cellular Endocrinology** 42:235–243.

Jegou, B., le Magueresse, B., Sourdaine, P., Pinneauc, Velez de la Calle, J.F., Garnier,

D.H., Guilloux, F. & Boisseau, C. Germ cell–Sertoli cell interactions in vertebrates. In: Cooke, B. & Sharpe, R., eds. **Molecular and Cellular Endocrinology of the Testis, Seromo Symposia Publications** 50:255–270.

Jutte, N.H.P.M., Grootegoed, J.A., Rommerts, F.F.G. & van der Molen, H.J. (1981). Exogenous lactate is essential for metabolic activities in isolated rat spermatocytes and spermatids. **Journal of Reproduction and Fertility** 65:399–405.

Kasson, B.G., Adashi, E.Y. & Hsueh, A.J.W. (1986). Arginine–vasopressin in the testis: an intragonadal peptide control system. **Endocrine Review** 7:156–168.

Khan, S.A., Hallin, P., Barlett, J., de Geyter, C. & Nieschlag, E. (1988). Characterization of a factor from human ovarian follicular fluid which stimulates Leydig cell testosterone production. **Acta Endocrinology** 118:283–293.

Khanum, A. & Dufau, M.L. (1988). Angiotensin II receptors and inhibitory actions in Leydig cells. **Journal of Biological Chemistry** 263:5070–5074.

Kleinman, H.K., Klebe, R.J. & Martin, G.R. (1981). Role of collagenous matrices in the adhesion and growth of cells. **Journal of Cellular Biology** 88:473–485.

Knecht, M., Feng, P. & Catt, K.J. (1987). Bifunctional role of transforming growth factor β during granulosa development. **Endocrinology** 120:123–1249.

Lawrence, D.A. (1985). Transforming growth factors: an overview. **Biology of the Cell** 53:93–98.

Lawrence, D.A., Pircher, R. & Jullien, P. (1985). Conversion of a high molecular weight latent β-TGF from chicken embryo fibroblasts into a low molecular weight active β-TGF under acidic conditions. **Biochemical and Biophysical Research Communications** 133:1026–1034.

Lawrence, D.A., Pircher, R., Krycee-Martinerie, C. & Jullien, P. (1984). Normal embryo fibroblasts release tranforming growth factors in a latent form. **Journal of Cellular Physiology** 121:184–188.

Lin, T., Blaisdell, J. & Haskell, J.F. (1987). Transforming growth factor β inhibits Leydig cell steroidogenesis in primary culture. **Biochemical and Biophysical Research Communications** 146:387–394.

Lin, T., Haskell, J., Vinson, N. & Terracio, L. (1986). Characterization of insulin and insulin-like growth factor 1 receptors in purified Leydig cells and their role in steroidogenesis in primary culture: a comparative study. **Endocrinology** 119:1641–1646.

Ling, N., Ying, S.W., Ueno, N., Shimasaki, B., Esch, F., Hotta, M. & Guillemin, R. (1986). Pituitary FSH is released by a heterodimer of the beta-subunits from the two forms of inhibin. **Nature** 321:779–782.

Lyons, R.M., Keski-Oja, J. & Moses, H. (1988). Proteolytic activation of latent transforming growth factor β from fibroblast-conditioned medium. **Journal of Cellular Biology** 106:1659–1665.

McLachlan, R.I., Robertson, D.M., de Kretser, D.M. & Burger, H.G. (1988). Advances in the physiology of inhibin and inhibin-related peptides. **Clinical Endocrinology** 29:77–114.

Mason, A.J., Hayflick, J.S., Ling, N., Esch, F., Ueno, N., Ying, S.-Y., Guillemin, R., Niall, H. & Seeburg, P.H. (1985). Complementary DNA sequences of ovarian follicular fluid show precursor structure and homology with transforming growth factor β. **Nature** 318:659–663.

Massague, J. (1987). The TGF-beta family of growth and differentiation factors. **Cell** 49:437–438.

Massague, J., Cheifetz, S., Ignotz, R.A. & Boyd, T.F. (1987). Multiple type β

transforming growth factors and their receptors. **Journal of Cellular Physiology**, Supplement 5:43–47.

Mather, J.P. & Philipps, (1984). Primary culture of testicular somatic cells. In: Barnes, D.W., Sirbasku, D.A. & Sato, G.H., eds. **Methods for Serum-Free Culture of Cells of the Endocrine System**, New York, Alan R. Liss, pp.29–45.

Meistrich, L.M., Longtin, J., Brock, W.A., Grimes, S.R. & Myles, L.M. (1981). Purification of rat spermatogenic cells and preliminary biochemical analysis of these cells. **Biological Reproduction** 25:1065–1077.

Mita, M., Price, J.M. & Hall, P.F. (1982). Stimulation by follicle-stimulating hormone of synthesis of lactate by Sertoli cell from rat testis. **Endocrinology** 110:1535–1541.

Morera, A.M., Benahmed, M., Cochet, C., Chauvin, M.A., Chambaz, E. & Revol, A. (1987a). A TGFβ-like peptide is a possible intratesticular modulator of steroidogenesis. In: Orgebin-Crist, M.C. & Danzo, B.J., eds. Cell Biology of The Testis and Epididymis. **Annals of the New York Academy of Sciences** 513:494–496.

Morera, A.M., Chauvin, M.A., de Peretti, E. & Benahmed, M. (1987b). SmC-IGF1: an intratesticular cytodifferentiative factor of Leydig cells? **Hormone Research** 28:50–57.

Morera, A.M., Cochet, C., Keramidas, M., Chauvin, M.A., de Peretti, E. & Benahmed, M. (1988). Direct regulating effects of transforming growth factor β on Leydig cell steroidogenesis. **Journal of Steroid Biochemistry** 30:443–447.

Neumann, H.C., Potts, G.O., Ryan, W.R. & Stonner, F.W. (1970). Steroidal heterocycles. XIII 4a, 5-epoxy = 5α-androst-2-eno-(2,3-d)isoxazoles and related compounds. **Journal of Medicinal Chemistry** 13:948–951.

Parvinen, M. (1982). Regulation of the seminiferous epithelium. **Endocrine Reviews** 3:404–417.

Payne, A.H., Chase, D.J. & O'Shaugnessy, P.J. (1982). Regulation of steroidogenesis in Leydig cells. In: Conn, M., ed. **Cellular Regulation of Secretion and Release** New York, Academic Press, pp.355–408.

Picard, J.Y., Benarous, R., Geurrier, D., Josso, N. & Kahn, A. (1986). Cloning and expresion of cDNA for anti-Mullerian hormone. **Proceedings of the National Academy of Sciences, USA** 83:5464–5468.

Pircher, R., Jullien, P. & Lawrence, D.A. (1984). Latent β-transforming growth factor in nontransformed and Kirten sarcoma virus-transformed normal rat kidney cells' clone 49F. **Cancer Research** 44:5538–5543.

Pircher, R., Jullien, P. & Lawrence, D.A. (1986). β-Transforming growth factor is stored in human blood platelets as a latent high-molecular-weight complex. **Biochemical and Biophysical Research Communications** 136:30–37.

Ritzen, E.M. (1983). Chemical messengers between Sertoli cells and neighboring cells. **Journal of Steroid Biochemistry** 19:499–504.

Rivier, C., Vale, W. & Rivier, J. (1987). Studies of the inhibin family of hormones: a review. **Hormone Research** 28:104–118.

Roberts, A.B., Flanders, K.C., Kondaiah, P., Thompson, N.L., van Obberghen-Schilling, E., Wakefield, L.M., Rossi, P., de Combrugghe, B., Heine, U. & Sporn, M.B. (1988). Transforming growth factor β; biochemistry and role in embryogenesis, tissue repair and remodelling and carcinogenesis. **Recent Progress in Hormone Research** 44:157–197.

Robinson, R. & Fritz, I.B. (1981). Metabolism of glucose by Sertoli cells in culture. **Biology of Reproduction** 24:1032-1041.

Rommerts, F.F.G., Hoogerbrugge, J.E. & van der Molen, H.J. (1986). Stimulation of steroid production in isolated rat Leydig cells by unknown factors in testicular fluid differs from the effects of LH and LH-releasing hormone. **Journal of Endocrinology** 109:111–117.

Rommerts, F.F.G., Molenaar, R. & van der Molen, H.J. (1985). Preparation of isolated Leydig cells. In: Birnbaumer, L. & O'Malley, eds. **Methods in Enzymology**, Vol. 109 **Hormone Action, Part 1, Peptide Hormones**, New York, Academic Press, pp.275–288.

Segarini, P.R. & Seyedin, S.M. (1988). High-molecular-weight receptor of transforming growth factor contains glycosaminoglycan chains. **Journal of Biological Chemistry** 263:8363–8370.

Sertoli, E. (1865). Dell'esistenza di particolari cellule ramificati nei canalicoli seminiferi del testiculo humano. **Morgani** 7:31–39.

Sharpe, R.M. (1984). Intratesticular factors controlling testicular function. **Biology of Reproduction** 30:29–49.

Sharpe, R.M. (1986). Paracrine control of the testis. **Clinical Endocrinology and Metabolism** 15:185–207.

Skinner, M.K. (1987). Cell–cell interactions in the testis. In: Orgebin-Crist, M.C. & Danzo, B.J., eds. Cell Biology of the Testis and Epididymis. **Annals of the New York Academy of Science** 513:158–171.

Skinner, M.K. & Fritz, I.B. (1984). Testicular peritubular cells secrete a protein under androgen control that modulates Sertoli cell function. **Proceedings of the National Academy of Sciences, USA** 82:116–117.

Skinner, M.K., Tung, P.S. & Fritz, I.B. (1985). Cooperativity between Sertoli cells and testicular peritubular cells in the production and deposition of extracellular matrix components. **Journal of Cellular Biology** 10:1941–1947.

Smith, E.P., Svoboda, M.E., van Wyk, J.J., Kierszenbaum, A.L. & Tres, L.L. (1987). Partial characterization of a somatomedin-like peptide from the medium of cultured rat Sertoli cells. **Endocrinology** 120:186–193.

Sordoillet, C., Chauvin, M.A., Revol, A., Morera, A.M. & Benahmed, M. (1988). Fibroblast growth factor is a regulator of testosterone secretion in cultured immature Leydig cells. **Molecular and Cellular Endocrinology** 58:283–286.

Sporn, M.B., Roberts, A.B., Wakefield, L.M. & Assoian, R.K. (1986). Tranforming growth factor-beta: biological function and chemical structure. **Science** 233:532–534.

Sporn, M.B., Roberts, A.B., Wakefield, L.M. & de Combrugghe, B. (1987). Some recent advances in the chemistry and biology of transforming growth factor β. **Journal of Cellular Biology** 1050:1039–1045.

Steinberger, E., Root, A., Ficher, M. & Smith, K.D. (1973). The role of androgen in the initiation of spermatogenesis in man. **Journal of Clinical Endocrinology and Metabolism** 37:746–751.

Syed, V., Khan, A. & Ritzen, E.M. (1985). Stage-specific inhibition of interstitial cell testosterone secretion by rat seminiferous tubules *in vitro*. **Molecular and Cellular Endocrinology** 40:257–264.

Tabone, E., Benahmed, M., Hartmann, D.J. & Morera, A.M. (1989). Interactions between Leydig, Sertoli and peritubular cells. *In vitro* detection of fibronectin, laminin and type IV collagen (submitted).

Tahri-Joutei, A. & Pointis, G. (1988). Time-related effects of arginine vasopressin on steroidogenesis in cultured mouse Leydig cells. **Journal of Reproduction and Fertility** 82:247–253.

Ten Dijke, P., Hansen, P., Iwata, K.K., Pierler, C. & Foulkes, J.G. (1988). Identification of another member of the transforming growth factor type β gene family. **Proceedings of the National Academy of Sciences, USA** 85:4715–4719.
Tsong, S.D., Phillips, D., Halmi, N., Liotta, A.S., Margoris, A., Bardin, C.W. & Krieger, D.T. (1982). ACTH and β endorphin-related peptides are present in multiple sites in the reproductive tract of the male rat. **Endocrinology** 110:2204–2206.
Tung, P.S. & Fritz, I.B. (1980). Interactions of Sertoli cells with myoid cells *in vitro*. **Biology of Reproduction** 23:207–217.
Ueno, N., Baird, A., Ling, N. & Guillemin, R. (1987). Isolation and partial characterization of fibroblast growth factor from bovine testis. **Molecular and Cellular Endocrinology** 49:189–194.
Vale, W., Rivier, J., Vaughan, J., McClintock, R., Corrigan, A., Woo, W., Karr, D. & Spiess, J. (1986). Purification and characterization of an FSH-releasing protein from porcine ovarian follicular fluid. **Nature** 231:776–778.
Van der Molen, H.J. & Rommerts, F.F.G. (1981). Testicular steroidogenesis. In: Burger, H. & de Kretser, D., eds. **The Testis**, New York, Raven Press, pp.213–238.
Verhoeven, G. & Cailleau, J. (1985). A factor in spent media from Sertoli cell-enriched cultures that stimulates steroidogenesis in Leydig cells. **Molecular and Cellular Endocrinology** 40:57–68.
Verhoeven, G. & Cailleau, J. (1986). Stimulatory effects of epidermal growth factor on steroidogenesis in Leydig cells. **Molecular and Cellular Endocrinology** 47:99–106.
Ying, S.Y. (1988). Inhibins, activins, and follistatins: gonadal proteins modulating the secretion of follicle-stimulating hormone. **Endocrine Reviews** 9:267–293.

Epidermal growth factor in human ovarian follicular fluid

L.G. WESTERGAARD AND C.Y. ANDERSEN

Laboratory of Reproductive Biology II, Department of Obstetrics and Gynecology, Rigshospitalet, University of Copenhagen, DK-2100 Copenhagen, Denmark.

Keywords

Epidermal growth factor, human, follicular fluid.

Introduction

In recent years considerable interest has focused on the possible role of polypeptide growth factors, such as epidermal growth factor (EGF), fibroblast growth factor (FGF), platelet-derived growth factor (PDGF), insulin-like growth factors (IGFs) and transforming growth factors (TGFs) as autocrine and/or paracrine regulators of ovarian follicular development and function. In addition to their well-known mitogenic effects, these growth factors have been shown to influence responsiveness to gonadotropins of and steroidogenesis in cultured granulosa and theca cells of various species, including the human (Gospodarowicz and Bialecki, 1979; Hsueh *et al.*, 1981; Adashi *et al.*, 1985; Tapanainen *et al.*, 1987). Moreover, growth factors have been shown to promote maturation of rat oocytes *in vitro* (Dekel and Scherizly, 1985; Feng *et al.*, 1988). Some recent data suggest that growth factors are present in the gonad and may be secreted and/or regulated locally (Hammond *et al.*, 1985; Neufeld *et al.*, 1987; Hsu *et al.*, 1987; Franks *et al.*, 1987, 1988).

If EGF and other growth factors play a major role in the local regulation of follicular steroidogenesis and oocyte meiosis *in vivo*, it would be reasonable to expect that intrafollicular levels of EGF are present in follicular fluid (FF), and also that intrafollicular levels of EGF vary among different follicles, which correspond to different stages of follicular development and oocyte meiosis. Previous studies have, in fact, demonstrated the presence of EGF in porcine FF (Hsu *et al.*, 1987) and, recently, Franks *et al.* (1987, 1988) reported high levels of EGF and FF from small follicles in women with polycystic ovary syndrome.

The aim of the present study was to cast light on the possible physiological role of EGF in the local control of human ovarian follicular development and oocyte meiosis. We measured concentrations of EGF and steroids in serum and FF aspirated from large (diameter above 15 mm) preovulatory follicles of women undergoing in-vitro fertilization (IVF)/embryo transfer (ET) and in serum and FF aspirated from small (diameter 2–4 mm) follicles of women undergoing elective caesarean section after term pregnancy.

Materials and methods

Preovulatory follicles

Follicular fluid was obtained by aspiration from 69 preovulatory follicles with diameters above 15 mm in 15 women undergoing transvaginal, ultrasound-guided recovery of oocytes for IVF and ET. Follicular development was stimulated by a combination of clomiphene citrate and human menopausal gonadotropins. Ovulation was triggered by an injection of 6000 i.u. human chorionic gonadotropin (hCG) 34 hours before aspiration of follicles and collection of oocytes. Immediately after each oocyte was transferred to culture *in vitro*, each aspirate of FF was centrifuged (1500xg) and the supernatants were stored individually at −20°C until analysis. Only clear aspirates of FF with no sign of blood admixture were included in the study. A sample of peripheral blood for analysis of serum was drawn from each woman at the time of follicle aspiration. The material for this study was selected from our stores of frozen FF and serum samples from patients who have undergone IVF; samples of FF and serum from women who did and from women who did not become pregnant were represented. Only FFs from follicles that yielded oocytes were included.

Small follicles

Aspirates of FF from 16 antral follicles with diameter from 2 mm to 4 mm were obtained from two women (eight samples of FF from each) who were undergoing elective caesarean section at term after they had given their informed consent. During the operation, and with the ovaries visible *in situ*, antral follicles were punctured with a 25-gauge needle (Butterfly 25 Short, Abbott Laboratories, Trorod, Denmark) and the FF was aspirated into a 1-ml syringe. After measurement of follicular diameter and the volume of the aspirated FF (Westergaard *et al*., 1985), the syringes were flushed with 200 μl of phosphate-buffered saline and the diluted aspirates of FF were centrifuged. The supernatants were stored at −20°C until analysis.

Radioimmunoassays

The concentration of EGF in FF and serum was determined by radioimmunoassay (Amersham) using human-r-EGF (Amersham) as standard. Standards, tracer, and samples were incubated with antibody (raised in rabbit), in a total volume of 0.4 ml, overnight at 5°C. Then rabbit-specific antibody raised in goat was added. The immunoprecipitate was collected by centrifugation and the radioactivity determined by gamma spectroscopy. With this assay the limit of detection of EGF was 0.5 ng/ml, and the intra-

Table 1. *Characterization of the women, follicles and oocytes*

Women	n	n	Follicles: Mean diameter in mm (range)	Follicles: Mean volume in ml (range)	Oocytes: Cleaved *in vitro*	Oocytes: Not cleaved *in vitro*
Pregnancy achieved	5	24	20 (15–24)	3.4 (1.5–6.5)	13 (54%)	11 (46%)
Pregnancy not achieved	10	45	19 (14–26)	3.5 (1.0–9.0)	22 (49%)	23 (51%)
Total	15	69			35 (51%)	34 (49%)

Table 2. *Concentration of EGF in serum of women who achieved and who did not achieve pregnancy after IVF/ET*

	n	EFG in ng/ml[a] mean ± S.E.M. (range)
Pregnancy achieved	5	2.13 ± 0.17 (1.60–2.65)
Pregnancy not achieved	10	2.00 ± 0.25 (1.20–3.75)
Total	15	2.04 ± 0.17 (1.20–3.75)

[a]No statistically significant difference between women achieving and not achieving pregnancy ($p \geqslant 0.10$).

assay coefficient of variation (n – 3) was 8% in a sample of serum that contained 1.55 ng EGF/ml. The preparation of antibody had 100% cross-reactivity with human EGF, 88% with mouse EGF, and 0% with rat TGF-α.

Levels of estradiol and progesterone were measured with a commercially available RIA-kit (Farmos, Finland). Statistical differences were evaluated using Students t-test and the Wilcoxon rank sum test for non-paired data.

Results

A total of 69 samples of FF and oocytes was aspirated from 15 women who were being treated for infertility with IVF/ET. Pregnancy was achieved in five of these women. Details regarding the number, size and volume of the follicles and rates of oocyte cleavage in the women who did and who did not achieve pregnancy are summarized in Table 1. Mean levels (± S.E.M.) of EGF in samples of serum at the time of follicle aspiration were around 2 ng/ml both in women who achieved pregnancy and in those who did not, as shown in Table 2. Table 3 shows that the mean levels of EGF in FF were around 1 ng/ml. The

Table 3. *Levels of EGF in follicular fluid, cleavage of oocytes and pregnancy*

		Number of follicles	EGF (ng/ml) mean ± S.E.M.
Pregnancy achieved	+ Oocyte cleavage	13	[a]1.03 ± 0.06 (0.60–1.35)
	− Oocyte cleavage	11	1.13 ± 0.09 (0.62–1.60)
No pregnancy	+ Oocyte cleavage	22	[a]1.11 ± 0.08 (0.66–1.87)
	− Oocyte cleavage	23	1.26 ± 0.10 (0.67–2.42)
	+ Oocyte cleavage	35	[a]1.08 ± 0.05 (0.60–1.87)
	− Oocyte cleavage	34	1.22 ± 0.08 (0.62–2.42)

[a]No statistical difference ($p > 0.10$).

levels of EGF in FF from follicles that yielded oocytes that cleaved *in vitro* were not significantly different from those in FF from follicles that yielded oocytes that remained unfertilized *in vitro*, independent of whether or not the woman became pregnant (Table 3). A significant linear correlation ($r = 0.77$, $p < 0.001$) between the mean concentration of EGF in FF and in serum was found, as shown in Figure 1. Levels of EGF in FF were not significantly correlated to the size of follicles (volume of FF), to levels of progesterone in FF, or to levels of estradiol in FF (data not shown).

A total of 16 samples of FF was aspirated from follicles of various diameters from two women during elective caesarean section at term. Seven follicles had a diameter of 2 mm, five of 3 mm, and four of 4 mm. The volume of FF aspirated from these follicles ranged between 20 μl and 60 μl. EGF was undetectable in FF from three follicles and levels of EGF varied between 10.5 ng/ml and 47.3 ng/ml in the remaining 13 cases, as shown in Figure 2. The mean ± S.E.M. concentration of EGF in FF from follicles of 2 mm in diameter (25.3 ± 6.0 ng/ml) was significantly higher than that in the follicles of 3 mm and 4 mm in diameter (9.2 ± 3.9 ng/ml and 11.5 ± 0.5 ng/ml, respectively), $p < 0.05$ (Fig. 2). The concentration of EGF in serum was only between 25% and 10% of the average levels of FF, being below the limits of detection in one of the women and 2.8 ng/ml in the other.

Discussion

Preovulatory follicles

This study is the first to demonstrate the presence of measurable quantities of EGF in antral fluid of human preovulatory follicles. The level of EGF in FF of these large follicles is rather low (ranging from 0.6 ng/ml to 2.4 ng/ml) and is about 60% of that in serum, with very little variability among follicles.

The site of production of intrafollicular EGF is unknown. The local production of EGF by the granulosa and/or theca cells is one possibility. The synthesis *de novo* of other growth factors, e.g. IGF-1 and FGF, has been

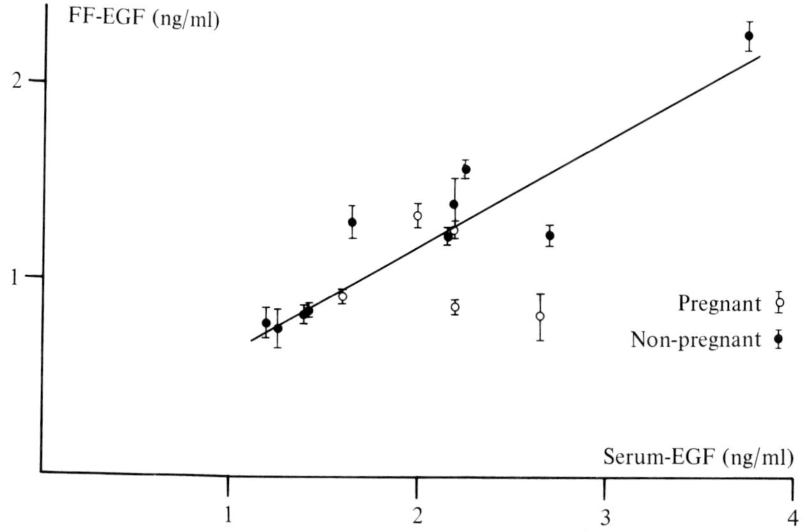

Fig. 1 Correlation between levels of EGF in FF and in serum (mean ± S.E.M.). ⚲ : mean ± S.E.M. of levels of EGF in women who achieved pregnancy. ⚲ : mean ± S.E.M. levels of EGF in women who did not achieve pregnancy.

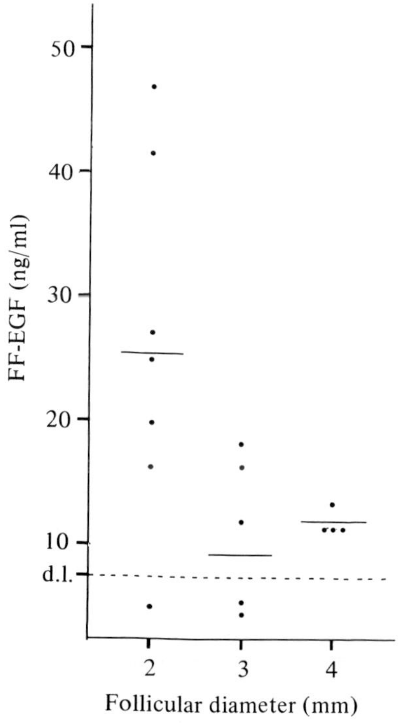

Fig. 2 Concentration of EGF (ng/ml) in FF aspirated from antral follicles with diameters of 2 mm, 3 mm and 4 mm in two women at term of pregnancy. d.l.: limit of detection. Horizontal bars represent the mean concentration of EGF in follicles of 2 mm, 3 mm and 4 mm in diameter.

shown in porcine (Hammond *et al.*, 1987) and bovine (Neufeld *et al.*, 1987) granulosa cells *in vitro*. A second possibility is that intrafollicular EGF is derived from the blood platelets (Oka and Orth, 1983) that may have contaminated FF during the aspiration procedure. Finally, it is possible that EGF in FF merely results from the passive diffusion of EGF from the circulation, via the theca vessels, into the antrum. The present results favor this third possibility, since a significant linear correlation between levels of EGF in serum and in FF and a constant concentration gradient of EGF from serum to FF were demonstrated. Moreover, the uniformity of the concentration of EGF in the FF of the different preovulatory follicles, which contained highly variable concentrations of steroids, argues against the local production of EGF by the granulosa/ theca cells or the contamination by blood platelets of the FF as sources of intrafollicular EGF.

A large number of studies have shown that EGF influences steroidogenesis in and the responsiveness to gonadotropins of granulosa cells and theca cells *in vitro* (Jones *et al.*, 1982; Knecht and Catt, 1983; Hsueh *et al.*, 1983; Tapanainen *et al.*, 1987). These studies suggest that EGF may possess important autocrine and/or paracrine functions in the ovary. In the present study we found no correlation between intrafollicular levels of EGF and levels of either progesterone or estradiol. These results indicate that EGF is not an important regulator of steroidogenesis in the human preovulatory follicle *in vivo*.

Previous studies have shown that EGF stimulates meiotic maturation of rat oocytes *in vitro* (Dekel and Scherizly, 1985; Feng *et al.*, 1988). These studies suggest that EGF might be one among a number of other intrafollicular, non-steroidal substances, such as oocyte maturation inhibitor (OMI; Channing *et al.*, 1978), meiosis-inducing substance (Westergaard *et al.*, 1984) and hypoxanthine (Downs *et al.*, 1986), which have been proposed as being involved in the local regulation of meiosis in the preovulatory oocyte. Thus, significant correlations between intrafollicular levels of OMI (Channing *et al.*, 1983) and meiosis-inducing substance (Westergaard *et al.*, 1985a) and the rates of cleavage of human oocytes *in vitro* and the rate of pregnancy after ET have been reported. In the present study no such correlation was found for levels of EGF, suggesting that a role for EGF in the local regulation of maturation of the human preovulatory oocyte is less likely.

We conclude from these results that the presence of EGF in the FF of the human preovulatory follicle is due to passive diffusion from the circulation. We also conclude that EGF is involved neither in the local regulation of steroidogenesis nor in oocyte meiosis at the preovulatory stage of human follicular development.

Small antral follicles

Levels of EGF in FF from small human antral follicles (diameter 2–4 mm) were up to 20 times higher than those in serum, and they showed considerable variation among follicles, ranging from below the limit of detection to 47.3 ng/ml. A significant inverse correlation between intrafollicular levels of EGF and follicular diameter (from 2 mm to 4 mm) was demonstrated. These findings are in agreement with results reported by Franks *et al.* (1987, 1988) on levels of EGF in FF from follicles of similar sizes from two women with polycystic ovary syndrome. From their results, Franks *et al.* (1988) proposed that the high levels of EGF in the follicles in polycystic ovaries might be responsible for the absence of follicular responsiveness to FSH in these women and, thus, might represent an aspect of the ovarian pathology in polycystic ovary syndrome. However, as also mentioned by Franks *et al.* (1988), the high intrafollicular levels of EGF in polycystic ovaries may merely reflect the small size of the follicles in these ovaries. Our results appear to support such an interpretation. From our present findings we propose that high intrafollicular levels of EGF may be a physiological phenomenon specific to the early stages of follicular development. We also propose that EGF is produced locally by the granulosa/theca cells in follicles with diameters of 4 mm and smaller, and that this local production gradually decreases as the follicle develops beyond 5–6 mm in diameter, and ceases when the preovulatory stage of development is reached.

It is generally accepted that intrafollicular estradiol is the major mitogen of granulosa cells in human antral follicles from 6 mm in diameter to preovulatory size (McNatty *et al.*, 1979). It has been shown that healthy, growing, human antral follicles with diameters below 6 mm invariably contain low levels of estradiol in the FF, and these levels are not different from those in atretic follicles (Westergaard *et al.*, 1985b). It seems, therefore, that proliferation of granulosa cells and growth of follicles depend on intrafollicular mitogens other than estradiol in follicles with diameters below 6 mm. On the basis of the present results we can only speculate as to whether intrafollicular EGF is a major regulator of human follicular growth during the early developmental stages. Further studies with larger numbers of small and medium-sized antral follicles are necessary to substantiate our findings.

Acknowledgements

The performance of the radioimmunoassays for progesterone and estradiol by Dr J. Kroll, Department of Clinical Chemistry, Rigshospitalet, and the excellent technical assistance of Vibeke K. Bjork are gratefully acknowledged. The financial support by the AG Louis Hansens Mindefond and the Lily B. Lunds Foundation is also gratefully acknowledged.

References

Adashi, E.Y., Resnick, C.E., D'Ercole, A.J., Svoboda, M.E. & Van Wyk, J.J. (1985). Insulin-like growth factors as intraovarian regulators of granulosa cell growth and function. **Endocrine Reviews** 6:400–420.

Channing, C.P., Chen-Quan, L., Seegar-Jones, G. & Jones, H. (1983). Decline of follicular oocyte maturation inhibitor coincident with maturation and achievement of fertilizability of oocytes recovered at midcycle of gonadotropin-treated women. **Proceedings of the National Academy of Sciences, USA** 80:4184–4188.

Channing, C.P., Hillensjo, T. & Schaerf, F.W. (1978). Hormonal control of oocyte meiosis, ovulation and luteinization in mammals. **Clinical Endocrinology and Metabolism** 7:601–624.

Dekel, N. & Scherizly, I. (1983). Epidermal growth factor induces maturation of rat follicle-enclosed oocytes. **Endocrinology** 116:406–409.

Downs, S.M., Coleman, D.L., Ward-Bailey, P.F. & Eppig, J.J. (1985). Hypoxanthine is the principal inhibitor of murine oocyte maturation in low molecular weight fraction of porcine follicular fluid. **Proceedings of the National Academy of Sciences, USA** 82:454–458.

Feng, P., Catt, K.J. & Knecht, M. (1988). Transforming growth factor beta stimulates meiotic maturation of the rat oocyte. **Endocrinology** 122:181–186.

Franks, S., Mason, H.D., Polson, D.W., Winston, R.M.L., Margara, R. & Reed, M.J. (1988). Mechanisms and management of ovulatory failure in women with polycystic ovary syndrome. **Human Reproduction** 3:531–534.

Franks, S., Neagle, G., Leake, R., Mason, H.D., Harlow, C., Winston, R., Margara, R. & Reed, M. (1987). Epidermal growth factor (EGF) concentrations in follicular fluid from normal and polycystic ovaries (PCO). **Journal of Endocrinology** (Suppl.) 112:Abstract 120.

Gospodarowicz, D. & Bialecki, H. (1979). Fibroblast and epidermal growth factors are mitogenic agents for cultured granulosa cells of rodent, porcine and human origin. **Endocrinology** 104:757–764.

Hammond, J.M., Baranao, J.L.S., Shaleris, D., Knight, A.B., Romaneus, J.A. & Rechler, M.M. (1985). Production of insulin-like growth factors by ovarian granulosa cells. **Endocrinology** 117:2553–2555.

Hsueh, A.J.W., Welsh, T.H. & Jones, P.C.B. (1981). Inhibition of ovarian and testicular steroidogenesis by epidermal growth factor. **Endocrinology** 108:2002–2004.

Hsu, C.-J., Holmes, S.D. & Hammond, J.M. (1987). Ovarian epidermal growth factor-like activity. Concentration in porcine follicular fluid during follicular enlargement. **Biochemical and Biophysical Research Communications** 147:242–247.

Jones, P.C.B., Welsh, T.H. & Hsueh, A.J.W. (1982). Regulation of ovarian progestin production by epidermal growth factor in cultured rat granulosa cells. **Journal of Biological Chemistry** 257:11268–11273.

Knecht, M. & Catt, K.J. (1983). Modulation of cAMP-mediated differentiation in ovarian granulosa cells by epidermal growth factor and platelet-derived growth factor. **Journal of Biological Chemistry** 258:2789–2794.

McNatty, K.P., Moore, Smith, D., Makris, A., Osathanondh, R. & Ryan, K. (1979). The microenvironment of the human antral follicle: interrelationships among the steroid level in antral fluid, the population of granulosa cells and the status of the oocyte *in vivo* and *in vitro*. **Journal of Clinical Endocrinology and Metabolism** 56:1022–1031.

Neufeld, G., Ferrara, N., Schwiegerer, L., Mitchell, R. & Gospodarowicz, D. (1987). Bovine granulosa cells produce basic fibroblastic growth factor. **Endocrinology** 121:597–603.

Oka, Y. & Orth, D.N. (1983). Human plasma epidermal growth factor/beta-urogastrone is associated with blood platelets. **Journal of Clinical Investigation** 72:249–259.

Tapanainen, J., Leionen, P.J. & Tapanainen, P. (1987). Regulation of human granulosa–luteal cell progesterone production and proliferation by gonadotropins and growth factors. **Fertility and Sterility** 48:576–580.

Westergaard, L., Byskov, A.G., Yding Andersen, C., Grinsted, J.U. & McNatty, K.P. (1984). Is resumption of meiosis in the human preovulatory oocyte triggered by a meiosis-inducing substance (MIS) in the follicular fluid? **Fertility and Sterility** 41:377–384.

Westergaard, L., Byskov, A.G., Van Look, P.F.A., Angell, R., Aitken, J., Swanston, I.A. & Templeton, A.A. (1985a). Meiosis-inducing substance in human preovulatory follicular fluid related to time of follicle aspiration and to the potential of the oocyte to fertilize and cleave *in vitro*. **Fertility and Sterility** 44:663–667.

Westergaard, L., McNatty, K.P. & Christensen, I.J. (1985b). Steroid concentrations in fluid from human ovarian antral follicles during pregnancy. **Journal of Endocrinology** 107:133–136.

The brain renin–angiotensin system and the secretion of anterior pituitary hormones in the rat

MARIANNE K. STEELE

Physiology Department, University of California, San Francisco, CA 94143-0444, USA.

Keywords

Angiotensin II, luteinizing hormone, prolactin, luteinizing hormone-releasing hormone, atrial natriuretic hormone, norepinephrine.

Introduction

Angiotensin II (AII) is a peptide of eight amino acids formed via an enzymatic cascade in which the substrate, angiotensinogen, is cleaved by the enzyme renin to form the decapeptide, angiotensin I. Angiotensin-converting enzyme then further reduces angiotensin I to AII. This cascade occurs in the bloodstream to maintain the circulating renin–angiotensin system, which classically has been implicated in the control of blood pressure, vascular reactivity, and fluid-electrolyte homeostasis.

In addition to the circulating AII system, research during the past 10 years has identified putative 'local', possibly intratissue, renin–angiotensin systems in a variety of organs including the brain, pituitary gland, adrenal gland, pineal, testis and ovary (for reviews, see Steele and Ganong, 1986b; Moffett *et al.*, 1987, Deschepper and Ganong, 1988).

The function of local tissue-generated AII may be similar to that of circulating AII, i.e. regulation of vascular tone and fluid/electrolyte shifts. However, other functions are also possible. For example, in the brain, as discussed in this chapter, AII acts as a neurotransmitter, affecting the release of other brain peptides intracerebrally. There is one report of angiogenesis after application of AII to the rabbit cornea (Fernandez *et al.*, 1985). Such data need to be confirmed and, if accurate, they raise the possibility that AII may play a role in angiogenesis in highly vascularized endocrine glands, such as the testis and ovary. A role for AII in the development of the ovarian follicle or corpora lutea or in follicular atresia has been postulated. Another possible action of local-tissue AII may be as a growth factor. AII has been reported to be a potent mitogen in bovine adrenocortical cells (Simonian and Gill, 1979) and to increase the synthesis of RNA in liver cells (Re and Parab, 1984). In addition to its potential role as a stimulus for steroidogenesis in the gonads (Pucell *et al.*, 1987), AII may be involved in cellular differentiation. The immature rat testis contains many more receptors for AII than are found in the adult testis, and these receptors appear to be localized on undifferentiated cells

(Millan and Aguilera, 1988). It is possible that the peptide may play a role in selection and growth of cells during testicular development.

Clearly, much work is needed in order to define and delineate the possible autocrine or paracrine functions of local, tissue-generated AII. At this time, two of the most intensively studied local systems are those in the brain and the ovary. This chapter focuses on the brain AII system, while the next chapter by Naftolin and his colleagues provides data on the ovarian AII system.

The brain renin–angiotensin system (Moffett *et al.*, 1987) participates in the control of a number of physiological functions, including blood pressure regulation, fluid and electrolyte balance, neuronal activity and secretion of hormones from the pituitary gland (Phillips, 1987). In addition to its effects upon the release of vasopressin, oxytocin and ACTH, brain-derived AII has been shown to influence the secretion of the reproductive hormones, luteinizing hormone (LH) and prolactin (PRL). This chapter includes a review of published data on the central role of AII in the regulation of LH and PRL release. In addition, new data are presented on the interactions of AII with other brain-peptide systems, namely LH-releasing hormone (LHRH) and atrial natriuretic peptide (ANP), in controlling the circulating levels of these anterior pituitary hormones.

What is the influence of gonadal hormones on the effects of AII on LH and PRL?

Initial studies demonstrated that intracerebroventricular (ICV) injection of high doses of AII increased plasma LH concentrations in ovariectomized rats pretreated with estradiol (Steele *et al.*, 1982). The increase was blocked by prior injection of saralasin, a blocker of AII receptors, which demonstrated the specificity of the AII effect on LH. AII also increased plasma LH levels in intact animals on the morning of proestrus (Steele *et al.*, 1983), a time when the brain has been 'primed' by increasing levels of endogenous estrogen on the preceding day.

The effects of ICV injection of AII on release of LH are not due to a direct effect of the peptide at the level of the pituitary gland. Although centrally administered AII might reach the adenohypophysis, the secretion of LH would not be affected since, *in vitro*, AII has no effect on gonadotropin release at doses that stimulate the secretion of PRL (Steele *et al.*, 1981).

The effects of ICV injection of AII on pulsatile secretion of LH in non-steroid-treated, ovariectomized rats have also been examined (Steele *et al.*, 1985). A continuous blood-sampling protocol was used to monitor pulses of LH before, during, and after ICV infusion of low doses of AII. In contrast to the stimulatory effect in intact rats, the data revealed a significant, dose-related inhibition of LH release by AII, which was abolished by co-infusion of saralasin. Saralasin, by itself, produced a small but significant increase in LH, as compared to levels in animals infused with artificial cerebrospinal fluid (aCSF), suggesting a role for endogenous AII in the control of LH secretion.

These same doses of AII did not modify levels of LH in animals pretreated with estradiol, but produced dose-related increases in LH in rats treated with estradiol and progesterone.

Taken together, these data reveal that ICV administration of low doses of AII selectively activates AII receptors in the brain to affect pituitary secretion of LH. The direction of this effect, stimulation or inhibition, is determined by an action of gonadal steroids. Similar steroid-induced reversals in the modulation of LH release have been observed with ICV administration of the catecholamine, norepinephrine (NE; Gallo and Drouva, 1979), raising the possibility of an AII–NE interaction in the brain. In the peripheral nervous system, AII has long been known to interact with NE (Westfall, 1980), and a similar situation may exist in the brain. Experiments testing this hypothesis are described below.

In contrast to release of LH, PRL secretion is consistently inhibited after ICV administration of AII, regardless of the steroid milieu of the animal. In ovariectomized rats, with or without treatment with estradiol and/or progesterone, ICV injection of AII in doses as low as 50 ng per rat inhibited the secretion of prolactin (Steele *et al.*, 1981; Myers and Steele, 1988) for up to 1 hour. Pretreatment of the animals with ICV injection of saralasin abolished the suppressive effects of AII on PRL release. In male rats, ICV injection of AII (50 ng per rat; Steele and Ganong, 1986a) or ICV administration of renin (Andersson *et al.*, 1982) reduced plasma levels of PRL. The effect of renin is mediated by AII, since treatment with a converting enzyme inhibitor prevented the suppressive effects on PRL (Andersson *et al.*, 1982).

To investigate whether the endogenous brain AII system participates in the suppression and maintenance of the low levels of PRL observed in ovariectomized animals, saralasin or sarthran, both blockers of AII receptors, were administered to such animals. In addition, the effects of an inhibitor of the synthesis of AII, enalaprilat, were investigated. None of these drugs, when administered into the third cerebral ventricle, produced an increase in plasma prolactin levels, compared to basal levels or to levels in control animals (Myers and Steele, unpublished data).

Taken together, these data show that, while the low plasma levels of prolactin observed in ovariectomized animals can be further suppressed by low doses of ICV–AII, endogenous brain AII is not tonically active in maintaining these low levels. In the future, we will be investigating the role of brain AII in the regulation of PRL release in other endocrine states, that is, during lactation and the estrous cycle.

Where in the brain does AII act to induce the release of LH and PRL?

To begin determining where AII acts in the brain to stimulate the secretion of LH, the effect of injection into hypothalamic tissue of angiotensins (I, II or III) was tested in ovariectomized rats pretreated with estradiol and progesterone

(Steele, 1987). Under these conditions, ICV infusion of AII stimulates the release of LH (Steele *et al.*, 1982, 1985). The animals were implanted with chronic bilateral brain cannulas, aimed either at the anterior hypothalamic–preoptic area or at the posterior hypothalamus. Additional animals received a single cannula aimed at the third cerebral ventricle. One microliter of aCSF or 1 μl of AII, AI, AIII or saralasin at various concentrations was injected through each of the bilateral tissue cannulas, or 2.0 μl of these various solutions were injected down the third ventricular cannula.

The data from these experiments showed that administration of 10^{-10} mol/l AII into the anterior hypothalamus–preoptic area resulted in a mean increase of 100% in blood LH levels within 10 minutes, while an equal volume and concentration of AII injected into the third ventricle or the posterior hypothalamus did not affect the levels of LH. Administration of 10^{-13} mol/l AII, injected into the rostral hypothalamus, produced a mean increase of 43% in blood LH concentrations, while administration of 10^{-16} mol/l AII or of aCSF did not significantly affect blood LH concentrations. Infusion of saralasin (10^{-11} mol/l) with AII (10^{-13} mol/l) abolished the effect of AII on the release in LH, without affecting levels of LH by itself. Compared to the increase in blood LH levels produced by injection of 10^{-10} mol/l AII into the anterior preoptic–anterior hypothalamic area, administration of equimolar concentrations of AI and AIII did not significantly affect LH levels.

The data from these experiments demonstrate that the anterior hypothalamic–preoptic area is particularly sensitive to the stimulatory actions of AII on the secretion of LH. These results suggest that the facilitatory effects of higher doses of AII – 150 ng/25 μl per hour infusion, 6 mmol/l (Steele *et al.*, 1985) – administered into the third ventricle were due to diffusion of the peptide to and its action in the rostral diencephalon.

The lack of responsiveness of levels of LH to AI and AIII suggests a degree of specificity attributable to AII alone. The absence of an effect of AI also suggests that, at this dose, there is insufficient conversion of the decapeptide to the active octapeptide AII in the anterior hypothalamic–preoptic region to affect the secretion of LH.

The exact area within the rostral hypothalamus in which AII acts to elicit the release of LH cannot be determined from these experiments. Although the medial preoptic area (MPOA) is a likely candidate as a mediator of this effect, the injected material undoubtedly spread beyond the limits of this nuclear region. The MPOA is an area of the brain that has been implicated in the phasic control of LH release (Barraclough and Wise, 1981); it contains AII receptors (Healy *et al.*, 1986) and is also an area in which catecholamine and LHRH neurons make synaptic connections (Hoffman, 1985).

What is the role of endogenous brain AII in controlling the release of LH in intact animals?

The observation that centrally administered AII stimulated the release of LH in steroid-treated ovariectomized rats (Steele *et al.*, 1982) and that it elevated plasma LH levels in intact, proestrous animals raised the possibility that AII synthesized within the brain might be involved in the normal, phasic, estrogen-induced release of LH seen during the afternoon of proestrus in intact rats (Steele *et al.*, 1983).

To test this hypothesis, female rats were injected ICV with saralasin, an AII receptor blocker, or with enalaprilat, an inhibitor of converting enzyme, or with saline, during the afternoon of proestrus. Blood samples were taken at hourly intervals, and on the following day the ova in the oviduct were counted.

Blockade of AII receptors in the brain abolished the preovulatory surge of LH and inhibited ovulation when values were compared to those from saline-injected animals. This effect was not mediated at the level of the median eminence, anterior pituitary gland or ovary, since these areas are outside the blood–brain barrier and intravenous administration of this dose of saralasin or a much larger dose did not affect the surge of LH or the extent of ovulation. In addition, centrally administered saralasin did not affect the LH response to a submaximal intravenous dose of LHRH, demonstrating that saralasin did not alter the responsiveness of the anterior pituitary gland.

Inhibition of converting-enzyme activity in the brain by enalaprilat also prevented the proestrous surge in LH and inhibited ovulation. Inspection of hormone profiles from individual rats showed that two animals had surges which were advanced relative to the timing seen in saline-injected animals, and two showed a 'normal' surge. In five animals, however, no surge of LH or ovulation was observed. Peripheral administration of enalaprilat had no significant effect on the LH surge or the frequency of ovulation.

Taken together, these data support an obligatory role for AII, manufactured in the brain, in the control of the secretion of LH and ovulation in intact female rats. The influence of local ovarian AII on ovarian function is discussed in the next chapter by Naftolin and his colleagues.

How do brain AII and norepinephrine interact in controlling the release of LH?

The effects of AII on LH release are undoubtedly mediated via the release of LHRH from the brain median eminence, passing through the pituitary portal vessels to act at the anterior pituitary gland. Therefore, we next examined whether AII acts directly on LHRH neurons or via another brain neurotransmitter system, for example that of NE. As mentioned above, AII has long been known either to potentiate the release of NE from nerve endings or to inhibit its re-uptake after secretion in the autonomic nervous system (Westfall, 1980).

Brain AII could act in a similar fashion to facilitate the release of brain NE to regulate release of LHRH and, subsequently, of LH. Further evidence for this hypothesis comes from reports that show that central administration of AII increases the turnover of catecholamines in certain areas of the brainstem (Printz *et al.*, 1982), in the median eminence, and in the hypothalamus (Sumners and Phillips, 1983).

To determine directly whether catecholamines mediate the stimulatory effects of AII on the secretion of LH, groups of ovariectomized rats pretreated with gonadal steroids were administered either diethyldithiocarbamate (DDC), an inhibitor of dopamine β-hydroxylase, to deplete hypothalamic stores of both NE and epinephrine, or with LY134046, a selective inhibitor of the synthesis of epinephrine. Treatment with DDC abolished the stimulatory effects of AII on the release of LH, and, in a separate group of rats, produced significant reductions in levels of both NE and epinephrine in the hypothalamus. LY134046 produced a comparable reduction in hypothalamic concentrations of epinephrine, with no effect upon levels of NE, and it did not inhibit the LH response to AII. Treatment with DDC did not affect the LH response to ICV infusion of NE or to intravenous LHRH, demonstrating that the drug did not modify adrenergic receptors or the responsiveness of the pituitary gland to stimulation (Steele and Ganong, 1986a).

In order to identify the type of adrenergic receptor which responded to the hypothalamic NE released by ICV injection of AII, animals were treated with either the α_1 blocking drug, prazosin, the α_2 blocking drug, yohimbine, or the mixed-β blocker, propranolol. Only administration of yohimbine blocked the stimulatory effects of ICV injection of AII (as well as those of ICV injection of NE) on the secretion of LH; prazosin did not affect the LH response to AII, while propranolol potentiated the effect of AII, as well as that of ICV-injected NE.

Taken together, this series of experiments demonstrates that the elevation in blood LH levels after ICV infusion of AII is mediated by the release of NE within the hypothalamus, which then acts at facilitatory α_2 receptors. Exogenous NE also acts at these receptors. The data regarding AII lend support to the hypothesis that at least some of the increase in catecholamine turnover associated with ICV administration of AII (Printz *et al.*, 1982; Sumners and Phillips, 1983) may be functionally related to the release of LH. The data regarding NE are also of interest since, previously, the only study demonstrating blockade of the facilitatory effect of NE on the release of LH in the steroid-treated ovariectomized animal had used the non-specific α blocker, phenoxybenzamine, which blocks both α_1 and α_2 receptors (Caceres and Taleisnik, 1982). Potentiation of the LH response to ICV-injected NE by propranolol has been reported previously (Caceres and Taleisnik, 1982). The fact that the LH response to ICV-injected AII is also potentiated in propranolol-treated animals provides further evidence that AII exerts its stimulatory effects on LH via the release of NE in the brain.

It is likely that the AII–NE interaction occurs within the rostral hypothalamus, perhaps within the MPOA. Ongoing experiments have been designed to monitor local release of hypothalamic NE after administration of AII. There is some evidence that brain AII stimulates the release of the brain catecholamine, dopamine (Andersson *et al.*, 1982; Sumners and Phillips, 1983). Such an effect, if real, may be related to the inhibitory effects of the peptide on the secretion of PRL.

Does AII affect the release of LHRH?

It is likely that the effects of ICV infusion or injection into tissue of AII on the release of LH are mediated ultimately by release of LHRH from the median eminence. In order to test whether AII affects the secretion of LHRH, we utilized an in-vitro system wherein whole blocks of hypothalamic tissue, including the preoptic area and median eminence, were perifused with various doses of AII (in a modified Krebs–Ringer buffer) and the LHRH in the effluent was measured by RIA (Steele and Levine, unpublished data).

The data obtained thus far show that AII (10^{-6} mol/l) stimulated the release of LHRH in four of six chambers which contained whole hypothalami from ovariectomized rats treated with ovarian steroids. At a concentration of 10^{-8} mol/l, AII did not affect the release of LHRH in four out of four chambers. Application of potassium ions at the end of the perifusion period elevated levels of LHRH in all chambers, attesting to the viability of the tissue through the end of the experiment.

Both the preoptic area and the median eminence contain AII terminals (Van Houten *et al.*, 1980; Lind *et al.*, 1985; Healy *et al.*, 1986) and receptors. In addition to an effect in the anterior forebrain (Steele, 1987), AII could act at the median eminence to affect the release of LHRH. Therefore, additional experiments were performed in which hypothalami without the median eminence or samples of median eminence alone were perfused with AII (10^{-6} mol/l).

The effluent from hypothalami without median eminence ($n=4$) contained little or no detectable LHRH, under either basal or AII-stimulated conditions; LHRH was detectable, however, during stimulation with K^+ ions. Levels of LHRH in the effluent from chambers that contained median eminence alone were as high as those seen previously with whole hypothalami and were not affected by administration of AII ($n=4$), as compared to levels in unstimulated chambers ($n=2$). Treatment with K^+ produced an increase in levels of LHRH in all chambers. These data are consistent with the hypothesis that the site of action for AII is within the anterior hypothalamus, probably within the preoptic area. Within this area, AII interacts with NE to affect LHRH cell bodies, such that LHRH is released at the median eminence.

What is the interaction between AII and ANP with respect to secretion of LH and PRL?

Atrial natriuretic peptide was originally isolated from cardiac extracts (de Bold *et al.*, 1981), in particular from the atria. However, recently ANP has also been localized in extracardiac tissues (McKenzie *et al.*, 1985), including specific areas of the central nervous system (Standaert *et al.*, 1988). The peripheral actions of ANP at the level of the kidney, adrenal gland and blood vasculature (Goetz, 1988) seem coordinated to oppose those of the circulating and tissue renin–angiotensin systems. For the most part, a similar situation exists within the central nervous system. Central administration of ANP inhibits the secretion of vasopressin (Samson *et al.*, 1987), the dehydration-induced intake of water (Katsuura *et al.*, 1986) and salt preference (Fitts *et al.*, 1985). In addition, ICV-injected ANP antagonizes the increase in blood pressure (Itoh *et al.*, 1986), water intake (Masotto and Negro-Vilar, 1985) and vasopressin secretion (Castro *et al.*, 1987) induced by ICV-injected AII.

A possible role for ANP in reproductive neuroendocrine function was suggested by the presence of immunoreactive ANP terminals and binding sites in the median eminence and cell bodies in the preoptic septal region. In fact, the highest concentration of ANP-like material in the brain has been found in the preoptic area and hypothalamus (Standaert *et al.*, 1988). Binding sites for ANP may also exist in the preoptic area, since iontophoresis or pressure injection of ANP into this area in ovariectomized rats produced a decrease in spontaneous neural firing (Wong *et al.*, 1986).

Recently, it was reported that high doses of ANP (ICV bolus, 3.0 μg or 6.0 μg in 2.0 μl saline per rat) suppressed plasma levels of LH and PRL in male rats (Samson *et al.*, 1988). The effects of ANP on plasma levels of LH and PRL are apparently mediated via the brain, since in these experiments, as well as in others (Simard *et al.*, 1986; Abou-Samra *et al.*, 1987), no direct effect of the peptide on the secretion of hormones by the anterior pituitary gland was observed. An action of the peptide at the median eminence is possible, although, *in vitro*, ANP did not affect basal release of LHRH from explants of median eminence.

The inhibitory actions of ANP on release of LH and PRL in male rats and ovariectomized female animals are similar to those seen after ICV administration of AII (Steele *et al.*, 1981, 1985). This observation raised the possibility that, in contrast to the antagonistic actions of central ANP and AII on fluid, electrolyte, and blood pressure homeostasis, the peptides may influence the secretion of LH and PRL in a similar direction.

In order to test this hypothesis, a study was initiated of the effects of ANP and/or AII on water intake and levels of LH and PRL in ovariectomized female rats pretreated with estradiol and progesterone (Steele, 1988). Ten minutes after administration of AII (50 ng), plasma LH values were increased by 100%, returning to baseline levels within 40 minutes of administration of

AII. Treatment with ANP (200 ng) produced a similar hormonal profile. Co-administration of AII with ANP resulted in a 200% increase in levels of LH, which remained elevated even 40 min after the injection, suggesting an additive effect of AII and ANP on the secretion of LH. Levels of PRL were not affected by either AII or ANP. However, co-injection of the peptides produced a significant suppression of levels of PRL. Water intake induced by injection of AII was attenuated by injection of ANP, which by itself did not stimulate water ingestion.

Taken together, these data suggest that AII and ANP interact differentially, depending on the variable being observed: the peptides are antagonistic in their effects on blood pressure, heart rate, renal nerve activity and fluid intake, and additive in their effects on the secretion of LH and PRL.

Conclusion

The data summarized in this review strongly support the hypothesis that hypothalamic AII is involved in the physiological control of the secretion of LH, especially in the process of ovulation. A role for AII in the release of PRL has been suggested. However, additional experiments need to be performed to define this function more clearly. With respect to LH, brain AII interacts with at least two other brain systems, those of NE and ANP, to affect the release of LHRH and ultimately the release of LH.

Traditionally, AII (as well as ANP) has been considered a cardiovascular and fluid-balance hormone, acting primarily within the circulation. The discovery of localized tissue AII systems, in addition to that in the brain, has raised the possibility that AII has actions beyond the regulation of blood pressure. A role for AII in reproductive physiology has now been established through identification of the reproductive role of AII in the brain and by the presence of the ovarian and testicular AII systems. It will be of interest in the future to investigate whether the brain and gonadal AII systems interact.

Acknowledgements

This work was supported by NIH grants HD18020, HL29714 and DK07265. I wish to thank W.F. Ganong, C.F. Deschepper, R. Gallo, L.S. Myers, J.E. Levine, D. San Juan and R. Shackelford for their exceptional assistance and encouragement during these studies.

References

Abou-Samra, A., Catt, K.J. & Aguilera, G. (1987). Synthetic atrial natriuretic factors stimulate cGMP production but not hormone release in rat pituitary cells. **Endocrinology** 120:18–24.

Andersson, K., Fuxe, K., Agnati, L.F., Ganten, D., Zini, F., Eneroth, P., Mascagni, F. & Infantillina, F. (1982). Intraventricular injections of renin increase amine turnover

in the tuberoinfundibular dopamine neurons and reduce the secretion of prolactin in the male rat. **Acta Physiologica Scandinavica** 116:317–320.
Barraclough, C.A. & Wise, P.M. (1981). The role of catecholamines in the regulation of pituitary lutenizing hormone and follicle-stimulating hormone release. **Endocrine Reviews** 3(1):91–119.
Caceres, A. & Taleisnik, S. (1982). Dissociation of the inhibitory and facilitory effects of norepinephrine on the release of LH by premammillary lesions. **Neuroendocrinology** 35:98–103.
Castro, R., Keiler, I., Schroeder, G. & Stock, G. (1987). Angiotensin-induced vasopressin release is attenuated by central atrial natriuretic factor. **Clinical and Experimental Hypertension: Theory and Practice** A9(1):81–94.
de Bold, A.J., Borenstein, H.B., Veress, A.T. & Sonnenberg, H. (1981). A rapid and potent natriuretic response to intravenous injection of atrial myocardial extract in rats. **Life Sciences** 28:89–94.
Deschepper, C.F. & Ganong, W.F. (1988). Renin and angiotensin in endocrine glands. In: Martini, L. & Ganong, W.F., eds. **Frontiers in Neuroendocrinology**, Vol. 10, New York, Raven Press, pp.79–98.
Fernandez, L.A., Turckler, J. & Mead, A. (1985). Neovascularization produced by angiotensin II. **Journal of Laboratory and Clinical Medicine** 105:141–145.
Fitts, D.A., Thundorst, R.L. & Simpson, J.B. (1985). Diuresis and reduction in salt appetite by lateral ventricular infusion of atriopeptin II. **Brain Research Bulletin** 348:118–122.
Gallo, R.V. & Drouva, S.V. (1979). Effect of intraventricular infusion of catecholamines on LH release in ovariectomized and ovariectomized, steroid-primed rats. **Neuroendocrinology** 29:149–162.
Goetz, K.L. (1988). Physiology and pathophysiology of atrial peptides. **American Journal of Physiology** 254:E1–E15.
Healy, D.P., Maciejewski, A.R. & Printz, M.P. (1986). Localization of central AII receptors with [^{125}I]-sar, ile^{8}-angiotensin II: periventricular sites of the anterior third ventricle. **Neuroendocrinology** 44:15–21.
Hoffman, G. (1985). Organization of LHRH cells: differential opposition to neurotensin, substance P and catecholamine axons. **Peptides** 6:439–461.
Itoh, H., Nakao, K., Morii, N., Yanada, T., Shiono, S., Sakamoto, M., Sugawara, A., Saito, Y., Katswera, G., Shiomi, G., Eigyo, M., Matsushita, A. & Imura, H. (1986). Central action of atrial natriuretic polypeptide on blood pressure in conscious rats. **Brain Research Bulletin** 16:745–751.
Kalra, S.P. & Kalra, P.S. (1983). Neural regulation of luteinizing hormone secretion in the rat. **Endocrine Reviews** 4:311–351.
Katsuura, G., Kakamura, M., Inouye, K., Kono, M., Nakao, K. & Imura, H. (1986). Regulatory role of atrial natriuretic polypeptide in water drinking in rats. **European Journal of Pharmacology** 121:285–289.
Lind, R.W., Swanson, L.W. & Ganten, D. (1985). Organization of angiotensin II immunoreactive cells and fibers in the rat central nervous system. **Neuroendocrinology** 40(1):2–24.
Masotto, C. & Negro-Vilar, A. (1985). Inhibition of spontaneous or angiotensin II-stimulated water intake by atrial natriuretic factor. **Brain Research Bulletin** 15:523–526.
McKenzie, J.C., Tanaka, I., Mosono, K. & Inagami, T. (1985). Immunocytochemical

localization of atrial natriuretic factor in kidney, adrenal medulla, pituitary and atrium of rat. **Journal of Histochemistry and Cytochemistry** 33:828–832.

Millan, M. & Aguilera, G. (1988). Angiotensin II receptors in testes. **Endocrinology** 122:1984–1990.

Moffett, R.B., Bumpus, M. & Husain, A. (1987). Minireview: cellular organization of the brain renin–angiotensin system. **Life Sciences** 41:1867–1879.

Myers, L.S. & Steele, M.K. (1988). Effect of angiotensin II (AII) and AII receptor blockers on prolactin secretion. **Society for Neuroscience** Abstract 14:147.

Phillips, M.I. (1987). Functions of angiotensin in the central nervous system. **Annual Review of Physiology** 49:413–435.

Printz, M.P., Ganten, D., Unger, T. & Phillips, M.I. (1982). Minireview: the brain renin angiotensin system. In: Ganten, D., Printz, M., Phillips, M.I. & Scholkens, B.A., eds. **The Renin Angiotensin System in the Brain**, New York, Springer-Verlag, pp.3–52.

Pucell, A.G., Bumpus, F.M. & Husain, A. (1987). Rat ovarian AII receptors: characterization and coupling to estrogen secretion. **Journal of Biological Chemistry** 262:7076–7080.

Re, R. & Parab, M. (1984). Effect of angiotensin II on RNA synthesis by isolated nuclei. **Life Sciences** 34:648–651.

Samson, W.K., Aguila, M.C. & Bianchi, R. (1988). Atrial natriuretic factor inhibits luteinizing hormone secretion in the rat: evidence for a hypothalamic site of action. **Endocrinology** 122:1573–1582.

Samson, W.K., Aguila, M.C., Martinovic, J., Antunes-Rodrigues, J. & Norris, M. (1987). Hypothalamic action of atrial natriuretic factor to inhibit vasopressin secretion. **Peptides** 8:449–451.

Simard, J., Hubert, F.F., Labrie, F., Assayag, G. & Heister, S. (1986). Atrial natriuretic factor-induced cGMP accumulation in rat anterior pituitary cells in culture is not coupled to hormonal secretion. **Regulatory Peptides** 15:269–274.

Simonian, M.H. & Gill, G.N. (1979). Regulation of deoxyribonucleic acid synthesis in bovine adrenocortical cells in culture. **Endocrinology** 104:588–595.

Standaert, D.G., Needleman, P. & Saper, C.B. (1988). Atriopeptin: neuromediator in the central regulation of cardiovascular function. In: Martini, L. & Ganong, W.F., eds. **Frontiers in Neuroendocrinology**, Vol. 10, New York, Raven Press, pp.63–78.

Steele, M.K. (1987). Effects of angiotensins injected into various brain areas on LH release in female rats. **Neuroendocrinology** 46:401–405.

Steele, M.K. (1988). Stimulatory effects of atrial natriuretic peptide and angiotensin II on LH release in female rats. **Society for Neuroscience** Abstract 14:146.

Steele, M.K., Gallo, R.V. & Ganong, W.F. (1983). A possible role for the brain renin–angiotensin system in the regulation of LH secretion. **American Journal of Physiology** 245:R805–R810.

Steele, M.K., Gallo, R.V. & Ganong, W.F. (1985). Stimulatory or inhibitory effects of angiotensin II upon LH secretion in ovariectomized rats: a function of gonadal steroids. **Neuroendocrinology** 40:210–216.

Steele, M.K. & Ganong, W.F. (1986a). Effects of catecholamine-depleting agents and receptor blockers on basal and angiotensin II- or norepinephrine-stimulated LH release in female rats. **Endocrinology** 119:2728–2736.

Steele, M.K. & Ganong, W.F. (1986b). Brain renin–angiotensin system and secretion of luteinizing hormone and prolactin. In: Ganong, W.F. & Martini, L., eds. **Frontiers in Neuroendocrinology**, Vol. 9, New York, Raven Press, pp.99–113.

Steele, M.K., McCann, S.M. & Negro-Vilar, A. (1982). Modulation by dopamine and estradiol of central effects of angiotensin II on anterior pituitary hormone release. **Endocrinology** 111:722–729.

Steele, M.K., Negro-Vilar, A. & McCann, S.M. (1981). Effect of angiotensin II on *in vivo* and *in vitro* release of anterior pituitary hormones in the female rat. **Endocrinology** 109:893–899.

Sumners, C. & Phillips, M.I. (1983). Central injection of AII alters catecholamine activity in rat brain. **American Journal of Physiology** 244:R257–R263.

Van Houten, M., Schiffrin, E.L., Mann, J., Posner, B.I. & Boucher, R. (1980). Radiographic localization of binding sites for blood-borne AII in the rat brain. **Brain Research Bulletin** 186:480–485.

Westfall, T.C. (1980). Neuroeffector mechanisms. **Annual Review of Physiology** 42:383–397.

Wong, M., Samson, W.K., Dudley, C.A. & Moss, R.L. (1986). Direct neuronal action of atrial natriuretic factor in the rat brain. **Neuroendocrinology** 44:49–53.

Renin and angiotensin formation and action in the ovary

M. ALAM, A. PALUMBO,[1] A. LIGHTMAN,[1] R. APA,[1] T. ZREIK,
P. ANDRADE-GORDON, A.H. DECHERNEY AND F. NAFTOLIN

[1]*Lalor Foundation Fellows, Department of Obstetrics and Gynecology, Yale University School of Medicine, New Haven, CT 06510, USA.*

Keywords

Renin, angiotensin, ovarian function, angiogenesis, oocyte maturation.

Renin–angiotensin systems in extrarenal tissues

The extrarenal renin–angiotensin system (RAS) in humans and animals has received a great deal of attention in recent years. There is evidence that a RAS exists in the brain, pituitary, adrenal cortex, liver, and reproductive systems, each system having a special role related to its site of origin (Naruse *et al.*, 1981, 1985; Brownfield *et al.*, 1983; Parmentier *et al.*, 1983; Ganong, 1984; Sarina *et al.*, 1985; Dechepper *et al.*, 1986). For example, Steele and others (Steele *et al.*, 1981, 1983; Aguilera *et al.*, 1982; Jones *et al.*, 1988) suggested that angiotensin II (AII), generated in the brain, may be involved in the regulation of secretion of prolactin (PRL), growth hormone (GH), TSH and luteinizing hormone (LH) from the pituitary.

Specific receptors for AII have been identified in the brain, adrenal glands and liver (Williams *et al.*, 1974; Goodfriend, 1983; Sarina *et al.*, 1985). AII has been shown to influence adrenal function, regulation of systemic blood pressure (Kotchen and Guthrie, 1980; Elliott *et al.*, 1982), synthesis and release of neurotransmitters (Khairallah, 1972; Chevillard *et al.*, 1979) and pituitary hormones (Steele *et al.*, 1981; Aguilera *et al.*, 1982), placental perfusion (Carter and Gothlin, 1970), neovascularization (Fernandez *et al.*, 1985), and various specific metabolic activities (Andersson, 1978). In the reproductive system, the testis (Dechepper *et al.*, 1986; Jackson *et al.*, 1988) and the uterus (Johnson *et al.*, 1984) have been shown to contain renin activity and converting enzyme (Dechepper *et al.*, 1986; Jackson *et al.*, 1988).

Sporadic reports of components of an ovarian RAS appeared prior to our measurements of high levels of renin-like activity and AII in human preovulatory follicular fluid (FF) (Fernandez *et al.*, 1985; Culler *et al.*, 1986; Lightman *et al.*, 1987) and the finding of prorenin in FF by the groups of Sealey and Derkx (Glorioso *et al.*, 1986; Derkx *et al.*, 1987). The latter authors have also indicated that the ovary may be the source of elevated levels of circulating prorenin during the mid- and late ovarian cycle and early pregnancy (Sealey *et al.*, 1985). The possibility that AII is generated locally and has intraovarian effects, such as regulation of steroidogenesis, control of blood flow and control of oocyte maturation, is exciting and has profound implications for the understanding and control of ovarian function and fertility.

Evidence for an ovarian RAS

Components of a RAS in FF

After some of the information described above became available, we looked for components of a RAS in the ovary and found levels of renin-like activity and AII immunoreactivity in FF from gonadotropin-stimulated women to be an order of magnitude higher than those levels in simultaneously drawn, circulating blood (Culler *et al.*, 1986; Fernandez *et al.*, 1985; Lightman *et al.*, 1987). At about the same time, Sealey's group reported levels of prorenin in FF to be 10- to 20-fold higher than in blood in gonadotropin-stimulated women (Glorioso *et al.*, 1986). Later, Derkx *et al.* (1987) observed similar results. While FF provides only a limited view of ovarian development and function, it is the fluid that bathes the cumulus and its developing ovum and, therefore, it is of great significance to fertility. The following evidence indicates the importance of measurements of AII in the FF, which is a natural reservoir and is endowed with the properties needed for a rapid increase in levels of AII: (1) stimulation by gonadotropin increases renin-like activity and levels of AII in FF; (2) theca and granulosa-lutein cells from preovulatory follicles are strongly immunopositive for renin and AII (Lightman *et al.*, 1986); (3) thecal cells (Paulson *et al.*, 1989), rat ovarian tissue (Husain *et al.*, 1987), and human granulosa-lutein cells in culture (Palumbo *et al.*, 1988) respond dramatically by increased steroidogenesis to levels of AII that are the same as those found in FF.

Localization and extent of the ovarian RAS

The presence of renin-like activity in the female genital tract, i.e. in the placenta, uterus, and oviducts of animals and humans, has been known for over 20 years (Johnson *et al.*, 1984; Wilkes *et al.*, 1985). The presence of this archetypal system in the reproductive tracts of primitive and complex animal species has important implications for the understanding and management of reproductive health and disease (Naftolin *et al.*, 1988). Eskildsen (1972) detected 'renin' in homogenates of rabbit ovaries without morphological localization. Recently, angiotensin-converting enzymatic activity was measured in human tissues, including the ovary, and was localized to the oocyte, among other ovarian compartments (VanSande *et al.*, 1985). We have examined the binding of renin- and AII-specific antisera to normal and stimulated ovaries from women and animals (Lightman *et al.*, 1986). Our ovarian immunohistochemical and in-vitro studies have demonstrated the presence of immunoreactive renin and AII in the cytoplasm of thecal, luteinized granulosa cells and in corpora lutea of both rat and human, indicating production of renin and AII *in situ* rather than concentration of these compounds from the blood. The presence in the rat ovary of mRNA specific for renin (Kim *et al.*, 1987) and angiotensinogen (Ohkubu *et al.*, 1986) has been found by in-situ hybridization and Northern blotting, respectively. Several groups have reported the presence of receptors for AII in the ovary (Pucell *et al.*, 1987; Husain *et al.*, 1987; Harwood and Hausdorff, 1987). In view of all the above data, the existence of an ovarian AII-generating system (OVRAS) and the role such a system might play in ovarian function have now become the focus of great interest.

Degree of autonomy of OVRAS

Although we have hypothesized the existence of an *intrinsic* ovarian renin–angiotensin system, the degree of autonomy of the system, i.e. the extent of its freedom from requirements for extraovarian precursors and actions, cannot be defined at this time. Indeed, complete physiologic autonomy is not a possibility, since the ovary is responsive to gonadotropins and other circulating materials, and since it receives renin substrate from the circulation. The significance of OVRAS will, therefore, not depend upon its autonomy; rather, it will hinge upon orchestration by extra- and intraovarian regulators of the production and actions of AII/AIII within the ovary.

Regulation of the ovarian RAS

It is not known whether the extrarenal and renal RAS are influenced by the same control mechanism(s). The direct stimulatory role of gonadotropins (Lightman *et al.*, 1987) seems unlikely to function via effects on organs other than the gonad; no receptors for gonadotropins have been found, for example, in the adrenal cortex. Control by gonadotropins could be direct, due to effects upon ovarian renin–angiotensin-generating cells; or it could be indirect, perhaps due to autocrine or paracrine agents, such as steroids and proteolytic enzymes (Boneher *et al.*, 1974; Wintroub *et al.*, 1984; Tang *et al.*, 1987; Liu *et al.*, 1987). This response to gonadotropin-induced steroids, for example, involves an increase in liver or ovarian production of AI from renin substrate through modulation of the activity of several ovarian enzymes that have renin-like activity and that cleave precursors to AI (Boneher *et al.*, 1974; Wintroub *et al.*, 1984; Tang *et al.*, 1987). The presence of AII immunoreactivity throughout the follicle wall and the luteal cells indicates a possible autocrine effect, since the AII-containing cells also produce steroids.

The ovary produces proteolytic enzymes, such as plasminogen activators (Liu *et al.*, 1987; O'Connell *et al.*, 1987), which could activate prorenin or cleave angiotensinogen directly to generate AII (Tang *et al.*, 1987). In addition to establishing local, i.e. cellular, autonomy in the control of the OVRAS, the presence in FF of plasminogen activators and inhibitors of plasminogen activators allows for the actions of OVRAS in the antrum, and especially on antral cells, independent of the presence of renin within ovarian cells. This model raises the possibility that two systems for formation of AII may exist: there may be a constitutive intracellular system, and there may also be a pool of precursors to AII and latent angiotensinogen-cleaving agents in the FF, which can be abruptly activated to produce dramatic increases in levels of AII, as occurs immediately before ovulation (Lightman *et al.*, 1989).

Association of ovarian RAS with ovarian function

The presence of receptors for AII in the ovary indicates a functional role for ovarian AII. Our autoradiographic data from studies *in vitro* (Lightman *et al.*, 1988) and the more extensive work of Husain *et al.* (1987), and Harwood and Hausdorff (1987) have demonstrated the presence of saralasin (Sar)-suppressible binding of AII in gonadotropin-stimulated compartments in the ovary. Binding of AII is associated in several organs with changes in phosphoinositol and calcium turnover rates, inositol triphosphate acting as the intracellular second messenger for the action of AII (Elliott *et al.*, 1982). Harwood's data are consistent with similar findings in the ovary (Harwood and Hausdorff, 1987). In addition, in a preliminary study, we have found that AII added to cultured luteal cells induces an increase in levels of prostaglandin F_{2a} in the medium (unpublished).

Effects of the RAS that might affect ovarian function

Steroidogenesis

AII is a specific ligand which controls secretion of aldosterone from adrenal glomerulosa cells. AII acts at more than one point in the biosynthesis of aldosterone. Several groups have demonstrated stimulatory responses of isolated glomerulosa cells to AII *in vitro*, and the suppressive effects of blockers of receptors for AII, such as Sar, on secretion of aldosterone (Crozet *et al.*, 1986). AII also enhances the action of ACTH on steroidogenesis in the fasciculata (Hepp *et al.*, 1977; Kotchen and Guthrie, 1980; Crozet *et al.*, 1986). Thus, the RAS might have a similar effect on ovarian steroidogenesis. Husain's group first reported increased secretion of estrogen by rat ovarian fragments cultured with added AII (Pucell *et al.*, 1987). We have carried out studies *in vitro*, using rat luteal cells in culture (unpublished) and washed human granulosa cells harvested from FSH/LH-stimulated women 36 hours after administration of human chorionic gonadotropin, cultured in the presence of AII and/or Sar^1 -Ala^5 angiotensin (saralasin). In all cases, AII induced increased secretion of steroids. This result was especially interesting in the case of cultures of human granulosa-lutein cells, since they showed differential regulation of steroidogenesis, with levels of progesterone and testosterone rising persistently while levels of estradiol rose in the presence of AII at levels found in preovulatory FF, but fell toward control levels at 10^{-9} mol/l AII or higher (Palumbo *et al.*, 1988). We have also found that levels of aromatase activity in human granulosa-lutein cells cultured in the presence of AII paralleled the biphasic changes in levels of estradiol (submitted for publication). Paulson and colleagues (1988) have reported the secretion of androgen from cultured ovarian theca cells, a result that is consistent with our own findings of increased secretion of androgens from cultured lutein cells (Palumbo *et al.*, 1988) and the AII immunopositivity of human ovarian hilus cells (Lightman *et al.*, 1986).

Arteriolar constriction

AII causes arteriolar constriction throughout the body (Page and Bumpus, 1974; Oliver and Sciacca, 1984) and has been shown to affect blood flow and its distribution in fetal lambs (Iwamoto and Rudolph, 1981). The ovary has an extensive blood supply and depends heavily upon regional blood flow. Direct effects of AII on this system could have dramatic consequences, but any conclusions are only speculative at present.

Angiogenesis

When blood flow to the kidney is impaired by constriction of the renal artery, angiotensin-dependent hypertension and the development of collateral circulation occur (Fernandez *et al.*, 1982; Okamura *et al.*, 1986). Studies by Fernandez *et al.* (1982) have demonstrated that renin, in the presence of appropriate substrate and converting enzyme for production of AII, can, by facilitating development of collateral circulation, increase the provision of blood to tissues that have been rendered ischemic (Fernandez *et al.*, 1982). It has also been shown that surgical implantation of AII in the rabbit cornea promotes the formation of new blood vessels (Fernandez *et al.*, 1982). This effect of AII could be of importance in other processes that require angiogenesis, such as the neovascularization that is fundamental to ovarian follicular development and formation of corpus luteum, since both require the development of new blood vessels, without which they could not exist.

Angiogenic capabilities were first attributed to the corpus luteum of the cow by Jakob *et al.* (1977) and subsequently demonstrated in corpora lutea and follicles from rabbits (Gospodarowicz and Tharkal, 1978), rats (Gaede *et al.*, 1985), and pigs (Frederick *et al.*, 1985). Makris *et al.* (1982) showed that extracts of porcine, whole non-luteal ovary and isolated theca stimulate the migration and proliferation of bovine endothelial cells. Frederick *et al.* (1984, 1985) injected purified fractions from human and porcine FF into rabbit corneas and showed striking angiogenesis. Thus, the available evidence suggests that follicles, as well as corpora lutea, produce angiogenic factor(s). At least part of this activity appears to be associated with a heat-labile, basic peptide whose stimulus for action is enhanced by treatment with gonadotropin (Sato *et al.*, 1982). The source of this ovarian angiogenic activity is both unclear and controversial; the follicular granulosa or theca cells seem likely, but not exclusive, sources. In a report by Frederick *et al.* (1985), porcine angiogenic activity was described as falling into two distinct molecular-weight ranges: 45–60 kDa and 1.5 kDa. These findings are consistent with angiogenic factors of low molecular weight, such as AII and AIII, which are octa- and septapeptides, respectively, although they may, perhaps, be combined with carrier proteins of higher molecular weight. In preliminary collaborative experiments with E. Lindenbaum using AII (unpublished), we have been able to stimulate angiogenesis in the chicken egg chorioallantoic membrane. However, even if these results prove to be consistent and specific to AII, it is too early to attempt to determine the mechanism of this action because, for example, a recent report by Sterling *et al.* (1989) indicates the possibility that, in luteal cells, AII induces mRNA for the angiogenic factor known as basic fibroblast growth factor.

The OVRAS as a possible marker of follicular development

No single clinical measurement of ovarian function is adequate for the study of fertility or the assessment of treatment. Perhaps the best indicator of follicular development is the concentration of estradiol in blood, especially when this measurement is combined with follicular measurement by ultrasound. However, even the combined approach is only partially successful in defining oocyte morphology and maturity (Pellicer *et al.*, 1987) The above-mentioned changes in levels of components of RAS in FF indicate that the OVRAS may be related to ovarian function and might be used as a marker of oocyte maturation. The work of Sealey *et al.* (1985) and others (Derkx *et al.*, 1987; Navot *et al.*, 1987), showing that blood prorenin levels in women rise at midcycle and during the luteal phase, indicates that prorenin may ultimately be an indicator of ovarian function, particularly in abnormal states.

The OVRAS in oocyte maturation

Blockade of OVRAS with Sar diminishes the percentage of oocytes with germinal vesicle breakdown after treatment with human chorionic gonadotropin (hCG) of immature rats primed with pregnant mare's serum gonadotropin (PMS). This effect is obviated by the concurrent administration of AII (Palumbo *et al.*, 1988).

Activity of OVRAS during ovulation

In view of the stimulatory role of gonadotropins on the OVRAS, the changes in renin-like activity and AII concentrations in FF displayed during the ovarian cycle and the effect of AII on steroidogenesis, we studied the effects on ovulation of Sar, a specific blocker of receptors for AII. The intraperitoneal administration of Sar to immature, gonadotropin-stimulated rats diminished hCG-induced ovulation. Simultaneous administration of receptor-saturating quantities of AII restored normal ovulatory rates (Pellicer *et al.*, 1988).

Pharmacologic control over the OVRAS

The need for new contraceptives stems from the complications associated with use of steroidal contraceptives (Masterson, 1988), and the recent withdrawal of intrauterine devices from the United States market because of complications due to infections. Thus, the ovarian renin–angiotensin system offers novel contraceptive possibilities at a particularly opportune time. Of equal interest is the possibility that manipulation of the OVRAS could enhance fertility. Since angiotensin has already been shown to affect steroidogenesis in every ovarian compartment, there is reason to expect that specifically targeted agonists or antagonists of the OVRAS could play a role in tailoring ovarian follicular development and subsequent events.

Prior to beginning our series of studies with Sar as a blocker of the OVRAS blocker, we tested the effects of orally administered inhibitors of angiotensin-converting enzyme (ACE) on reproduction. We found no consistent effects of these agents on ovarian cyclicity, rates of induced pseudopregnancy, pregnancy rates, or on the offspring of rats treated during the cycle. Similar findings have been reported in abstract by Peterson *et al.* (1989). The explanation for these findings appears to be the failure of inhibitors of ACE to block formation of AII entirely: our immunohistochemical studies of ovaries from rats treated with inhibitors of ACE showed the continued presence of immunoreactive AII (unpublished observations).

Saralasin exerts an inhibitory effect on synthesis of both aldosterone and corticosterone in rat and human adrenal tissue in culture (Crozet *et al.*, 1986). This result indicates that AII might normally be produced locally and control production of adrenal steroids. Such a possibility in another steroid-producing organ, the ovary, seems to be logical and fits with our pilot data on drugs active in the RAS. Several clinically available drugs block formation of AII (Moursi *et al.*, 1986; Sakagude *et al.*, 1988,) but no indications of their effects on reproduction have been recorded. In addition to possible fortuitous effects upon the OVRAS, these drugs or their derivatives raise the possibility of purposeful manipulation of the OVRAS for enhancement of fertility or contraception.

Acknowledgement

This work was supported by NIH-HD22970 (F.N.) and the Andrew Mellon Foundation.

References

Aguilera, G., Hyde, C.L. & Catt, K.J. (1982). Angiotensin II receptors and prolactin release in pituitary lactotrophs. **Endocrinology** 111:1045–1950.

Andersson, B. (1978). Regulation of water intake. **Physiological Review** 58:582–603.

Boneher, R., Asselin, J. & Genest, J. (1974). A new enzyme leading to the direct formation of angiotensin II. **Circulation Research** Suppl. I 203–209.

Brownfield, M.S., Reid, I.A., Ganten, D. & Ganong, W.F. (1983). Differential distribution of immunoreactive angiotensin and angiotensin-converting enzyme in rat brain. **Neuroscience** 7:1759–1769.

Carter, A.M. & Gothlin, J. (1970). Effects of angiotensin, oxytocin and vasopressin on placental circulation. An angiographic study in rabbits. **Investigative Radiology** 2:86–91.

Chevillard, C., Duchenne, N., Pasquier, R. & Alexandre, J.M. (1979). Relation of the centrally evoked pressor effect of angiotensin II to central noradrenaline in the rabbit. **European Journal of Pharmacology** 58:203–206.

Crozet, A., Penhoat, A. & Saez, J.M. (1986). Processing of angiotensin II and (Sar, Ala)AII by cultured bovine adrenocortical cells. **Endocrinology** 118:2312–2318.

Culler, M.D., Tarlatzis, B.C., Lightman, A., Fernandez, L.A., DeCherney, A.H., Negro-Vilar, A. & Naftolin, F. (1986). Angiotensin II immunoreactivity in human ovarian follicular fluid. **Journal of Clinical Endocrinology and Metabolism** 62:613–615.

Dechepper, C.F., Mellon, S.H., Cumin, F., Baxter, J.D. & Ganong, W.F. (1986). Analysis by immunocytochemistry and *in situ* hybridization of renin and its mRNA in the kidney, testis, adrenal and pituitary glands of the rat. **Proceedings of the National Academy of Sciences, USA** 83:7552–7558.

Derkx, F.H.M., Alberda, A.T., Zeilmaker, G.H. & Schalekamp, M.A.D.H. (1987). High concentrations of immunoreactive renin, prorenin and enzymatically active renin in human ovarian follicular fluid. **British Journal of Obstetrics and Gynaecology** 94:4–9.

Do, Y.S., Sherrod, A., Lobo, R.A., Paulson, R.J., Shinagawa, T., Chen, S.W., Kjos, S. & Hsueh, W. (1988). Human ovarian theca cells are a source of renin. **Proceedings of the National Academy of Sciences, USA** 85:1957–1961.

Elliott, M.E., Alexander, R.C. & Goodfriend, T.K.L. (1982). Aspects of angiotensin action in the adrenal. Key roles for calcium and phosphatidyl inositol. **Hypertension** Suppl. II 4:53–58.

Eskildsen, P.C. (1972). Location of renin in rabbit uterus by help of microdissection. **Acta Pathologica Microbiologica Scandinavica** 80:241–252.

Fernandez, L.A., Caride, V.J., Twickler, J. & Galarde, R.E. (1982). Renin–angiotensin and development of collateral circulation and renal ischemia. **American Journal of Physiology** 243:869–876.

Fernandez, L.A., Tarlatzis, B.C., Rzasa, P.F., Caride, V.J., Laufer, N., Negro-Vilar, A.F., DeCherney, A.H. & Naftolin, F. (1985a). Renin-like activity in ovarian follicular fluid. **Fertility and Sterility** 44:219.

Fernandez, L.A., Twickler, J. & Mead, A. (1985b). Neovascularization produced by angiotensin II. **Journal of Laboratory and Clinical Medicine** 105:141–145.

Frederick, J.L., Hoa, N., Preston, D.S., Frederick, J.J., Campeau, J.D., Ono, T. & DiZerega, G.H. (1985). Initiation of angiogenesis by porcine follicular fluid. **American Journal of Obstetrics and Gynecology** 152:1073–1078.

Frederick, J.L., Shimanuki, T. & DiZerega, G.S. (1984). Initiation of angiogenesis by human follicular fluid. **Science** 24:389–390.

Gaede, S.D., Sholley, M.M. & Quattropani, S.L. (1985). Endothelial mitosis during the initial stages of corpus luteum neovascularization in the cycling adult rat. **American Journal of Anatomy** 172:173–180.

Ganong, W.F. (1984). The brain renin angiotensin system. **Annual Review of Physiology** 46:17–31.

Gill, G.N., Ill, C.R. & Simonian, M.H. (1977). Angiotensin stimulation of bovine adrenocortical cell growth. **Proceedings of the National Academy of Sciences, USA** 74:5569–5573.

Glorioso, N., Atlas, S.A., Laragh, J.H., Jewelwicz, R. & Sealy, J.E. (1986). Prorenin in high concentrations in human ovarian follicular fluid. **Science** 23:1422–1424.

Goodfriend, T.L. (1983). Angiotensin receptors and specific functions of angiotensin I, II and III. In: Genest, J., Kuchel, O., Hamet, P. & Cantin, M., eds. **Hypertension,** New York, McGraw-Hill, p.271.

Gospodarowicz, D. & Tharkal, K.K. (1978). Production of a corpus luteum angiogenic factor responsible for proliferation of capillaries and neovascularization of the corpus luteum. **Proceedings of the National Academy of Sciences, USA** 75:847–851.

Harwood, J.P. & Hausdorff, W.P. (1987). Angiotensin II receptors in the ovary: characterization and linkage of calcium metabolism. In: **Proceedings of the Sixty-Ninth Annual Meeting of the Endocrine Society**, Indianapolis, p.227.

Hepp, R., Grillet, C., Peytremann, A. *et al.* (1977). Stimulation of corticosteroid synthesis by angiotensin II in bovine adrenal fasciculata cells. **Endocrinology** 101:717–725.

Husain, A., Bumpus, F.M., Desilva, P. & Speth, R.C. (1987). Localization of angiotensin II receptors in ovarian follicles and the identification of angiotensin II in rat ovaries. **Proceedings of the National Academy of Sciences, USA** 84:2489–2494.

Iwamoto, H.S. & Rudolph, A. (1981). Effects of angiotensin on the blood flow and its distribution in fetal lamb. **Circulatory Research** 48:183–189.

Jackson, B., Cubela, R.B., Sakaguchi, K. & Johnston, C.I. (1988). Characterization of angiotensin-converting enzyme (ACE) in the testis and assessment of the *in vivo* effects of the ACE inhibitor perindopril. **Endocrinology** 123:50–55.

Jakob, W., Jentzsch, K.D., Mauersberger, B. & Oehme, P. (1977). Demonstration of angiogenesis activity in the corpus luteum of cattle. **Experimental Pathology (Jena)** 13:231–236.

Johnson, J., Johnson, I.R., Fonau, J.E. & Craven, D.J. (1984). The site of renin in the human uterus. **Histopathology** 8:273–278.

Jones, T.H., Brown, B.L. & Dobson, P.R.M. (1988). Evidence that angiotensin II is a paracrine agent mediating gonadotropin-releasing hormone stimulated inositol phosphate production and prolactin secretion in the rat. **Journal of Endocrinology** 116:367–371.

Khairallah, P.A. (1972). Action of angiotensin on adrenergic nerve endings: inhibition of NE uptake. **Federation Proceedings** 31:1351–1357.

Kim, S.J., Shinjo, M., Fakamizu, A., Miyasaki, H., Usuki, S. & Mukrami, K. (1987). Identification of renin and renin mRNA sequence in rat ovary and uterus. **Biochemical and Biophysical Research Communications** 142:169–175.

Kochen, T. & Guthrie, G. (1980). Renin–angiotensin–aldosterone and hypertension. **Endocrinology Reviews** 1:78–80.

Lightman, A., Jones, C., Fernandez, L.A., Boyers, S., Decherney, A.H. & Naftolin, F.

(1986). OVRAS: The ovarian renin angiotensin system: immunohistochemical localization of renin and angiotensin II immunoreactivity in human and rat ovary. In: **Proceedings of the 68th Annual Meeting of the Endocrine Society**, Anahlem. Abstract No.25, p.34.

Lightman, A., Jones, C., Maclusky, N.J., Palumbo, A., DeCherney, A.H. & Naftolin, F. (1988). Immunocytochemical localization of angiotensin II – immunoreactivity and demonstration of angiotensin II binding in the rat ovary. **American Journal of Obstetrics and Gynecology** 159:526–530.

Lightman, A., Palumbo, A., DeCherney, A.H. & Naftolin, F. (1989). The ovarian renin–angiotensin system. In: Adashi, E.Y., ed. **Seminars in Reproductive Endocrinology**, New York, Thieme-Stratton, pp.79–87.

Lightman, A., Tarlatzis, B.C., Rzasa, P.F., Culler, M.D., Caride, V.J., Negro-Vilar, A.F., Lennard, D., DeCherney, A.H. & Naftolin, F. (1987). The ovarian renin angiotensin system: renin-like activity and angiotensin II/III immunoreactivity in gonadotropin-stimulated and unstimulated human follicular fluid. **American Journal of Obstetrics and Gynecology** 156:808–815.

Liu, Y., Cajander, S.B., Kristensen, P. & Hsueh, A.J.W. (1987). Gonadotropin regulation of tissue-type and urokinase-type plasminogen activators in rat granulosa and theca interstitial cells during the preovulatory period. **Molecular and Cellular Endocrinology** 54:221–229.

Makris, A., Ryan, K.J., Yasumizu, I., Hill, K. & Zetter, B. (1982). The non-luteal porcine ovary as a source of angiogenesis factor. **Journal of Cell Biology** 95:193–198.

Masterson, B.J. (1988). Oral contraceptive agents; current status. **American Journal of Surgery** 155:619–627.

Moursi, M., Ganten, D., Lang, R. & Unger, T. (1986). Antihypertensive action and inhibition of tissue converting enzyme (CE) by three pro-drug CE inhibitors, Enalopril, Ramipril and Perindopril in stroke-prone spontaneously hypertensive rats. **Journal of Hypertension** 4:S495–S498.

Naftolin, F., Lavy, G., Palumbo, A. & DeCherney, A.H. (1988). Poissons, grenouilles, femmes et hommes: the appropriation and retention of fundamental cellular mechanisms for reproduction. **Gynecology and Endocrinology** 2:265–273.

Naruse, M., Naruse, K., Kurinoto, F., Sakurai, H., Yoshida, S., Toma, H., Ishii, T., Obana, K., Demura, H., Inagami, T. & Shizume, K. (1985). Evidence for the existence of des-asp-angiotensin II in human uterine and adrenal tissues. **Journal of Clinical Endocrinology and Metabolism** 61:480–483.

Naruse, M., Takii, Y. & Inagami, T. (1981). Renin exists in high concentration in the rat adrenal gland. **Biomedical Research** 2:583–586.

Navot, D., Margolioth, E.J., Laufer, N. *et al.* (1987). Direct correlation between plasma renin activity and severity of the ovarian hyperstimulation syndrome. **Fertility and Sterility** 48:57–63.

O'Connell, M.L., Canipari, R. & Strickland, S. (1987). Hormonal regulation of tissue plasminogen activator secretion and mRNA levels in rat granulosa cells. **Journal of Biological Chemistry** 262:2339–2344.

Ohkubo, H., Nakayama, K., Tanaka, T. & Nakanishi, S. (1986). Tissue distribution of rat angiotensinogen mRNA and structural analysis of its heterogeneity. **Journal of Biological Chemistry** 261:319–323.

Okamura, T., Miyazaki, M., Inagami, T. & Toda, N. (1986). Vascular renin–

angiotensin system in two-kidney, one-clip, hypertensive rats. **Hypertension** 8:560–565.

Oliver, J.A. & Sciacca, R.R. (1984). Local generation of AII as a mechanism of regulation of peripheral vascular tone in the rat. **Journal of Clinical Investigation** 74:1247–1251.

Page, I.H. & Bumpus, F.M., eds. (1974). **Angiotensin: Handbook of Experimental Pharmacology**, Vol. 37, New York, Springer.

Palumbo, A., Alam, M., Lightman, A., MacLusky, N., DeCherney, A.H. & Naftolin, F. (1988a). Angiotensin II effects *in vitro* steroidogenesis by human granulosa lutein cells in culture. In: **Proceedings of the 70th Annual Meeting of the Endocrine Society**, New Orleans, Louisiana. Abstract No.1075, p.289.

Palumbo, A., Pelliger, A., Decherney, A.H. & Naftolin, F. (1988b). Angiotensin action in oocyte maturation in the rat. Abstract presented at the 1988 meeting of the Society for Gynecological Investigation. Abstract No.107.

Parmentier, M., Inagami, T., Pochet, R. & Desclin, J.C. (1983). Pituitary-dependent renin-like immunoreactivity in the rat testis. **Endocrinology** 112:1318–1323.

Paulson, R.J., Do, Y.S., Hsueh, W.A., Eggena, P. & Lobo, R.A. (1989). Ovarian renin production *in vitro* and *in vivo*: characterization and clinical correlation. **Fertility and Sterility** 51:634–638.

Pellicer, A., Diamond, M.P., DeCherney, A.H. & Naftolin, F. (1987). Intra-ovarian markers of follicular and oocyte maturation. **Journal of In Vitro Fertilization and Embryo Transfer** 4:205–217.

Pellicer, A., Palumbo, A., DeCherney, A.H. & Naftolin, F. (1988). Blockage of ovulation by an angiotensin antagonist. **Science** 240:1660–1661.

Peterson, C.M., Morioka, N., Zhu, C. & Lemaire, W. (1989). The action of angiotensin-converting enzyme inhibition of ovulation in the rat. **Society for Gynecologic Investigation**, 36th Annual Meeting, San Diego, Abstract 282.

Pucell, A.G., Bumpus, F.M. & Husain, A. (1987). Rat ovarian angiotensin II receptors. Characterization and coupling to estrogen secretion. **Journal of Biological Chemistry** 262:7076–7080.

Sakagude, K., Chai, S.Y., Jackson, B., Johnston, C. & Mendelsohn, F. (1988). Inhibition of tissue ACE; quantification by autoradiography. **Hypertension** 11:230–238.

Sarina, C., Sinton, L., Thomas, W.G. & Pascoe, W. (1985). Liver angiotensin II receptors in the rat: binding properties and regulation by dietary NA and angiotensin II. **Journal of Endocrinology** 106:103–111.

Sato, E., Ishibashi, T. & Koide, S.S. (1982). Inducement of blood vessel formation by ovarian extracts from mice injected with gonadotropins. **Experientia** 8:1248–1249.

Sealey, J.E., Atlas, S.A., Glorioso, N., Manapat, H. & Laragh, J.H. (1985a). Cyclical secretion of prorenin during the menstrual cycle: synchronization with LH and progesterone. **Proceedings of the National Academy of Sciences, USA** 84:8705–8709.

Sealey, J.E., McCord, D., Taufield, P.A. *et al.* (1985b). Plasma prorenin in first trimester pregnancy: relationship to changes in human chorionic gonadotropin. **American Journal of Obstetrics and Gynecology** 153:514–519.

Steele, M.K., Gallo, R.V. & Ganong, W.F. (1983). A possible role for the brain renin–angiotensin system in the regulation of LH secretion. **American Journal of Physiology** 245:R805–R810.

Steele, M.K., Negro-Vilar, A. & McCann, S.M. (1981). Effect of AII on *in vivo* and *in vitro* release of anterior pituitary hormones in the female rat. **Endocrinology** 109:893–899.

Sterling, D., Stone, R., Magness, R.R., Waterman, M.R. & Simpson, E.R. (1989). Angiotensin II (AII) inhibits LH-stimulated expression of mRNA encoding cholesterol side-chain cleavage ($P450_{scc}$), and stimulates expression of mRNA encoding basic fibroblast growth factor in bovine luteal cells in primary culture. **Society for Gynecologic Investigation**, 36th Annual Meeting, San Diego, Abstract 248.

Tang, S.-S., Loscalzo, J. & Dzau, V.J. (1987). Tissue plasminogen activator activates renin angiotensin *in vitro*. **High Blood Pressure Council Meeting** Abstract 2.

VanSande, M.E., Scharpe, S.L., Neels, H.M. & Vancamp, K.O. (1985). Distribution of angiotensin converting enzyme in human tissues. **Clinica Chimica Acta** 147:255–260.

Wilkes, B., Krim, E. & Mento, P. (1985). Evidence for a functional renin–angiotensin system in the full-term fetoplacental unit. **American Journal Physiology** 249:E366–373.

Williams, G.H., McDonnel, L.M., Raux, M.C. & Hollenberg, N.K. (1974). Evidence for different angiotensin II receptors in rat adrenal glomerulosa and rabbit vascular smooth muscle cells. **Circulation Research** 34:384–390.

Wintroub, B.U., Klickstein, L.B., Dzau, V.J. & Watt, K.W. (1984). Granulocyte–angiotensin system: identification of angiotensinogen as the plasma protein substrate of leukocyte cathepsin G. **Biochemistry** 23:227–232.

IV Extracellular matrix and cell differentiation

The influence of extracellular matrix and cell–cell interactions on the secretory activity of Sertoli cells

A. STEINBERGER, A. JANECKI AND E. CASTELLON-VERA

Department of Obstetrics, Gynecology and Reproductive Sciences, The University of Texas Medical School at Houston, Houston, TX 77030, USA.

Keywords

Sertoli cells, peritubular myoid cells, germ cells, extracellular matrix, polarized secretion, androgen-binding protein, transferrin, inhibin, co-culture.

Introduction

The mammalian testis is a complex organ composed of two major components: avascular seminiferous tubules in which the process of spermatogenesis takes place, and interstitial tissue containing blood vessels, lymphatics, and the major steroid-producing cells – the Leydig cells. In addition to germ cells at various stages of differentiation, the seminiferous tubules also contain somatic epithelial cells – the Sertoli cells. In his original description of their unique cell structure, Sertoli (1865) postulated that these cells provide physical support and perform a 'nursing' function for the developing germ cells. This concept is still generally accepted although, despite intensive investigations, the precise nature of the Sertoli cells' 'nursing' function remains elusive.

Remarkable progress has been made in the last decade with respect to Sertoli cell functions and their regulation (see reviews by Parvinen, 1982; Sanborn *et al.*, 1983; Sharpe, 1983). Over 50 glycoproteins have been shown to be secreted by the Sertoli cells. Some of these glycoproteins are similar to serum proteins (e.g. plasminogen activator, ceruloplasmin, transferrin), whereas others appear to be Sertoli-cell specific (e.g. androgen-binding protein (ABP), inhibin). Since most of these substances are regulated by follicle-stimulating hormone (FSH) and/or testosterone, which are known to be essential for spermatogenesis, it is assumed that secretions from Sertoli cells play a critical role in mediating the hormonal effects and providing essential energy substrates and nutrients to the germ cells. There are several observations that support this assumption. Since germ cells do not possess receptors for androgens or for FSH, they cannot respond directly to these hormones. Also, because of the existence of the 'blood–testis' barrier, the more advanced germ cells have no free access to circulating substances and must depend mainly on the microenvironment that is controlled by the Sertoli cells.

The morphological features of the blood–testis barrier have been well characterized (Dym and Fawcett, 1970; Fawcett, 1975; Setchell and Waites,

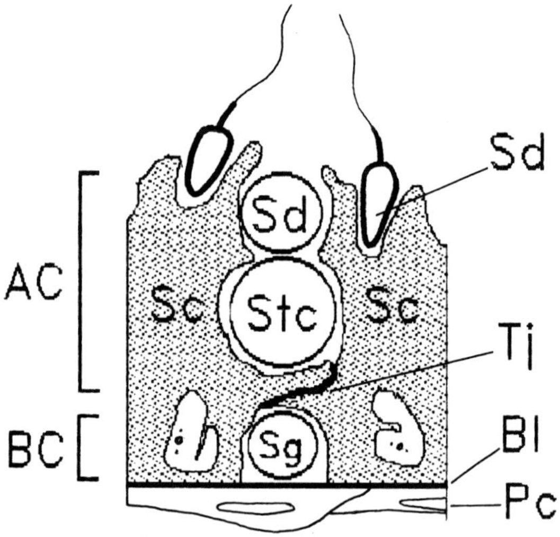

Fig. 1 Main structural features of rat seminiferous tubules. Bl, basal lamina; Pc, peritubular myoid cells; Sc, Sertoli cells; Sg, spermatogonia; Stc, pachytene spermatocytes; Sd, spermatids. The presence of tight junctions (Tj) between neighboring Sc separate the basal (BC) and apical (AC) compartments.

1975; Waites and Gladwell, 1982; Russell *et al.*, 1983). The specialized tight junctions formed between adjacent Sertoli cells during postnatal development create a physical barrier to macromolecules from the circulation and divide the seminiferous tubular space into a basal and adluminal compartment. During the differentiation of germ cells, spermatocytes are transported across the tight junctions into the adluminal compartment where the completion of meiosis and maturation of spermatids take place. Germ cells located in the adluminal compartment can be presumed to be those most dependent on Sertoli cell function (Fig. 1). Recently, using two-compartment cultures, it has been demonstrated that Sertoli cell secretions (e.g. ABP, transferrin and inhibin) are bidirectional and differentially regulated by hormones (Janecki and Steinberger, 1986, 1987a; Steinberger *et al.*, 1988). Furthermore, ABP appears to be secreted bidirectionally *in vivo* also (Mather *et al.*, 1983).

It is reasonable to assume that substances secreted by the Sertoli cells apically into the tubule fluid would have the greatest impact on the differentiation of germ cells, whereas those elaborated basally are more likely to affect the peritubular cells and Leydig cells. Indeed, certain products of Sertoli cells (e.g. gonadotropin-releasing hormone (GnRH)-like peptide, estradiol, inhibin, etc.) have been shown to modulate steroidogenesis in and responsiveness to hormones of Leydig cells. There is also considerable evidence, however, to suggest that Sertoli cell functions, besides being regulated by FSH and androgens, can be significantly influenced by products elaborated by other testicular cells (see Fig. 12), as well as by the extracellular matrix (ECM).

The testis is one of most actively proliferating tissues in the body which also continually undergoes differentiation. Embryologically, it originates from three major tissue sources: mesoderm (Sertoli cells), gonocytes (germ cells) and mesenchyme (peritubular and interstitial cells). As is the case in other organs, the morphogenesis and functions of its components are dependent on endocrine factors and various local signals for the control and coordination of integrated functions and gene expression of these cells. The cell–cell interactions may include signals transmitted via intercellular gap junctions, paracrine mechanisms involving locally secreted products, ECM, etc. Although the overall importance of mesenchymal–epithelial interactions in morphogenesis and organ function has been recognized for a long time (Grobstein, 1954; Hay, 1981; Bissell *et al.*, 1982; Yamada, 1983), the importance of these interactions in the testis has been intensively investigated only within the last decade.

Most cells capable of replication and long-term survival are associated with a basement membrane formed by secretory products of both epithelial and mesenchymal cells. The major components of the ECM are collagens, elastin, proteoglycans, glycoprotein fibrils and anchorage proteins such as fibronectin and laminin, but the precise composition of the ECM varies in different tissues (Kleinman *et al.*, 1981). The role of the ECM in regulating and maintaining differentiated cellular functions received considerable attention when culture methods were developed that allowed long-term survival of differentiated cells in chemically defined media *in vitro*. The availability of purified components of the ECM (e.g. collagens I and IV, laminin) made it possible to investigate their relative importance in the regulation of gene expression in specific cell types. The main shortcoming of such an approach, however, is that it does not take into account the structural complexity of ECM and the overall effects that result from interactions of its various components. Another approach was to use crude tissue or organ extracts that contained insoluble cross-linked components of the ECM ('biomatrix') as substratum for culturing cells *in vitro*. Such use of ECM showed considerable tissue specificity and was found to improve the morphology, survival and functional integrity of epithelial cells in culture (Gospodarowicz *et al.*, 1980; Gatmaitan *et al.*, 1983).

It has been postulated, and limited indirect evidence supports the hypothesis, that ECM may exert its influence by stabilizing hormones and growth factors that interact with receptors on the cell membrane or with the cytoskeleton (Reid and Jefferson, 1984). It is noteworthy that 'biomatrix' derived from a transplantable mouse tumor line which secretes basement membrane components (Orkin *et al.*, 1977) provides a more effective substratum for the differentiation of epithelial cells in culture than does 'biomatrix' from normal tissues. The combined use of 'biomatrix', hormones and growth factors often eliminates the need for serum in cultures of functionally competent cells. Although much has been learned about the overall importance of ECM in gene expression, the role of its individual components or mechanism of action remains unclear.

The modulatory effects of ECM and cell–cell interactions on the secretory activity of Sertoli cells *in vitro* are the subjects of this chapter. Recent results from our laboratory are presented in the light of existing knowledge and relevant findings reported by other investigators. Since no extensive review of the literature on this subject was intended, many important contributions to this field may not have been cited.

Materials and methods

Isolation and culture of cells

Sertoli cell

Sertoli cells (75–95% pure) were isolated from testes of rats of different ages (10–32 day old) by the enzymatic method described previously (Janecki and Steinberger, 1987a). The cells (>95% viable) were plated either in plastic dishes (Figs. 2a and 2b) or on Millipore filters in two-compartment culture chambers (Figs. 2c and 2d). To examine the effects of components of the ECM on Sertoli cell function, the cell support was covered with a dry film of collagen IV plus laminin, collagen I, or Matrigel (Collaborative Research) diluted 1:1 with culture medium (Janecki and Steinberger, 1987b). The cultures were maintained at 34°C in basal, chemically defined medium (Dulbecco MEM:Ham's F12, 1:1), or in medium that contained FSH (200 ng/ml), testosterone (10^{-6} mol/l), FSH plus testosterone, or 2–5% fetal bovine serum (FBS). In some experiments the monolayers were treated with a hypotonic solution 20 mmol/l Tris–HCl (pH 7.4), as described by Wagle *et al.* (1986) to eliminate residual germ cells. The hypotonic treatment *per se* does not significantly affect Sertoli cell function (Wagle *et al.*, 1986).

Peritubular myoid cells

The peritubular myoid cells (Pc) were isolated from testes of 14-day-old rats, as described previously (Janecki and Steinberger, 1987b), and cultured in plastic dishes for 3 days in Dulbecco MEM:Ham's F12 (1:1) supplemented with 10% FBS. The cells were then removed enzymatically and replated on the lower side of Millipore filters in inverted two-compartment chambers. After 48 hours, freshly isolated Sertoli cells were placed on the upper side of the filters and the co-cultures were reincubated in appropriate media at 34°C (Fig. 2d). For control purposes, the Sertoli cells were co-cultured with fibroblasts from testicular tunica albuginea, as described for Pc.

Germ cells

The germ cells (>95% viable) were isolated from testes of 26-day-old rats by the collagenase/trypsin method, as described in detail elsewhere (Janecki *et al.*,

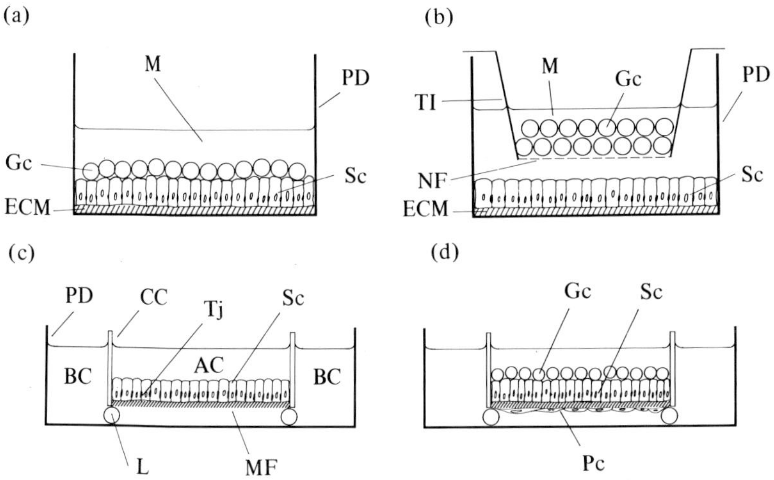

Fig. 2 Schematic representations (without correct proportions) of culture systems used in our studies. (a) *Direct* co-culture of germ cells (Gc) and Sertoli cells (Sc) in a single culture chamber. The Sc (2×10^6 cells) were maintained in appropriate medium (M) on Matrigel-coated (ECM) plastic dishes (PD). The Gc (>80% pachytene spermatocytes) were added directly on top of Sc monolayers. (b) *Indirect* Sc–Gc co-culture. The monolayer of Sc was cultured as described in (a). A transwell insert (TI) and nucleopore filter (NF) were used to maintain the Gc separated from the Sc and to allow exchange of soluble products without direct contact between cells of different types. (c) Two-compartment culture. The monolayer of Sc is supported by a Millipore filter (MF) which forms the bottom of the culture chamber (CC). The culture chamber rests on silicone rubber 'legs' (L) in a larger plastic dish (PD). The intercellular tight junctions (Tj) formed by the Sc create an apical (AC) and basal (BC) compartment which correspond to the adluminal and basal compartment in the seminiferous tubule. Thus, products of the Sc can be secreted bidirectionally and measured independently in AC and BC. (d) Co-culture of Sc with Gc and/or peritubular myoid cells (Pc). The Pc are cultured on the lower side of the filter allowing free exchange of soluble products, whereas the Gc are placed directly on top of the Sc monolayer.

1988). The resulting population consisted of approximately 85% mid- and late-pachytene spermatocytes, 10% round spermatids, and 5% other types of cell. For direct co-culture, the germ cells were placed on top of 1–4-day-old monolayers of Sertoli cells, as shown in Figures 2a and 2d. For indirect co-cultures, the germ cells were contained in Transwell culture inserts (Costar), above the monolayers of Sertoli cell, and separated from the monolayers by Nucleopore membranes (Fig. 2b). For control purposes, the germ cells were cultured alone or were replaced by rat thymus lymphocytes.

Permeability of monolayers of Sertoli cells to [^{3}H]-inulin

To assess the 'tightness' of Sertoli cell monolayers, the rate of diffusion of [^{3}H]-inulin (specific activity: 260 mCi/g) from the basal to the apical compartment during incubation for 3.5 hours was measured after various culture times, as described previously (Janecki and Steinberger, 1987a).

Assay of ABP, transferrin and inhibin in the culture media

ABP was measured by radioimmunoassay (RIA), as described previously (Janecki and Steinberger, 1987b). Most reagents were provided by NIDDK, and the antibody by Dr G. Gunsalus, Population Research Center. Transferrin (Trf) in the media was measured by specific RIA, according to the method of Skinner and Griswold (1982). The rat Trf and Trf-specific antibodies were supplied by Cappel Labs, Cochranville. Inhibin in the medium was measured by RIA, using antibody raised against a synthetic 30-amino acid sequence from the N-terminal portion of the α-chain of porcine inhibin (kindly provided by Dr B. Schanbacher). The antigen was a generous gift from Dr R. Guillemin (Salk Institute, California) and was used for iodination and as a standard in the RIA, which was a modification of that described by Ying *et al.* (1987).

Analysis of the data

Secretion of products in the two-compartment culture chambers was expressed either as total secretion [combined amounts in the basal (BC) and apical (AC) compartments], or as the ratio of the amounts secreted into the two compartments (BC:AC). A minimum of three cultures was used per treatment, and each experiment was repeated two to three times. All numerical data were analyzed by Student's t-test or analysis of variance, and by Duncan's new multiple-range test.

Results and discussion

Effects of ECM on morphology and function of Sertoli cells in vitro

In rat seminiferous tubules, the Sertoli cells are in contact with the basement membrane of the boundary tissue which has been described as consisting of an innermost, homogeneous basal lamina; collagen fibers; and a more peripheral, denser layer, which is surrounded by a single layer of Pc (Dym and Fawcett, 1970). The morphology and function of Sertoli cells *in vitro* are dramatically influenced by the substratum on which they are cultured. If plated on plastic or glass, the cells appear flat and dedifferentiated, whereas on reconstituted basement membrane (Matrigel, Collaborative Research) or on collagen IV and laminin, they assume a tall, polarized morphology similar to that seen *in vivo* (Suarez-Quian *et al.*, 1984; Hadley *et al.*, 1985). Analysis of culture conditions suggests that both Sertoli cells and Pc participate in the formation of basal lamina (Tung and Fritz, 1980; Tung *et al.*, 1984). The Sertoli cells secrete type IV collagen, laminin, and proteoglycans that contain chondroitin sulfate, whereas the Pc secrete collagen IV and I, fibronectin, and heparin sulfate glucosaminoglycans. The Pc and Sertoli cells appear to form structural ECM *in vitro* only when co-cultured with direct contact between cells (Skinner *et al.*, 1985). The interaction of peritubular and Sertoli cells, in addition to enhancing their morphogenetic expression, also prolongs their survival in serum-free media and increases the secretions from Sertoli cells (Fritz and Tung, 1986; Tung and Fritz, 1986).

Effects of components of the ECM on polarized secretions from Sertoli cells in vitro

In 1979, Handler and colleagues described a two-compartment culture chamber with a Millipore filter as substrate for investigation of the polarized transport through urinary bladder epithelium. Modifications of this chamber were later adapted for investigations of polarized functions of rat Sertoli cells *in vitro* (Janecki *et al.*, 1988; Byers *et al.*, 1986). A schematic diagram of the chamber used in our laboratory is shown in Figure 2c.

When plated at relatively high density (2–3x10^6 cells/cm^2) on Millipore filters in the two-compartment chambers, the Sertoli cells formed a confluent, highly polarized monolayer with intercellular tight junctions which dramatically decreased the passage of [^{3}H]-inulin. In these cultures, ABP and Trf were secreted bidirectionally. Neither testosterone nor FSH significantly changed the polarity of secretion of either of these glycoproteins, whereas the presence of FBS in the medium dramatically increased the ratio of BC:AC (Janecki and Steinberger, 1987a). These observations suggested that some serum component(s) might be involved in the regulation of polarized secretions from Sertoli cells. One possibility is through the deposition of testis-specific ECM components, since serum has been reported to enhance this process (Skinner *et al.*, 1985). There is considerable evidence to indicate that components of the ECM can affect both the morphology and secretory function of Sertoli cells *in vitro*. When cultured on testis-derived 'biomatrix' (Tung and Fritz, 1984), ECM deposited by Pc (Mather *et al.*, 1984), collagen IV plus laminin (Suarez–Quian *et al.*, 1984) or a preparation of reconstituted basement membrane (Hadley *et al.*, 1984), rat Sertoli cells displayed polarized morphology similar to that seen *in vivo*, in sharp contrast to the flattened appearance of these cells on glass or plastic. Some preparations of ECM which have been used to coat plastic dishes also enhanced the secretory activity of Sertoli cells *in vitro* (Mather *et al.*, 1984; Hadley *et al.*, 1985). In many cases, however, the morphology of Sertoli cells maintained on ECM-coated dishes was not significantly different from that observed when these cells were cultured at high density on Millipore filters in two-compartment culture chambers.

Table 1. *Effect of substratum on the attachment of Sertoli cells from rats of different ages*

Substratum	Age of animal 14 days		18 days		26 days	
	Unattached cells (percent of plated) Plastic	filter	Plastic	filter	Plastic	filter
Untreated	21 ± 5	13 ± 3[b]	10 ± 3	7 ± 2	8 ± 3	6 ± 2
Coated with collagen I	5 ± 3[a]	6 ± 2[a]	5 ± 2[a]	5 ± 3	7 ± 4	4 ± 2
Coated with Matrigel	6 ± 3[a]	5 ± 3[a]	4 ± 3[a]	4 ± 2	6 ± 2	6 ± 4

Sertoli cells were plated on treated or untreated plastic or Millipore filters (0.45μ) at a density of 2 x 10^6 cells/cm^2. After 5 h, the media were collected and spun at 100 x g for 10 min. The sedimented cells were dissociated with 0.5% trypsin and counted using a hemocytometer. The values are percentages of initially plated cells and represent means ± S.D. of results from triplicate cultures in two separate experiments.
[a]Significantly ($p < 0.05$) different from corresponding untreated controls.
[b]Significantly ($p < 0.05$) different from corresponding value for cells plated on plastic.

Moreover, there are some discrepancies between reported results concerning the polarity secretion of ABP and Trf which appeared to depend on whether or not the filters were coated with ECM (Hadley *et al.*, 1987).

We investigated the role of components of the ECM in the attachment, spreading and monolayer permeability of Sertoli cells, as well as in the secretion of proteins, using conventional plastic dishes in addition to two-compartment culture chambers. The cells attached better in serum- free media when plated on collagen I or Matrigel-coated plastic than when plated on plain plastic (Table 1), although cells plated on collagen I remained aggregated for at least 4 days and slowly spread out thereafter, as reported by others (Tung and Fritz, 1986; Borland *et al.*, 1986). The attachment and spreading of cells in the absence of Matrigel declined with age. More than 20% of Sertoli cells from 14-day-old rats failed to attach to plastic in serum-free medium within 5 hours, and monolayer confluency was reached only after 48 hours. In contrast, about 6% of cells remained unattached after 5 hours, and confluency was reached within 18 hours when the cells were plated on Matrigel-coated dishes. Little difference in attachment and spreading was observed with Sertoli cells from 18- and 26-day-old rats (Table 1). Although these differences were much less pronounced if the monolayers were maintained on Millipore filters, these results confirm the postulated role of ECM in enhancing attachment of cultured epithelial cells to the substratum (Salas *et al.*, 1987).

We investigated the effect of collagen IV plus laminin (CL) and Matrigel on the total secretion (combined amounts in the apical and basal compartments) of ABP and Trf in two-compartment cultures. Coating the Millipore filter with CL or Matrigel significantly increased the total secretion of both glycoproteins (Fig. 3). Matrigel was more effective than CL in enhancing secretion of ABP,

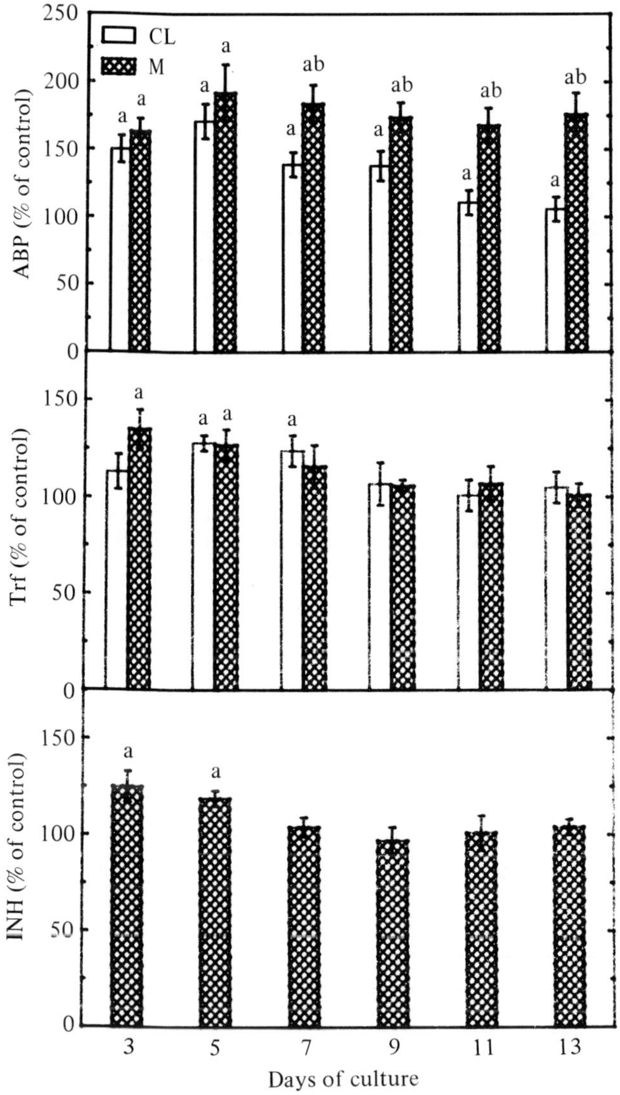

Fig. 3 Effects of coating Millipore filters with collagen IV plus laminin (CL) or with Matrigel (M) on the total secretion of androgen binding protein (ABP), transferrin (Trf) and inhibin (INH) by Sertoli cells (Sc) obtained from 18-day-old rats. The cells were plated in two-compartment chambers at a density 2.5×10^6 cells/cm^2, and cultured in chemically defined medium that contained FSH (200 ng/ml) and testosterone (10^{-6} mol/l). The amount of ABP, Trf and INH in the medium was evaluated by specific radioimmunoassays. The results are expressed as percent of values observed in control cultures on uncoated filters, and represent mean results ± S.D. from six cultures. (a) Significantly different ($p < 0.05$) from control cultures, maintained on plain Millipore filters. (b) Significantly different ($p < 0.05$) from corresponding CL value (figure modified from Janecki *et al.*, 1987b).

whereas the extent of secretion of Trf was, in most cases, similar for cells attached to either substratum. Moreover, the effect of Matrigel on the secretion of ABP was always more pronounced than that on Trf. In fact, in serum-free media, no effect of Matrigel on secretion of Trf was noted after 5 days of culture, whereas the secretion of ABP was enhanced by approximately 70% up to day 13. Similarly to secretion of Trf, the secretion of inhibin was only slightly elevated in the presence of Matrigel, and the effect was usually noted only during the initial 4–5 days of culture (Fig. 3). These results are consistent with the data published by Mather *et al.* (1984), who noted that complex preparations of ECM were more effective in stimulating the secretion of ABP and Trf than individual components of the ECM, and that the effect of ECM on secretion of ABP was more pronounced than its effect on secretion on Trf. Hadley *et al.* (1985) also reported enhanced secretion of ABP when Sertoli cells were cultured on Matrigel-coated plastic. In contrast, Ailenberg and colleagues (Ailenberg and Fritz, 1988; Ailenberg *et al.*, 1988) found no effect of Matrigel on total secretion of Trf and plasminogen activator by Sertoli cells maintained in two-compartment chambers in serum-free medium, although Matrigel stimulated the secretion of Trf in the presence of 10% FBS. The reason for these discrepancies is not clear, but they could be due to differences in composition of media and pretreatment of Millipore filters. Our data and most results published by others tend to indicate that ECM enhances the secretory activity of Sertoli cells in culture. However, the secretion of some proteins (e.g. ABP) is apparently affected to a greater extent than that of others (e.g. Trf or inhibin), suggesting that the ECM may differentially regulate the expression of various genes.

The effect of components of the ECM on the polarity of secretion of ABP, Trf and inhibin was investigated in two-compartment chambers using Millipore filters coated with CL or Matrigel. Neither CL nor Matrigel significantly changed the polarity (BC:AC) of secretion of ABP, Trf or inhibin, either in the presence of FSH plus testosterone (Fig. 4) or with basal medium alone (not shown). It is noteworthy that Matrigel slightly, but significantly, decreased the permeability of monolayers of Sertoli cells to [^{3}H]-inulin (Janecki and Steinberger, 1987b), a result that suggests that components of the ECM may enhance the formation of tight junctions. Alternatively, the decreased permeability of monolayers might be the result of better attachment and spreading of cells. Although the effect of Matrigel on the attachment and spreading of cells was related to the age of donor animals (see Table 1), Matrigel had no influence on the polarity of secretion of ABP and Trf by cells isolated from 14–32-day-old rats (not shown). These data do not exclude the possibility that ECM may affect the polarity of secretion of other Sertoli cell proteins, or that the absence of an effect in our experiments may have been due to use of non-specific preparations of ECM. It is well known that many effects of ECM on epithelial cell morphology and metabolic activity depend on the tissue-specific composition of the matrix (Reid *et al.*, 1981). Matrigel is a

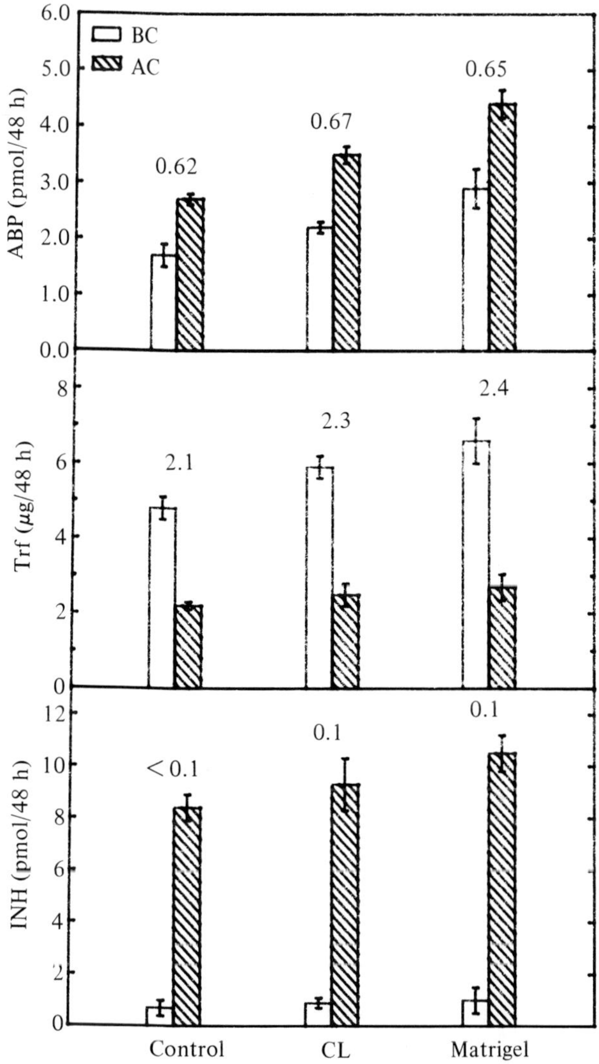

Fig. 4 Polarized secretion of ABP, Trf and INH by Sertoli cells cultured on either untreated Millipore filters (control), filters coated with collagen IV plus laminin (CL) or with Matrigel. The amount of each glycoprotein secreted between days 5 and 7 of culture was determined in media collected separately from the apical (AC) and basal compartment (BC). The culture conditions were the same as described in the legend to Fig. 3. The values represent means ± S.D. of results from six cultures in two separate experiments. The numbers above the bars indicate the ratio of BC:AC.

product of EHS tumor cells and contains collagen IV, laminin, heparin sulfate proteoglycans, entactin and nidogen (Kleinman *et al.*, 1986), which may be different from the components of testis-specific ECM. It is also possible that preparations of Sertoli cells, which may be contaminated with peritubular cells, develop functional polarity via the cooperative secretion of essential components of the ECM, thereby eliminating the need for addition of an ECM to the substratum. It has been shown that cultured Sertoli cells already secrete collagen IV at a high rate within the initial 48 hours after plating. Moreover, when co-cultured with peritubular cells, the Sertoli cells secrete considerable amounts of laminin (Skinner *et al.*, 1985).

Nitsch and Wollman (1980) reported that suspensions of thyroid epithelial cells, cultured in the presence of 0.5% FBS, formed vesicles and were 'physiologically' polarized for several days, whereas an increase in the concentration of serum to 5% resulted in a slow reversal of the polarity. Chambard and colleagues (1984) noted a change in polarity of thyroid vesicles maintained in media that contained 5–20% FBS. In this regard, it seems noteworthy that we also observed a reversal of the polarity of secretion of ABP by Sertoli cells cultured on untreated Millipore filters in the presence of 2–5% FBS (Janecki and Steinberger, 1987a, 1987b). However, it is not clear whether, in this case, the reversal of polarity was due to a direct effect of serum on Sertoli cells or to the serum-stimulated proliferation of peritubular cells which, in turn, can affect this process (see below).

Cell–cell interaction in the regulation of Sertoli cell function in vitro

Interactions between germ cells and Sertoli cells

There is increasing evidence that germ cells can modulate the function of Sertoli cells. A functional interaction could be anticipated on the basis of the structure of the seminiferous epithelium. All germ cells within the epithelium are in direct contact with the plasmalemma of Sertoli cells, and retain this contact as they divide and differentiate (Russell and Peterson, 1985). Moreover, cyclical changes in several properties of Sertoli cells (e.g. number of hormone receptors, accumulation of lipids, secretion of proteins) are synchronous with changes in the population of germ cells in the seminiferous epithelium, suggesting some influence of germ cells on the morphology and function of the Sertoli cells (Parvinen, 1982; Sharpe, 1986). Selective depletion of germ cells *in vivo* has also indicated that germ cells may affect not only the magnitude but also the polarity of secretion of various proteins from Sertoli cells (Mather *et al.*, 1983; Sharpe, 1982, 1988).

Studies *in vitro* have shown that direct co-culture of Sertoli cells with germ cells increases the secretion of ABP (Galdieri *et al.*, 1984; le Magueresse *et al.*, 1986) and estradiol-17β, and that stimulation of protein phosphorylation may be involved in this process (Welsh *et al.*, 1984). All of these observations have raised many additional questions. Is direct contact between cells essential for

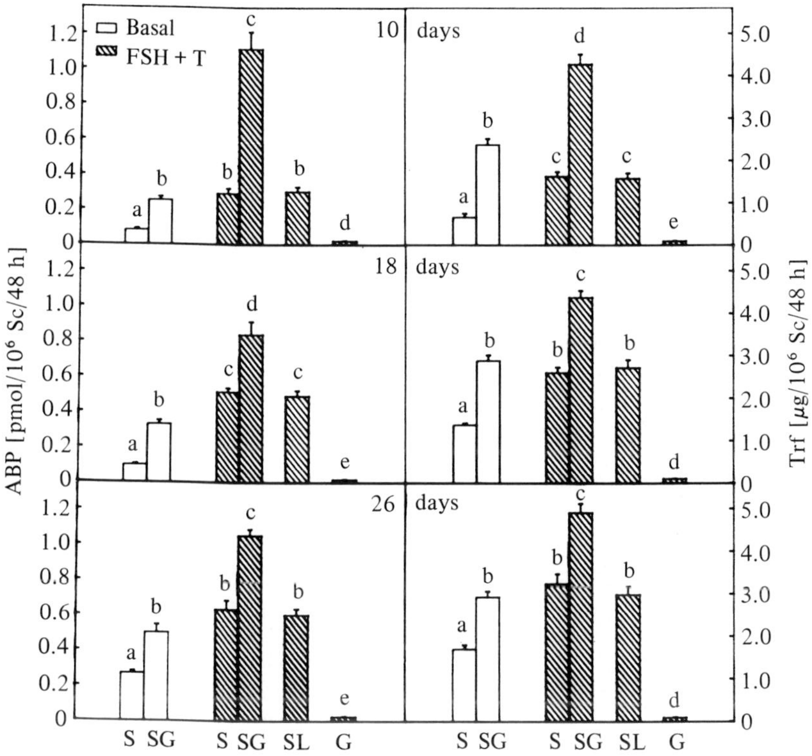

Fig. 5 Secretion of ABP and Trf during direct co-culture of Sertoli cells (S) from rats of different ages. Germ cells (G) or lymphocytes (L) were added on top of 2-day-old monolayers, 8 hours after hypotonic treatment, and were co-cultured for 4 days in either basal medium (BASAL) or medium supplemented with FSH (200 ng/ml) + 10^{-6} mol/l testosterone (FSH + T). The media were changed every other day and the glycoproteins were measured in media collected after the final 48-hour period. The bars represent means ± S.D. of values from triplicate cultures. Different superscripts indicate significant ($p<0.05$) differences within the same age group.

this communication? Do germ cells affect Sertoli cells through paracrine interaction? To what extent are maturational changes in the Sertoli cells *in vivo* dependent on the appearance of differentiating germ cells? Do germ cells regulate the polarity of secretion of proteins from Sertoli cells? What is the physiological significance of this local regulation?

Some of these questions were explored using various techniques (see Fig. 2). We evaluated the effect of germ cells (>80% pachytene spermatocytes) on the secretion of ABP and Trf by Sertoli cells obtained from 10-, 18-, and 26-day-old rats (Figs. 5 and 6). Addition of germ cells directly to monolayers of Sertoli

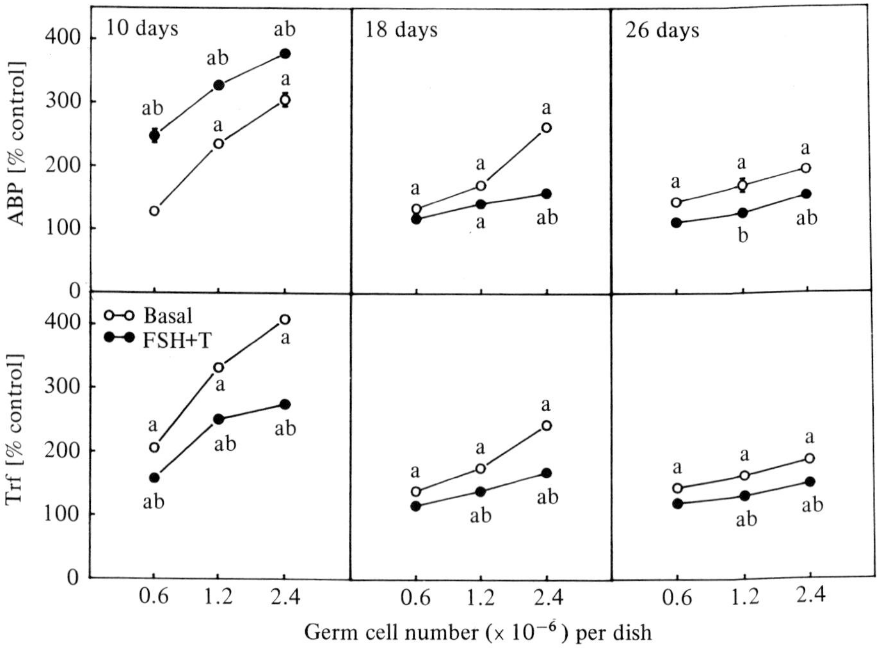

Fig. 6 Relationship between number of germ cells and the secretion of ABP and Trf in *direct* co-cultures maintained in either basal medium (BASAL) or in medium that contained FSH (200 ng/ml) + 10^{-6} mol/l testosterone (FSH + T). The results are expressed as percent of control values from cultures of Sertoli cells by themselves. (a) Significantly ($p < 0.05$) different from control. (b) Significantly ($p < 0.05$) different from values for corresponding co-cultures in basal medium.

cells significantly increased the secretion of both ABP and Trf from cells from rats at all three ages; Sertoli cells from 10-day-old rats showed the greatest response (Fig. 5). The degree of enhancement was related to the number of germ cells added, but decreased with the age of donor rats (Fig. 6). In cultures of Sertoli cells from 10-day-old rats, the relative increase in secretion of ABP was higher in the presence of FSH plus testosterone, whereas the opposite was found for secretion of Trf. Furthermore, with Sertoli cells from older animals, the percent increase in secretion of ABP and Trf was always higher in the absence of FSH and testosterone. As shown in Figure 7, there was no difference between direct and indirect stimulatory effects of germ cells on the secretion of ABP and Trf by Sertoli cells from 10-day-old rats. However, with Sertoli cells from older animals, the indirect co-culture proved less stimulatory than the direct co-culture of cells. Moreover, removal of germ cells from the co-cultures caused decreased secretion of both glycoproteins from cells taken from rats at all ages. In the Sertoli cells from the 18- and 26-day-old rats,

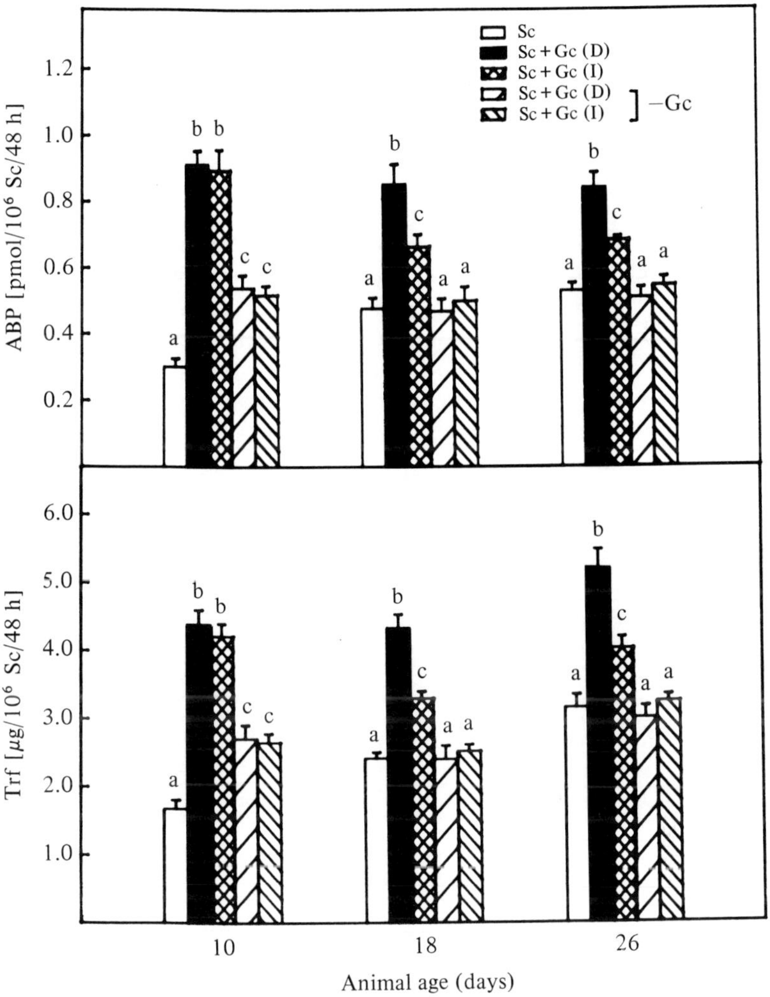

Fig. 7 Reversibility of the effect of germ cells (Gc) on secretions from Sertoli cells (Sc). The Gc (1.8×10^6) were added to hypotonically treated 2-day-old monolayers of Sc. After 48 hours, the Gc were removed by hypotonic treatment (direct co-cultures), or by elimination of the inner chambers (indirect co-cultures), and the monolayers of Sc were reincubated for an additional 48 hours in the presence of FSH (200 ng/ml) and testosterone (10^{-6} mol/l). ABP and TRF were measured in the media by radioimmunoassay. Open squares: control Sc-only cultures; closed squares: direct co-cultures; crossed squares: indirect co-culture; squares with single diagonal: direct co-cultures after removal of Gc; squares with double diagonal: indirect co-cultures after removal of Gc. Values are means ± S.D. of results from triplicate cultures. Within each age group, different superscripts indicate significant differences ($p < 0.01$).

secretions declined to the level found in control of Sertoli cells by themselves. Several conclusions can be drawn from the above-mentioned results. Sertoli cells respond to pachytene spermatocytes with increased secretion of both ABP and Trf. This effect appears to be cell specific and related to the number of added germ cells; it is most pronounced in Sertoli cells from 10-day-old rats in which pachytene spermatocytes have not yet appeared in the seminiferous epithelium. These results are in general agreement with other reported data (Galdieri *et al.*, 1984; le Magueresse *et al.*, 1986; le Magueresse and Jégou, 1988), although le Magueresse and Jégou (1988) found Sertoli cells from 10-day-old rats to be less responsive to germ cells. The reason for this discrepancy is not clear. Finally, exposure to pachytene spermatocytes *in vitro* affects secretions from Sertoli cells through both direct contacts between cells and soluble factors. However, direct contact between cells appears to play a much more major role after the appearance of pachytene spermatocytes in the seminiferous epithelium.

To determine whether germ cells affect the polarity of secretions from Sertoli cells, as was suggested by experiments *in vivo* (Mather *et al.*, 1983), we co-cultured enriched populations of pachytene spermatocytes with Sertoli cells from 14-day-old rats in two-compartment culture chambers (Janecki *et al.*, 1988). Addition of germ cells directly to the monolayer of Sertoli cells reduced the ratio of BC:AC for ABP from 2.0 to 0.6. This effect was most pronounced 2 days after the germ cells were added directly to 2-day-old monolayers of Sertoli cells (Fig. 8) and was noted only in the presence of FSH (Fig. 9). In contrast to results for ABP, the polarity of secretion of Trf was not significantly altered. In other experiments, the Sertoli cells were isolated from 32-day-old rats in such a way that many original germ cells were included in the preparation. After 2 days of culture, most contaminating germ cells were removed from the experimental chambers by hypotonic treatment. As seen in Figure 10, removal of germ cells resulted in a gradual, FSH-independent increase of the BC:AC ratio of ABP (from 0.6 to 1.4) but there was no significant change in the polarity of secretion of Trf. Note that the BC:AC ratio of 0.6 for ABP secreted in control cultures, which were not exposed to hypotonic treatment, indicates that about 62% of the total ABP was secreted apically. This value is similar to that obtained indirectly from experiments *in vivo* (Mather *et al.*, 1983). Removal of the germ cells increased the BC:AC ratio to 1.4, a value close to that associated with cultures of Sertoli cells from 14-day-old rats (see Fig. 8), which were isolated essentially free of pachytene spermatocytes. These results strongly suggest that germ cells may be involved in regulating the polarity of some of the secretions from Sertoli cells (e.g. ABP) without affecting the polarity of secretion of other products (e.g. Trf). It also seems that FSH may be necessary for the expression of the effect of germ cells on the polarity of secretion of ABP in rats at 14 days of age, when pachytene spermatocytes begin to appear in the seminiferous epithelium. By contrast, in more mature Sertoli cells the regulatory function of pachytene spermatocytes

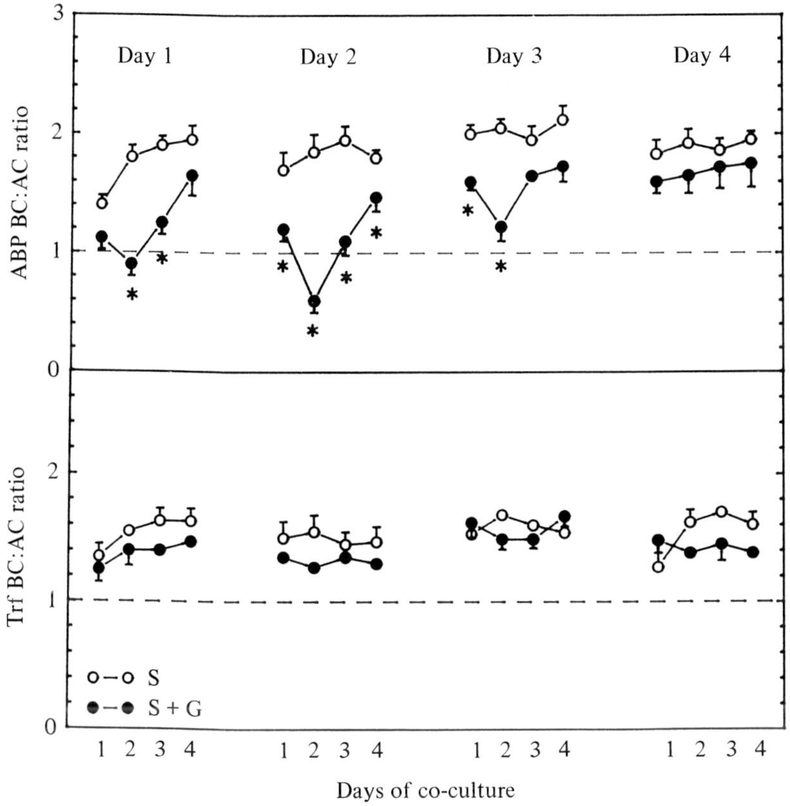

Fig. 8 The BC:AC ratio of ABP and Trf in cultures of Sertoli cells without (S) or with germ cells (S + G). Germ cells (1.6×10^6) were added on top of 1–4-day-old monolayers of Sertoli cells (indicated at top of figure) and co-cultured in medium that contained FSH (200 ng/ml) for an additional 4 days. The values are means ± S.D. of results from four cultures in one representative experiment. *Significantly different ($p < 0.01$) from values for cultures of Sertoli cells alone (modified from Janecki *et al.*, 1988).

appears to be FSH independent. All of these results support the hypothesis that the appearance of pachytene spermatocytes in the seminiferous epithelium during sexual maturation alters the secretory activity of Sertoli cells, as well as the polarity of secretion of at least some of the secretory products. The details of the mechanism involved in this process still remain obscure and require further extensive studies.

Interactions between peritubular myoid cells and Sertoli cells

The close topographic proximity of Pc and Sertoli cells in the seminiferous tubules suggests a functional interaction between these two types of cell. The

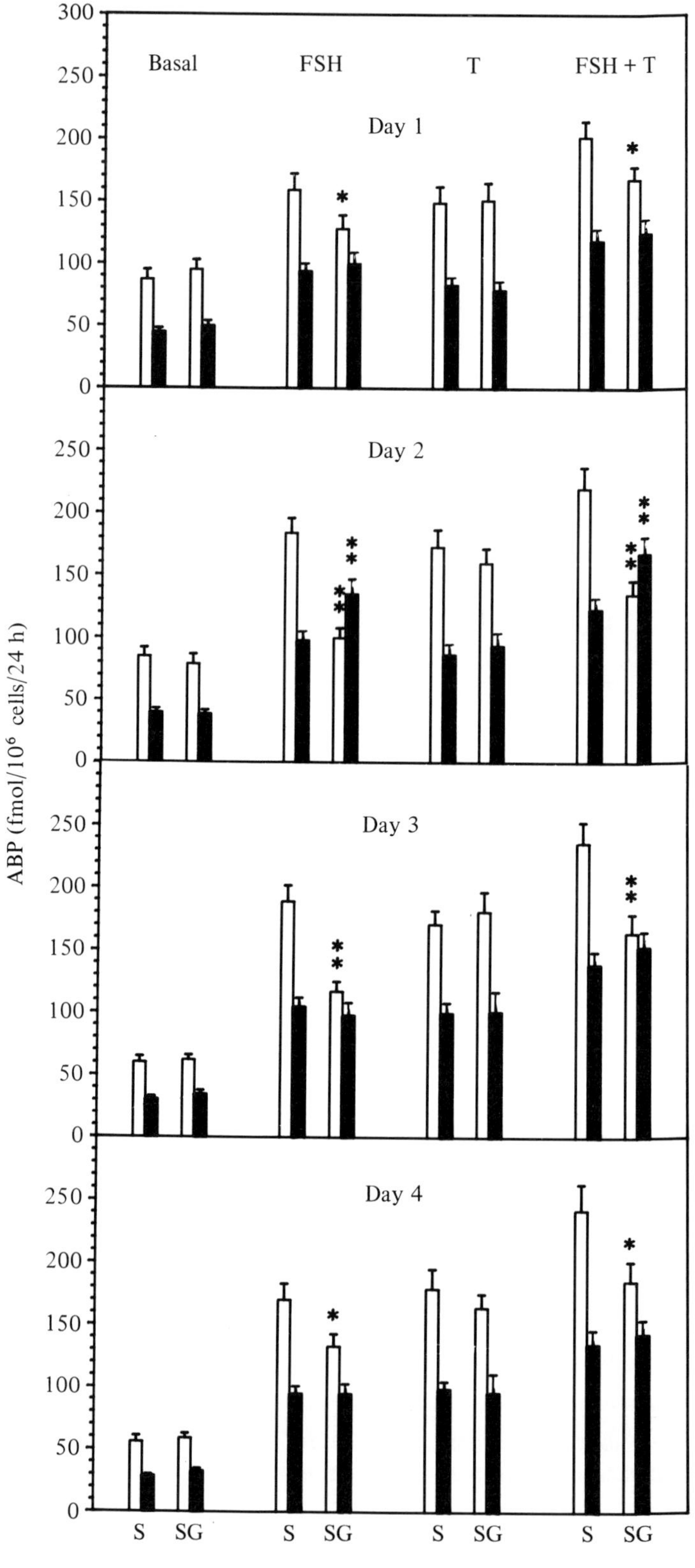
ABP (fmol/10^6 cells/24 h)
Basal
FSH
T
FSH + T
Day 1
Day 2
Day 3
Day 4
300
250
200
150
100
50
0
S
SG
S
SG
S
SG
S
SG

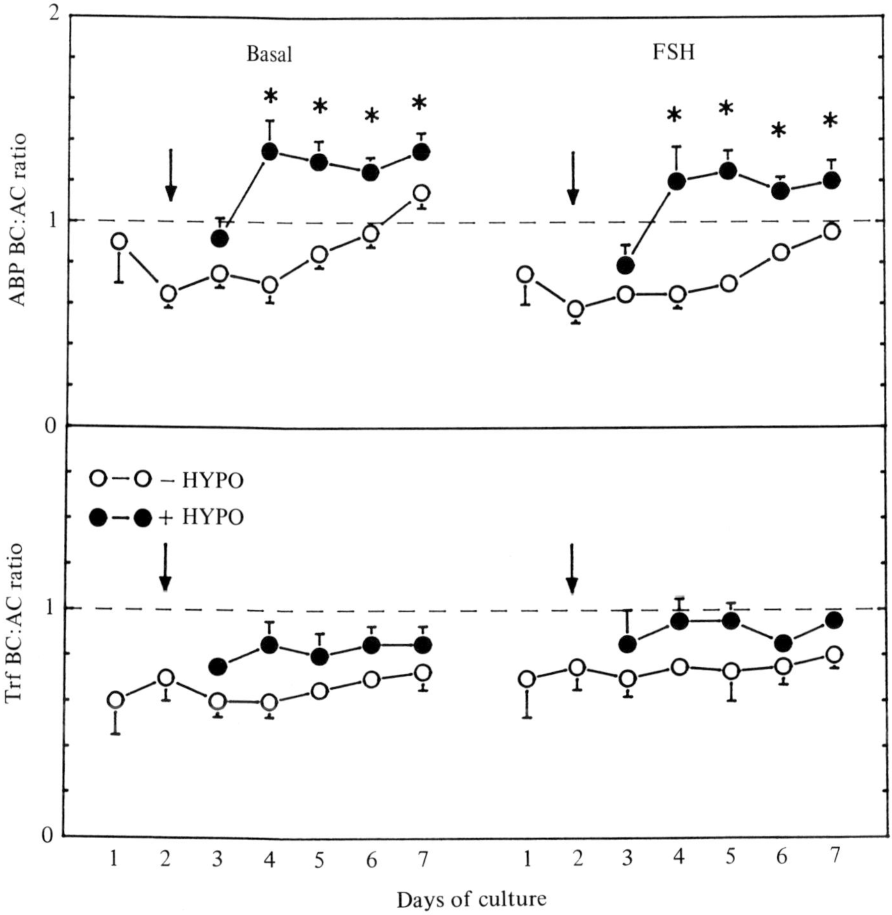

Fig. 10 The effect of removal of germ cells (hypotonic treatment) on the ratios of BC:AC for ABP and Trf secreted by Sertoli cells from 32-day-old rats. The cultures (5x10⁶ cells) were maintained for 7 days in either basal medium or medium supplemented with FSH (200 ng/ml). After 2 days, some cultures were treated with hypotonic buffer (+HYPO). Untreated cultures served as controls (−HYPO). *Significantly different ($p<0.05$) from corresponding control value.

Fig. 9 Amounts of ABP secreted during consecutive 24-hour periods into the apical compartment (open bars) and basal compartment (closed bars). Two-day-old monolayers of Sertoli cells from 14-day-old rats were cultured for 4 days in basal medium (BASAL) or in medium supplemented with FSH (200 ng/ml), 10^{-6} mol/l testosterone (T), or FSH+T, either alone (S) or in direct contact with 2×10^{6} germ cells (SG). The data are means ±S.D. of results from three separate culture chambers of a representative experiment. *$p<0.05$, **$p<0.01$ with respect to values from corresponding cultures of Sertoli cells alone (modified from Janecki *et al.*, 1988).

role of Pc in modulating the function of Sertoli cells was investigated only recently in co-cultures *in vitro*. It has been demonstrated that Pc cooperate with Sertoli cells in the deposition of components of the ECM and the formation of basal lamina (Tung *et al.*, 1984; Skinner *et al.*, 1985), a process believed to play a role in tubulogenesis and phenotypic differentiation of Sertoli cells *in vivo* (Tung and Fritz, 1986). It has been demonstrated also that Sertoli cells co-cultured with Pc engage in increased secretion of ABP, although there is some discrepancy with respect to the necessity for direct contacts between cells for elicitation of this effect (Tung and Fritz, 1980; Hutson and Stocco, 1981). Recently, Skinner and Fritz (1985, 1986) reported that, *in vitro*, Pc secrete several factors which influence the secretory activity of Sertoli cells. One such factor is P-Mod-S protein (molecular weight 70 kDa), the level of which is regulated by testosterone, and which stimulates the secretion of ABP, Trf and several other proteins from Sertoli cells *in vitro*. Another factor originating in the Pc is the recently characterized inhibitor of plasminogen activator (Hettle *et al.*, 1988). Thus, Pc seems to affect the functions of Sertoli cells in at least two ways: by participating in the formation of the basal lamina, and through paracrine mechanisms via the secretion of regulatory factors. It has been suggested that the effects of testosterone on the functions of Sertoli cells might, at least in part, be mediated by the Pc (Skinner and Fritz, 1985).

We investigated the effect of Pc on the polarity of secretions from Sertoli cells *in vitro*. The Pc and Sertoli cells (from 14- and 18-day-old rats, respectively), were co-cultured on opposite sides of the Millipore filter in two-compartment chambers (Janecki and Steinberger, 1987b). This arrangement prevented direct contact between the two types of cell but permitted exposure of Sertoli cells to secretory products of the Pc. The results of these experiments are shown in Figure 11. In the absence of Pc or serum, ABP was secreted predominantly apically (BC:AC ratio 0.6) whereas most Trf was secreted basolaterally (BC:AC ratio 2.0), results consistent with those in a previous report (Janecki and Steinberger, 1987a). Co-culture with Pc resulted in dramatically increased BC:AC ratios for both ABP and Trf, although the effect on secretion of ABP was significantly more pronounced. In the presence of 2% serum (without Pc) the BC:AC ratio for both ABP and Trf was approximately 3.0, and was further increased by co-culture with Pc. Testosterone enhanced the effects of Pc, although by itself it did not change the polarity of secretion. These data indicate that Pc can affect the polarity of secretion from Sertoli cells through soluble factor(s) which appear to be regulated by testosterone. At present we do not know whether the observed effect was due to P-Mod-S (Skinner and Fritz, 1985), other paracrine factors, or some soluble, testis-specific components of the ECM. It is also not clear whether the effects of serum were due to stimulated replication of Pc. It is possible that serum alone can change the polarity of secretion of ABP and Trf, as was reported for thyroid cells in culture (Nitsch and Wollman, 1980).

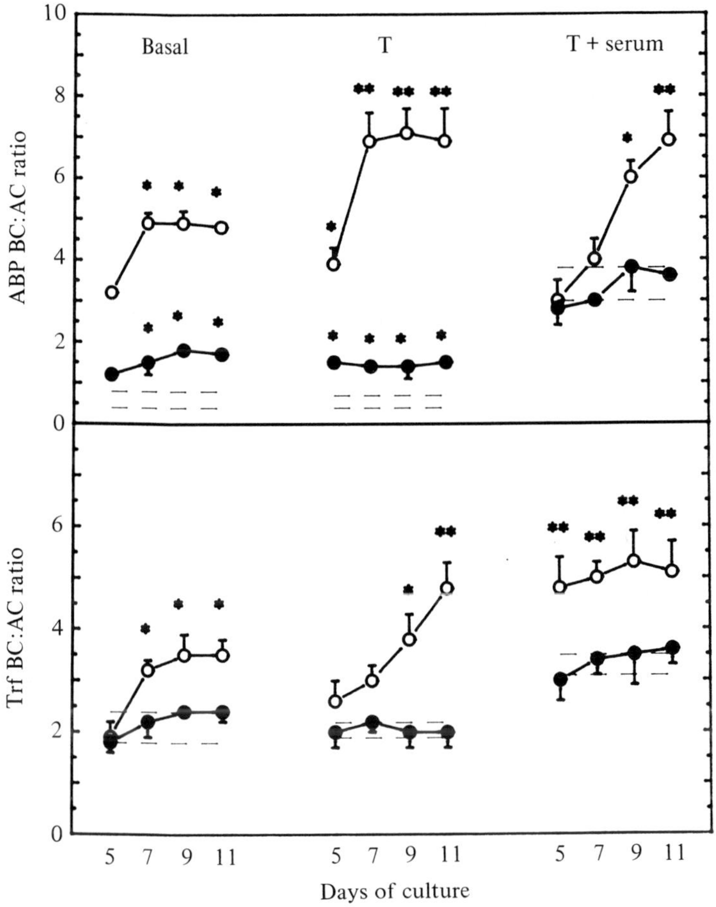

Fig. 11 Effects of testosterone (T) and serum on the polarized secretion of ABP and Trf by Sertoli cells co-cultured with peritubular myoid cells (open circles) or testicular fibroblasts (closed circles). The cells were maintained either in basal medium, in medium that contained 10^{-6} mol/l testosterone (T), or in medium that contained T plus 2% FBS. The areas within dashed lines represent means ± S.D. of values from control cultures of Sertoli cells by themselves. *Significantly different ($p < 0.01$) from control values. **Significantly different ($p < 0.01$) from values for cells in basal medium on the corresponding day of culture (modified from Janecki *et al.*, 1987b).

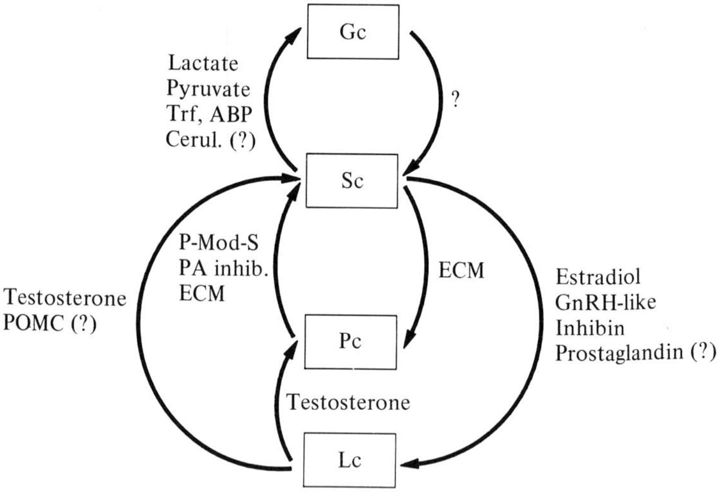

Fig. 12 Current concept of intercellular interactions in the rat testis. Gc, germ cells; Sc, Sertoli cells; Pc, peritubular myoid cells; Lc, Leydig cells; Trf, transferrin; ABP, androgen-binding protein; Cerul., ceruloplasmin; PA inhib., inhibitor of plasminogen activator; POMC, derivatives of pro-opiomelanocortin; ECM, extracellular matrix.

However, absence of any additive effect of serum and Pc in our experiments suggests a predominant role for Pc in the observed phenomenon. The effect of Pc appears to be cell specific, since testicular fibroblasts influenced the polarity of ABP secretion only slightly and had no effect at all on the secretion of Trf. Recently, Ueda *et al.* (1988) reported that direct co-culture of Sertoli cells with Pc in a two-compartment chamber resulted in a 2.5-fold increase in basolateral secretion of SP 1 protein, but they found no effect of Pc on the polarity of secretion of Trf. Similarly, Ailenberg and colleagues (Ailenberg *et al.*, 1988) found no significant effect of Pc on the polarity of secretion of Trf during 4 days of co-culture. This apparent discrepancy might be due to the fact that, in our experiments, maximal effects of Pc were observed after 7 days of co-culture, so that 4 days of co-culture may have been too short a time for a conspicuous effect of Pc on the polarity of secretion of Trf to be observed. Clearly, more studies are needed to clarify the physiological importance of Pc in the regulation of secretions from Sertoli cells and the physiology of seminiferous tubules.

Acknowledgements

This work was supported in part by NIH Grant HD 17802 and funds from WHO.

References

Ailenberg, M. & Fritz, I.B. (1988). Control of levels of plasminogen activator activity secreted by Sertoli cells maintained in a two-chamber assembly. **Endocrinology** 122:2613–2618.

Ailenberg, M., Tung, P.S., Pelletier, M. & Fritz, I.B. (1988). Modulation of Sertoli cell functions in the two-chamber assembly by peritubular cells and extracellular matrix. **Endocrinology** 122:2604–2612.

Bissell, M.J., Hall, G.H. & Parry, G. (1982). How does the extracellular matrix direct gene expression? **Journal of Theoretical Biology** 99:31–68.

Borland, K., Ehrlich, H.P., Muffly, K., Dillis, W.L. & Hall, P.F. (1986). Interaction of rat Sertoli cells with a collagen lattice *in vitro*. **In Vitro Cell Development Biology** 22(11):661–669.

Byers, S.W., Hadley, M.A., Djakiew, D. & Dym, M. (1986). Growth and characterization of polarized monolayers of epidydimal epithelial cells and Sertoli cells in dual environment culture chambers. **Journal of Andrology** 7:59–68.

Chambard, M., Verrier, B., Gabrion, J. & Mauchamp, J. (1984). Polarity reversal of inside-out thyroid follicles cultured within collagen gel: reexpression of specific function. **Biologie Cellulaire** 51:315–326.

Dym, M. & Fawcett, D.W. (1970). The blood–testis barrier in the rat and the physiological compartmentation of the seminiferous epithelium. **Biology of Reproduction** 3:308–326.

Fawcett, D.W. (1975). Ultrastructure and function of the Sertoli cells. In: Greep, R.O. & Astwood, E.B., eds. **Handbook of Physiology, 5** Section 7, Washington DC, American Physiology Society, pp.21–55.

Fritz, I.B. & Tung, P.S. (1986). Role of interactions between peritubular cells and Sertoli cells in mammalian testicular functions. In: Gall, J.G., ed. **Gametogenesis and the Early Embryo** New York, Allan R. Liss, pp.151–173.

Galdieri, M., Monaco, L. & Stefanini, M. (1984). Secretion of androgen-binding protein by Sertoli cells is influenced by contact with germ cells. **Journal of Andrology** 5:409–416.

Gatmaitan, Z., Jefferson, D.M., Ruiz-Opazo, N., Biempica, L., Arias, I., Dudas, G., Leinwand, L. & Reid, L.M. (1983). Regulation of growth and differentiation of a rat hepatoma cell line by the synergistic interactions of hormones and collagenous substrata. **Journal of Cell Biology** 97:1179–1190.

Gospodarowicz, D., Vlodavsky, I. & Savion, N. (1980). Permissive effect of the extracellular matrix on cell proliferation *in vitro*. **Proceedings of the National Academy of Sciences, USA** 77:4094–4098.

Grobstein, C. (1954). Tissue interaction in the morphogenesis of mouse embryonic rudiments *in vitro*. In: Rudrik, D., ed. **Aspects of Synthesis and Order in Growth**, New Jersey, University Press, pp.233–256.

Hadley, M.A., Byers, S.W., Suarez-Quian, C.A., Kleinman, H.K. & Dym, M. (1985). Extracellular matrix regulates Sertoli cell differentiation, testicular cord formation, and germ cell development. **Journal of Cell Biology** 101:1511–1522.

Hadley, M.A., Djakiew, D., Byers, S.W. & Dym, M. (1987). Polarized secretion of androgen-binding protein and transferrin by Sertoli cells grown in a bicameral culture system. **Endocrinology** 120:1097–1103.

Hay, E.D. (1981). Collagen and embryonic development. In: Hay, E.D., ed. **Cell**

Biology of Extracellular Matrix, New York, Plenum Press, pp.379–409.

Hettle, J.A., Balekjian, E., Tung, P.S. & Fritz, I.B. (1988). Rat testicular peritubular cells in culture secrete, an inhibitor of plasminogen activator activity. **Biology of Reproduction** 38:359–371.

Hutson, J.C. & Stocco, D.M. (1981). Peritubular cell influence on the efficiency of androgen-binding protein secretion by Sertoli cells in culture. **Endocrinology** 108:1362–1368.

Janecki, A., Jakubowiak, A. & Steinberger, A. (1988). Effect of germ cells on vectorial secretion of androgen-binding protein and transferrin by immature rat Sertoli cells *in vitro*. **Journal of Andrology** 9:126–132.

Janecki, A. & Steinberger, A. (1986). Polarized Sertoli cell functions in a new two-compartment culture system. **Journal of Andrology** 7:69–71.

Janecki, A. & Steinberger, A. (1987a). Bipolar secretion of androgen-binding protein and transferrin by Sertoli cells cultured in a two-compartment culture chamber. **Endocrinology** 120:291–298.

Janecki, A. & Steinberger, A. (1987b). Vectorial secretion of transferrin and androgen-binding protein in Sertoli cell cultures: effect of extracellular matrix, peritubular myoid cells and medium composition. **Molecular and Cellular Endocrinology** 52:125–136.

Kleinman, H.K., Klebe, R.J. & Martin, G.R. (1981). Role of collagenous matrices in the adhesion and growth of cells. **Journal of Cell Biology** 88:473–485.

Kleinman, H.K., McGarvey, M.L., Hassel, J.R., Star, V.L., Cannon, F.B., Laurie, G.W. & Martin, G.R. (1986). Basement membrane complexes with biological activity. **Biochemistry** 25:312–318.

Le Magueresse, B. & Jégou, B. (1986). Possible involvement of germ cells in regulation of estradiol-17-beta and ABP secretion by immature rat Sertoli cells: *in vitro* studies. **Biochemical and Biophysical Research Communications** 141:861–869.

Le Magueresse, B. & Jégou, B. (1988). *In vitro* effects of germ cells on the secretory activity of Sertoli cells recovered from rats of different ages. **Endocrinology** 122:1672–1680.

Le Magueresse, B., Le Gac, F., Loir, M. & Jégou, B. (1986). Stimulation of rat Sertoli cell secretory activity *in vitro* by germ cells and residual bodies. **Journal of Reproduction and Fertility** 77:489–498.

Mather, J.P., Gunsalus, G.L., Musto, N.A., Cheng, C.Y., Parvinen, M., Wright, W., Perez-Infante, V., Margioris, A., Liotta, A., Becker, R., Krieger, D.T. & Bardin, C.W. (1983). The hormonal and cellular control of Sertoli cell secretion. **Journal of Steroid Biochemistry** 19(1):41–51.

Mather, J.P., Wolpe, S.D., Gunsalus, G.L., Bardin, C.W. & Phillips, D.M. (1984). Effect of purified and cell-produced extracellular matrix components on Sertoli cell function. In: Catt, K.J. & Dufau, M.L., eds. Hormone Action and Testicular Function **Annals of the New York Academy of Science** 438:572–576.

Nitsch, L. & Wollman, S.H. (1980). Ultrastructure of intermediate states in polarity reversal of thyroid epithelium in follicles in suspension culture. **Journal of Cell Biology** 86:875–880.

Orkin, R.W., Gehron, P., McGoodwin, E.B., Martin, G.R., Valentine, T. & Swarm, R. (1977). A murine tumor producing a matrix of basement membrane. **Journal of Experimental Medicine** 145:204–220.

Parvinen, M. (1982). Regulation of the seminiferous epithelium. **Endocrine Reviews** 3:404–417.

Reid, L.M. & Jefferson, D.M. (1984). Cell culture studies using extracts of extracellular matrix to study growth and differentiation in mammalian cells. In: Mather, J.P., ed. **Mammalian Cell Culture**, New York and London, Plenum Press, pp.239–280.

Reid, L., Morrow, B., Jubinsky, P., Schwartz, E. & Gatmaitan, Z. (1981). Regulation of growth and differentiation of epithelial cells by hormones, growth factors, and substrates of extracellular matrix. **Annals of the New York Academy of Sciences, USA** 372:354–371.

Russell, L.D. & Peterson, R.N. (1985). Sertoli cell junctions: morphological and functional correlates. **International Review of Cytology** 94:177–211.

Russell, L.D., Tallon-Doran, M., Weber, J.E., Wong, V. & Peterson, R.N. (1983). Three-dimensional reconstruction of rat stage V Sertoli cell: III. A study of specific cellular relationships. **American Journal of Anatomy** 167:181–192.

Salas, P.J.I., Vega-Salas, D. & Rodriguez-Boulan, E. (1987). Collagen receptors mediate early events in the attachment of epithelial (MDCK) cells. **Journal of Membrane Biology** 98:223–236.

Sanborn, B., Wagle, J.R., Steinberger, A. & Lamb, D.J. (1983). Sertoli cell as an androgen target. In: D'Agata, R., Lipsett, M.B., Polosa, P. & Van der Molen, H.J., eds. **Recent Advances in Male Reproduction: Molecular Basis and Clinical Implications**, New York, Raven Press, pp.69–78.

Setchell, B.P. & Waites, G.M.H. (1975). The blood–testis barrier. In: Greep, R.O. & Astwood, A.B., eds. **Handbook of Physiology** Vol. 5, Washington, DC, American Physiology Society, pp.143–172.

Sertoli, E. (1865). Dell'esistenzia di particolari cellule ramificate nei canalicoli seminiferi del testicolo umano. **Morgagni** 7:31–40.

Sharpe, R.M. (1983). Local control of testicular function. **Journal of Experimental Physiology** 68:265–287.

Sharpe, R.M. (1986). Paracrine control of the testis. **Clinical Endocrinology and Metabolism** 15:185–207.

Sharpe, R.M. (1988). Bidirectional secretion by the Sertoli cell. **International Journal of Andrology** 11:87–91.

Skinner, M.K. & Fritz, I.B. (1985). Testicular peritubular cells secrete a protein under androgen contact that modulates Sertoli cell functions. **Proceedings of the National Academy of Sciences, USA** 82:114–118.

Skinner, M.K. & Fritz, I.B. (1986). Identification of a non-mitogenic paracrine factor involved in mesenchymal–epithelial cell interactions between testicular peritubular cells and Sertoli cells. **Molecular and Cellular Endocrinology** 44:85–97.

Skinner, M.K. & Griswold, M.D. (1982). Secretion of testicular transferrin by cultured Sertoli cells is regulated by hormones and retinoids. **Biology of Reproduction** 27:211–221.

Skinner, M.K., Tung, P.S. & Fritz, I.B. (1985). Cooperativity between Sertoli cells and testicular peritubular cells in the production and deposition of extracellular matrix components. **Journal of Cell Biology** 100:1938–1941.

Steinberger, A., Janecki, A. & Jakubowiak, A. (1988). New experimental approaches to the study of inhibin physiology *in vitro*. In: Burger, H.G., Findlay, J.K., DeKretser, D.M. & Igarashi, M., eds. **Inhibin – Non-Steroidal Regulation of Follicle-Stimulating Hormone Secretion**, New York, Raven Press, pp.163–179.

Suarez-Quian, C.A., Hadley, M.A. & Dym, M. (1984). Effects of substrate on the shape of Sertoli cells *in vitro*. In: Catt, K.J. & Dufau, M.L., eds. Hormone Action and Testicular Function **Annals of the New York Academy of Sciences** 438:417–435.

Tung, P.S. & Fritz, I.B. (1980). Interactions of Sertoli cells with myoid cells *in vitro.* **Biology of Reproduction** 23:207–217.

Tung, P.S. & Fritz, J.B. (1984). Extracellular matrix promotes rat Sertoli cell histotypic expression *in vitro.* **Biology of Reproduction** 30:213–229.

Tung, P.S. & Fritz, I.B. (1986). Extracellular matrix component and testicular peritubular cells influence the rate and pattern of Sertoli cell migration *in vitro.* **Developmental Biology** 113:119–134.

Tung, P.S., Skinner, M.K. & Fritz, I.B. (1984). Cooperativity between Sertoli cells and peritubular myoid cells in the formation of the basal lamina in the seminiferous tubule. In: Catt, K.J. & Dufau, M.L., eds. Hormone Action and Testicular Function **Annals of the New York Academy of Sciences** 438:435–446.

Ueda, H., Tres, L.L. & Kierszenbaum, A.L. (1988). Culture patterns and sorting of rat Sertoli cell secretory proteins. **Journal of Cell Science** 89(2):175–188.

Wagle, J.R., Heindel, J.J., Sanborn, B.M. & Steinberger, A. (1986). Effect of hypotonic treatment on Sertoli cell purity and function in culture. **In Vitro** 22:325–331.

Waites, G.M.H. & Gladwell, R.T. (1982). Physiological significance of fluid secretion in the testis and blood–testis barrier. **Physiology Review** 62(2):624–671.

Welsh, M.J., Ireland, M.E. & Treisman, G.J. (1984). Sertoli cell adenylyl cyclase is stimulated by a factor associated with germ cells. In: Catt, K.J. & Dufau, M.L., eds. Hormone Action and Testicular Function **Annals of the New York Academy of Sciences** 438:576–579.

Yamada, K.M. (1983). **Cell Interactions and Development** New York, Wiley Interscience.

Ying, S.Y., Czvik, J., Becker, A., Ling, N., Ueno, N. & Guillemin, R. (1987). Secretion of follicle-stimulating hormone and production of inhibin are reciprocally related. **Proceedings of the National Academy of Sciences, USA** 84(13):4631–4635.

The influence of ovarian granulosa cell factors on the proliferation and differentiation of endothelial cells

R.D. KOOS

Department of Physiology, University of Maryland School of Medicine, Baltimore, MD, USA.

Keywords

Angiogenesis, granulosa cells, endothelial cells, follicles, mitogens, heparin-binding growth factors, fibroblast growth factors, angiogenesis *in vitro*, non-mitogenic angiogenic factors.

Introduction

Growth of the ovarian follicle and corpus luteum is accompanied by the development of rich, new vascular networks that provide the necessary nourishment for these tissues to carry out the vital reproductive functions of gamete and steroid production. This vascular development is noteworthy for its rapidity and extent, especially since angiogenesis is a rare phenomenon in the normal, uninjured body, and occurs for the most part only in the ovary and in the uterine endometrium. In other organs and tissues, endothelial cells are nearly quiescent (D'Amore and Thompson, 1987). By contrast, numerous diseases are characterized by active angiogenesis (Folkman and Klagsbrun, 1987). It is, therefore, of some importance to elucidate how angiogenesis is regulated in the female reproductive tract.

Angiogenesis occurs when a tissue is deprived of an adequate blood supply, either as a result of wounding or inflammation or when hyperplasia or neoplasia gives rise to new tissue that cannot be nourished by existing vessels. In the ovary, the granulosa layer of the follicle and early corpus luteum, which undergoes tremendous hyperplasia in a short period of time, provides an example of such a situation. Like epithelial carcinomas *in situ*, the granulosa layer is separated from stromal blood vessels (in the thecal layer) by a basement membrane until ovulation occurs. Tumors have long been known to recruit new blood vessels through the release of diffusible angiogenic factors (Folkman and Klagsbrun, 1987); it seems reasonable to assume that granulosa cells are the source of similar angiogenic factors. To validate this assumption, the effects on endothelial cells of factors released from cultured rat granulosa cells were investigated. These studies have revealed that granulosa cells are, indeed, the source of several factors that can promote the proliferation and migration of endothelial cells and capillary morphogenesis.

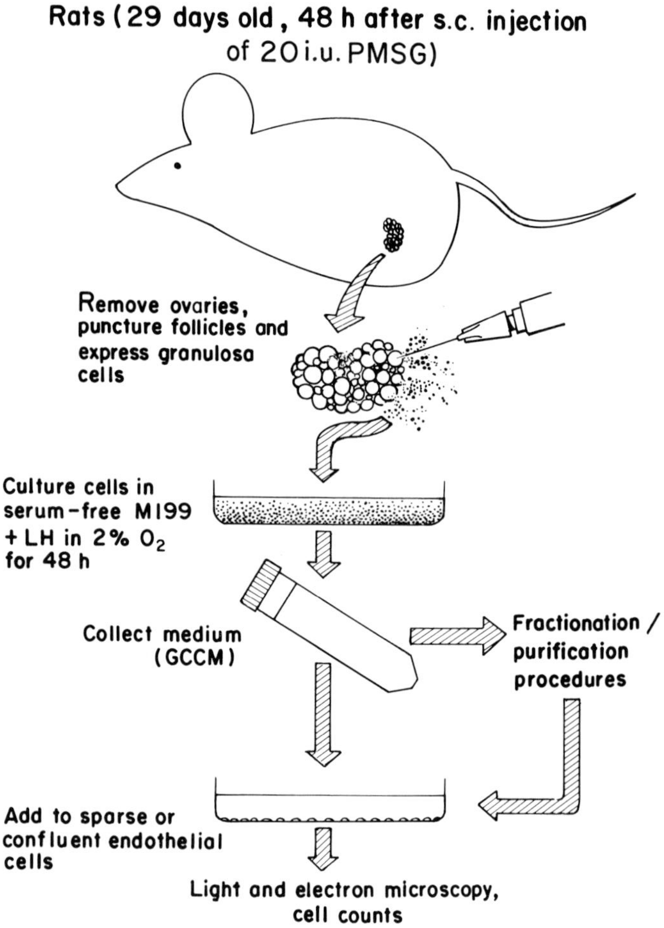

Fig. 1 Method for the production of granulosa cell-conditioned medium (GCCM).

Materials and methods

Culture of granulosa cells

Granulosa cells were obtained from immature Sprague–Dawley rats (29 days old) 48 hours after injection (s.c.) of 20 i.u. of pregnant mare's serum gonadotropin (PMSG), as described earlier (Koos, 1986; Fig. 1). Two million viable cells were cultured in 3 ml of serum-free Medium 199 (M199; Gibco, Grand Island, NY) that contained 10 ng/ml luteinizing hormone (LH: oLH-23, National Hormone and Pituitary Program) for 48 hours. The cultures were incubated in an atmosphere of 93% N_2, 2% O_2, and 5% CO_2. The conditioned medium (granulosa cell-conditioned medium, GCCM) was collected, centrifuged to remove any cells and cellular debris, and stored frozen at −90°C.

Ultrafiltration

For some studies, GCCM was fractionated by centrifugal ultrafiltration through Centricon 10 and/or Centricon 30 microconcentrators (Amicon, Danvers, MA).

Heparin-affinity chromatography

To determine if granulosa cells release a heparin-binding growth factor, GCCM was chromatographed on a heparin-affinity column (Klagsbrun *et al.*, 1987; Neufeld *et al.*, 1987). GCCM (100 ml) was first concentrated by ultrafiltration in a stirred cell using a membrane with a nominal cut-off of 8 kDa. The retentate was loaded onto a 1-ml column of heparin–Sepharose (Pharmacia, Piscataway, NJ). The column was washed extensively with 0.2 mol/l NaCl in 0.01 mol/l Tris–HCl, pH 7. Bound material was eluted stepwise with 0.6, 0.8, 1.0, 1.25, 1.5, 2.0, and 2.5 mol/l NaCl in the same buffer. The fractions were concentrated and the elution buffer exchanged with fresh M199 (2 ml M199x2) by centrifugal ultrafiltration (Centricon 10 Microconcentrators, Amicon, Danvers, MA). After the second wash with M199, the retentate was reconstituted with M199 to 1 ml and filter-sterilized. An aliquot of 0.1 ml of this solution was added to a 2-cm well in a culture dish that contained a sparse distribution of endothelial cells, prepared as described below. In each experiment, each fraction from the column was assayed in triplicate. Each assay well also received 0.4 ml of M199 that contained 0.625% serum (to give a final volume of 0.5 ml and a concentration of serum of 0.5%). Control cultures were treated with 0.5 ml of fresh M199 that contained 0.5% serum.

Western blot analysis

Samples of GCCM were fractionated by ultrafiltration (8-kDa cut-off membrane) and the concentrated retentate subjected to electrophoresis on an SDS–polyacrylamide gel (12.5%). The separated proteins were electroeluted to Immobilon membranes (Millipore, Bedford, MA) and incubated with an affinity-purified antibody raised against basic fibroblast growth factor (bFGF) (Amgen, Thousand Oaks, CA) or normal rabbit IgG. Blots were developed using an avidin–biotin–alkaline phosphatase system (Vector Laboratories, Burlingame, CA); as little as 1 ng of standard bFGF could be detected in this system.

Culture of endothelial cells

Endothelial cells from fetal bovine aorta were cultured as described earlier (Koos, 1986).

Assay for mitogenesis

Aliquots of GCCM fractions obtained by ultrafiltration or heparin-affinity chromatography were added to sparse cultures of endothelial cells (10^4 cells/well). Controls consisted of fresh M199 that contained a low (0.5% or 1%) or high (10%) level of serum (fetal bovine serum or a 1:1 mixture of fetal bovine serum and iron-supplemented calf serum; HyClone, Logan, UT). After 96 hours, cell nuclei were counted (Koos, 1986).

Assay for angiogenesis in vitro

GCCM was filtered through a membrane with a 30-kDa cut-off and various dilutions of the concentrated retentate were added to confluent endothelial cells grown either directly on plastic or on a collagen gel. In the latter case, Vitrogen 100 (Collagen Corporation, Palo Alto, CA) was used. The solution of Vitrogen was mixed with 0.1 mol/l NaOH and 2x Medium 199 (Gibco, Grand Island, NY) at a ratio of 8:1:9. This solution (200 μl) was added to 2-cm culture wells and incubated at 37°C until it gelled. Each well was rinsed with 300 μl of culture medium before the cells were plated. After the cells reached confluence, the growth medium was removed and various concentrations of the >30-kDa retenate of the preparation of GCCM were added. Cells were observed daily under a phase-contrast microscope. After 96 hours, the cultures were fixed and processed for light and electron microscopy (Montesano *et al.*, 1986).

Results

GCCM contains two distinct endothelial cell mitogens

GCCM is a potent stimulator of the proliferation of endothelial cells (Koos, 1986). To determine the nature of the mitogenic activity, GCCM was sequentially filtered through 10- and 30-kDa ultrafiltration membranes. As shown in Table 1, mitogenic activity was found in two of the three resulting fractions: the <10-kDa and the >30-kDa fraction. There was no significant mitogenic activity in the 10–30-kDa fraction. The low-molecular-weight activity was not affected by heating to 100°C for 4 minutes. By contrast, heat destroyed all mitogenic activity in the high-molecular-weight fraction, suggesting that the active factor in this fraction might be a protein. It is noteworthy that the endothelial cells treated with the low- and high-molecular-weight fractions differed markedly in morphology (see below).

Since bFGF is produced by bovine granulosa cells (Neufeld *et al.*, 1987) and is a potent inducer of the proliferation of endothelial cells (Gospodarowicz *et al.*, 1986), it seemed possible that the high-molecular-weight mitogenic activity in GCCM was due to bFGF. To examine this possibility, GCCM was chromatographed over heparin–Sepharose and the resulting fractions tested for mitogenic activity. There was significant mitogenic activity in the fraction

Table 1. *Mitogenic activity of fractions of GCCM obtained by ultrafiltration*

Treatment[a]	Endothelial cells/well (x10³) Before heating	After heating at 100°C, 4 min
Control[b]	8.1 ± 2.3	ND[c]
GCCM[d]	78.5 ± 10.5	27.9 ± 6.4
GCCM fractions[e] (kD)		
<10	50.0 ± 3.4	44.8 ± 11.3
>10, <30	13.5 ± 1.3	ND
>30	33.1 ± 2.1	6.1 ± 1.3

[a]Volume = 1 ml.
[b]Fresh M199 + 1% fetal bovine serum only.
[c]ND, not determined.
[d]50% GCCM/50% fresh M199 + 2% fetal bovine serum (final serum concentration was 1%).
[e]The concentrated retentates were washed and reconstituted to the original volume with fresh M199. All three ultrafiltration fractions were then diluted 1:1 with fresh M199 plus 2% serum (final concentration of serum was 1%).

eluted with 1.0 mol/l NaCl (Fig. 2). The mitogenic effect was completely blocked by the addition of 90 μg/ml heparin (data not shown). Similar effects of heparin on bFGF-stimulated proliferation of endothelial cells have been reported (Gospodarowicz *et al.*, 1986). The presence of the mitogenic activity in the fraction eluted with 1.0 mol/l NaCl indicated that the active factor is probably not bFGF, which is typically eluted from heparin–Sepharose by 1.5 mol/l NaCl (Klagsbrun *et al.*, 1987). GCCM was also evaluated for the presence of bFGF by Western blot analysis with a specific, affinity-purified antibody. No bFGF was detected in GCCM by this method. Rat granulosa cells (approximately 5×10^7) were also extracted and analyzed; again, no bFGF was found. However, bFGF was readily detected in extracts of an equivalent number of endothelial cells from fetal bovine aorta (data not shown), which have been shown to produce this factor (Schweigerer *et al.*, 1987). Thus, the heparin-binding endothelial cell mitogen in GCCM does not appear to be bFGF.

Fractions of GCCM eluting from heparin at 0.6–0.8 mol/l NaCl appeared to cause small increases in numbers of endothelial cells, as determined by counts of nuclei (Fig. 2). Examination of the cells during the culture period showed, however, that 10–40% of the endothelial cells in these treated groups were binucleate. This observation indicates that GCCM may contain another interesting and novel growth factor.

GCCM contains a factor that stimulates elongation and migration of endothelial cells and angiogenesis in vitro

In addition to its mitogenic activity, GCCM contains a distinct factor that induces elongation of the endothelial cells (Koos, 1986). The elongation-

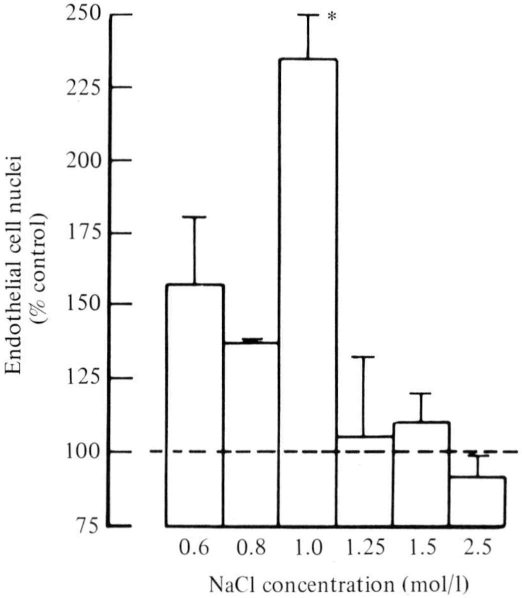

Fig. 2 Proliferation of endothelial cells in response to GCCM fractionated by affinity chromatography on heparin–Sepharose. Each bar represents the mean (±S.E.) of results from three experiments with three different batches of GCCM. Additional methodological details are described in Materials and methods. *p<0.001.

inducing activity appears to be associated with a factor of relatively high molecular weight (>30 kDa). This approximate size was confirmed during the sequential ultrafiltration studies described above. Cultures treated with the <10-kDa fraction of GCCM had the cobblestone appearance typical of endothelial cells. By contrast, endothelial cells treated with the >30-kDa fraction became elongated, with cellular projections typical of migrating cells. Furthermore, when GCCM was added to confluent cultures of endothelial cells that displayed the cobblestone appearance, the cells became elongated and aligned with one another within 24 hours. Within 48 hours, the migration of cells under the original monolayer of cells was apparent. Within 96 hours, an extensive network of anastomosing, capillary-like 'tubules' had formed beneath the original monolayer of cells. The >30-kDa fraction of GCCM had the same effect as unfractionated GCCM, but the <30-kDa fraction did not induce formation of capillaries. Control cultures of endothelial cells, treated with only 1% or 10% fetal bovine serum, maintained their characteristic cobblestone morphology throughout the 96-hour culture period.

The effects of this in-vitro angiogenic factor on endothelial cells grown on a collagen substrate, rather than directly on plastic, were also examined. Within 48 hours after treatment with the >30-kDa fraction of GCCM (8x), many endothelial cells had elongated and reorganized to form a complex network of capillary-like cords under the original monolayer (Fig. 3); branches of these structures could be seen deep within the collagen gel. Many of the multicellular branches appeared to contain lumens (Fig. 4), as confirmed by electron microscopy (data not shown). The ability of this in-vitro angiogenic factor to promote the migration and differentiation of endothelial cells suggests that it may play an important role in the angiogenic process.

Dose–response, time-course, and analytical studies were carried out on the factor in GCCM that induces angiogenesis *in vitro* (Blake and Koos, 1987). Various dilutions of the concentrated >30-kDa retentate of GCCM (8x, 4x, 2x, 1x in fresh M199 + 1% fetal bovine serum) were added to confluent endothelial cells (on plastic). Within 6 hours, the 8x dose had caused a marked elongation of the cells. Within 24 hours, a complex, anastomosing network of capillary-like tubules had formed. The interval until tubules were formed increased and the magnitude of the response decreased as the concentration of the >30-kDa retentate was decreased. Samples of the 8x concentrated fraction of GCCM were treated with trypsin, acidified (with HCl to 1 mol/l), or heated (100°C, 4 minutes). The heated >30-kDa fraction stimulated the formation of tubules as strongly as the untreated material. By contrast, trypsin and acid almost completely destroyed the tubule-inducing activity. These results suggest that the GCCM factor that induces angiogenesis *in vitro* is a heat-stable protein.

Discussion

A significant portion of the mitogenic activity in GCCM is associated with material that has a relatively low molecular weight and is resistant to heating. It is quite possible, therefore, that this factor is not a protein. This conclusion is supported by the observation that only part of the mitogenic activity in GCCM is sensitive to trypsin (Koos, 1986). Low-molecular-weight (<1 kDa) mitogenic factors have been extracted from tumors (Fenselau *et al.*, 1981) and other tissues (reviewed in Folkman and Klagsbrun, 1987; D'Amore and Thompson, 1987). Recently, a similar type of factor was reported to be present in medium conditioned by vascular smooth-muscle cells (Hoover *et al.*, 1989). These low-molecular-weight endothelial cell mitogens have not been further characterized and their role in angiogenesis, if any, remains to be determined.

The higher-molecular-weight mitogenic activity in GCCM is retained by an ultrafiltration membrane with a nominal cut-off of 30 kDa. This property would appear to make it distinct from the FGFs that have molecular weights of approximately 16–19 kDa (Klagsbrun *et al.*, 1987). However, heparin-affinity chromatography revealed the presence of a heparin-binding mitogen in GCCM. This factor was eluted from heparin–Sepharose by 1.0 mol/l NaCl,

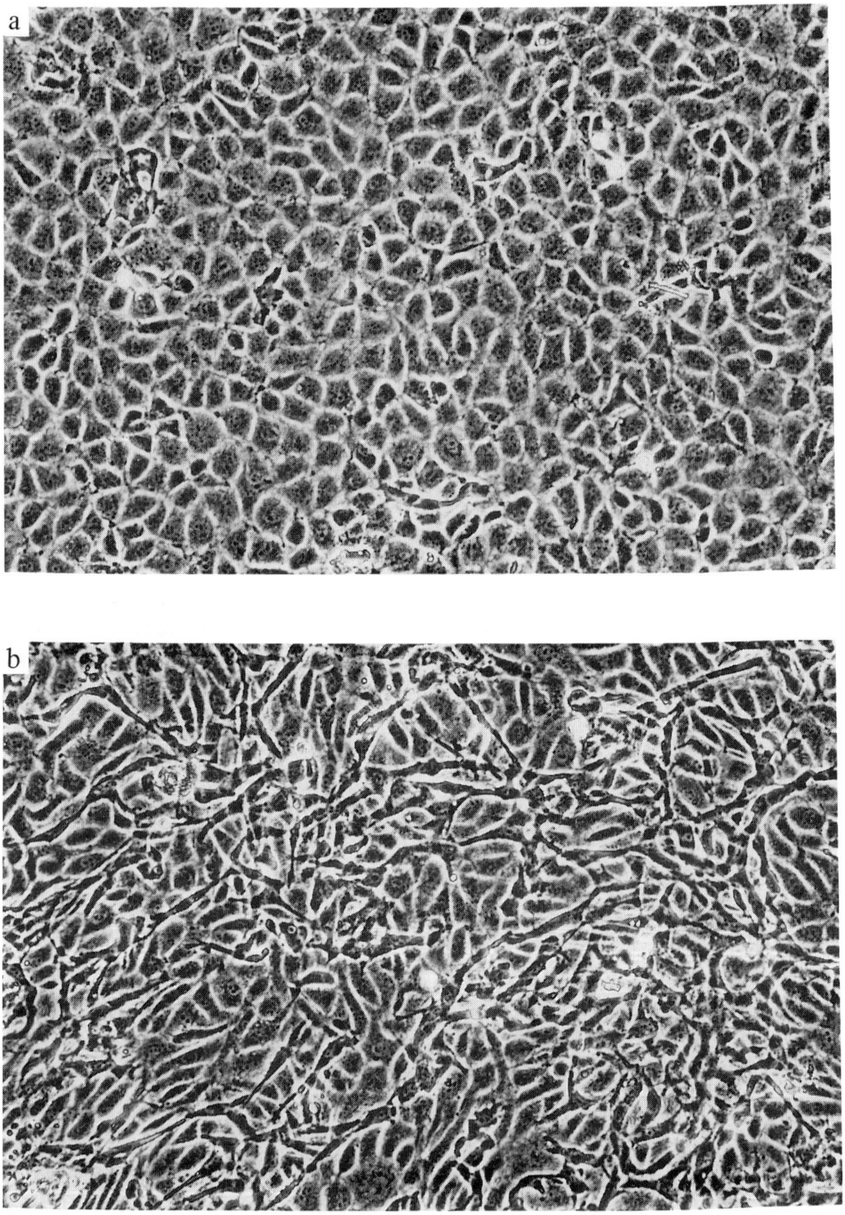

Fig. 3 Endothelial cells grown to confluence on a collagen gel and then treated for 48 hours with (A) 1% serum in M199 (control), or (**B**) the concentrated (8x) >30-kDa fraction of GCCM (phase-contrast; x220).

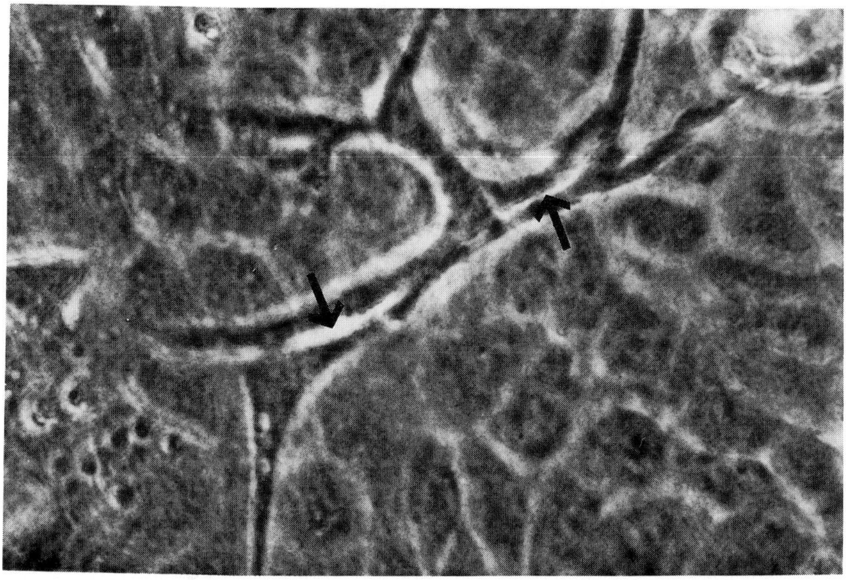

Fig. 4 A capillary-like endothelial cell sprout in a collagen gel (phase-contrast). Lumens are visible within the sprout (arrows) (x660).

the same concentration of NaCl as that which elutes acidic FGF (aFGF). The inconsistency in terms of size might be explained if the granulosa cell factor is bound to other materials in conditioned medium. The activity is heat labile, as are the FGFs (Gospodarowicz and Cheng, 1986). It has been reported that bFGF is produced by cultured bovine granulosa cells (Neufeld *et al.*, 1987). However, bFGF is eluted from heparin by 1.5 mol/l NaCl. Western blot analysis failed to show any bFGF in GCCM or in extracts of granulosa cells. Shimasaki *et al.* (1989) recently reported that they were unable to detect mRNA specific for bFGF in the rat ovary by Northern blot analysis with a cDNA probe made from a rat ovarian library. It is somewhat surprising to find FGF-like activity in conditioned medium, since the precursors to both aFGF and bFGF apparently lack signal sequences (Gospodarowicz *et al.*, 1987). It is possible that an FGF could be released from dead or damaged granulosa cells during the conditioning period. Acidic FGF has been found largely in neural tissue, but more recently it was also identified in kidney (Gautschi-Sova *et al.*, 1987) and heart (Speir *et al.*, 1988); it may turn out to be more widely distributed than was originally thought. It is possible that the heparin-binding growth factor in GCCM is aFGF.

It is also possible that the heparin-binding growth factor in GCCM could be related to one of the recently identified products of oncogenes that code for FGF-like factors – int-2, hst/KS3, and FGF-5. The *int*-2 gene is expressed in mammary tumors induced by the mouse mammary tumor virus; it is also expressed during early embryonic development in the mouse (Wilkinson *et al.*, 1988). The predicted product of the *int*-2 gene has considerable similarity to bFGF (45% identity) and somewhat less to aFGF (35%). The *hst/KS3* oncogene was isolated from a human stomach tumor (Taira *et al.*, 1987) and from a Kaposi's sarcoma (Delli Bovi *et al.*, 1987). It potentially codes for a protein of 206 amino acids, a portion of which would have 43% and 37% identity with bFGF and aFGF, respectively; there is, in addition, a large number of conservative amino acid substitutions. Unlike aFGF and bFGF, the predicted *hst/KS3* product contains a sequence of 24 hydrophobic or neutral amino acids similar to a typical signal sequence, which indicates that the hst/KS3 protein is probably secreted. This hypothesis is supported by the observation that medium conditioned by cells transfected with this gene caused significant stimulation of growth of NIH 3T3 cells (Delli Bovi *et al.*, 1987). The human *FGF-5* oncogene codes for a protein of 267 amino acids which contains a region of 122 residues with 40–50% identity to aFGF, bFGF, int-2, and hst/KS3 (Zhan *et al.*, 1988). This gene was found to be expressed not only in three lines of human tumor cells, but also in the human neonatal brain. Like *hst/KS3*, the predicted product of the *FGF-5* gene contains a region that resembles a hydrophobic signal sequence. Furthermore, medium conditioned by cells transformed with the *FGF-5* gene is strongly mitogenic for both 3T3 cells and endothelial cells from the fetal bovine heart. Like aFGF, FGF-5 is eluted from heparin–Sepharose by 1.0 mol/l NaCl (Zhan *et al.*, 1988).

The high-molecular-weight factor that induces angiogenesis *in vitro* is clearly distinct from the heparin-binding growth factor from GCCM. It is heat stable, while the high-molecular-weight mitogenic activity of GCCM is heat labile. Furthermore, its level in GCCM is enhanced when the granulosa cells are cultured in a low-oxygen atmosphere (Koos, 1986). In contrast to this result, hypoxic culture did not affect the overall mitogenic activity of GCCM. It does seem likely that the factor is a protein; treatment with trypsin and with acid destroys the activity (Blake and Koos, 1987). It has been reported that bFGF can induce angiogenesis *in vitro*, but this induction required a minimum dose of 3 ng/ml, ten times the dose that maximally stimulated mitogenesis (Montesano *et al.*, 1986). As discussed above, there is no evidence at all for the presence of bFGF in GCCM, let alone at such high levels. Maciag (1984) has reported that the acidic heparin-binding factor endothelial cell growth factor (ECGF) does not enhance angiogenesis *in vitro*.

In a preliminary report, Rone *et al.* (1988) described the isolation of a non-mitogenic chemotactic factor from rat corpus luteum. Non-mitogenic angiogenic factors have also been isolated from lines of melanoma cells (Osthoff *et al.*, 1987) and monocytes (Höckel *et al.*, 1987). Knighton *et al.* (1983) reported that macrophages secrete a non-mitogenic angiogenic factor, but only when cultured under hypoxic conditions. This observation is in agreement with the observation that the factor in GCCM that induces angiogenesis *in vitro* is produced when the granulosa cells are cultured in a low-oxygen environment (Koos, 1986). The possibility that such non-mitogenic factors are cell-attachment molecules, components of the extracellular matrix, or proteases rather than hormonal-type factors cannot be ruled out at this time. Nevertheless, all of these classes of compounds are thought to play important roles in angiogenesis (Folkman and Klagsbrun, 1987; D'Amore and Thompson, 1987).

Whatever the identity of the in-vitro angiogenic factor in GCCM, it could potentially play a key role in the angiogenic process. Several observations indicate that migration, rather than proliferation, is the primal event in the angiogenic process. For example, growth of new blood vessels occurs in the corneas of rabbits irradiated to prevent cell division (Sholley *et al.*, 1984). The vessels are limited in length, but functional. The mitogenic component of capillary growth may result from the initiation of migration.

In summary, granulosa cells are capable of stimulating all three recognized events in the angiogenic process: (1) proliferation of endothelial cells; (2) migration of endothelial cells; and (3) protease production by endothelial cells (as demonstrated by the ability of the endothelial cells to invade a collagen gel). Studies of granulosa cells promise new insights into both normal and pathological angiogenesis.

Acknowledgements

This work was supported by grants HD17999 and CA45055 from NIH. I would like to thank Dr Barry J. Sugarman and Dr Michael Fox of Amgen, Thousand Oaks, CA, for their generous gift of reagents used in these studies. I also wish to thank Erik Olson for his excellent assistance with studies described in this paper. PMSG and LH were provided by the National Hormone and Pituitary Program.

Note added in proof: Subsequent to the submission of this paper, the author has published two reports on the expression of the genes for bFGF and aFGF in the rat ovary.

Koos, R.D. & Olson, C.E. (1989). Expression of basic fibroblast growth factor in the rat ovary: Detection of mRNA using reverse transcription–polymerase chain reaction amplification. **Molecular Endocrinology** 3:2041–2048.

Koos, R.D. & Olson, C.E. (1989). Detection of acidic fibroblast growth factor mRNA in the rat ovary using reverse transcription–polymerase chain reaction amplification. **Biochemical and Biophysical Research Communications** 165:82–88.

References

Blake, A.G. & Koos, R.D. (1987). Characterization of a factor in granulosa cell-conditioned medium that induces angiogenesis *in vitro*. **Biology of Reproduction** 36(Suppl. 1), No. 34.

D'Amore, P.A. & Thompson, R.W. (1987). Mechanisms of angiogenesis. **Annual Review of Physiology** 49:453–464.

Delli Bovi, P., Curatola, A.M., Kern, F.G., Greco, A., Ittman, M. & Basilico, C. (1987). An oncogene isolated by transfection of Kaposi's sarcoma DNA encodes growth factor that is a member of the FGF family. **Cell** 50:729–737.

Fenselau, A., Watt, S. & Mello, R.J. (1981). Tumor angiogenic factor purification from the Walker 256 rat tumor. **Journal of Biological Chemistry** 256:9605–9611.

Folkman, J. & Klagsbrun, M. (1987). Angiogenic factors. **Science** 235:442–447.

Gautschi-Sova, P., Jiang, Z., Frater-Schroder, M. & Bohlen, P. (1987). Acidic fibroblast growth factor is present in non-neural tissue: isolation and chemical characterization from bovine kidney. **Biochemistry** 26:5844–5847.

Gospodarowicz, D. & Cheng, J. (1986). Heparin protects basic and acidic FGF from inactivation. **Journal of Cellular Physiology** 128:475–484.

Gospodarowicz, D., Massoglia, S., Cheng, J. & Fujii, D.K. (1986). Effect of fibroblast growth factor and lipoproteins on the proliferation of endothelial cells derived from bovine adrenal cortex, brain cortex, and corpus luteum capillaries. **Journal of Cellular Physiology** 127:121–136.

Gospodarowicz, D., Neufeld, G. & Schweigerer, (1987). Fibroblast growth factor: structural and biological properties. **Journal of Cellular Physiology** Supplement 5:15–26.

Höckel, M., Sasse, J. & Wissler, J.H. (1987). Purified monocyte-derived angiogenic substance (angiotropin) stimulates migration, phenotypic changes, and 'tube formation' but not proliferation of capillary endothelial cells *in vitro*. **Journal of Cellular Physiology** 133:1–13.

Hoover, G.A., McCormick, S. & Kalant, N. (1989). Effects of porcine aortic smooth muscle cell conditioned medium on endothelial cell replication. **Arteriosclerosis** 9:76–83.

Klagsbrun, M., Sullivan, R., Smith, S., Rybka, R. & Shing, Y. (1987). Purification of endothelial cell growth factors by heparin affinity chromatography. **Methods in Enzymology** 147B:95–105.

Knighton, D.R., Hunt, T.K., Scheuenstuhl, H., Halliday, B.J., Werb, Z. & Banda, M.U. (1983). Oxygen tension regulates the expression of angiogenesis factor by macrophages. **Science** 221:1283–1285.

Koos, R.D. (1986). Stimulation of endothelial cell proliferation by rat granulosa cell-conditioned medium. **Endocrinology** 119:481–489.

Koos, R.D. & Lemaire, W.J. (1983). Evidence for an angiogenic factor from rat follicles. In: Greenwald, G.S. & Terranova, P.F., eds. **Factors Regulating Ovarian Function**, New York, Raven Press, pp.191–195.

Maciag, T. (1984). Angiogenesis. **Progress in Hemostasis and Thrombosis** 7:167–182.

Montesano, R., Vassalli, J.D., Baird, A., Guillemin, R. & Orci, L. (1986). Basic fibroblast growth factor induces angiogenesis *in vitro*. **Proceedings of the National Academy of Sciences, USA** 83:7297–7301.

Neufeld, G., Ferrara, N., Schweigerer, L., Mitchell, R. & Gospodarowicz, D. (1987). Bovine granulosa cells produce basic fibroblast growth factor. **Endocrinology** 121:597–603.

Osthoff, K.S., Frühbeis, B., Overwien, B., Hilbig, B. & Sorg, C. (1987). Purification and characterization of a novel human angiogenic factor (h-AF). **Biochemical and Biophysical Research Communications** 146:945–952.

Rone, J.D., Kanayama, M. & Goodman, A.L. (1988). Rat luteal angiogenic factor: preliminary characterization. **70th Annual Meeting of the Endocrine Society** No. 1122.

Schweigerer, L., Neufeld, G., Friedman, J., Abraham, J.A., Fiddes, J.C. & Gospodarowicz, D. (1987). Capillary endothelial cells express basic fibroblast growth factor, a mitogen that promotes their own growth. **Nature** 325:257–259.

Shimasaki, S., Emoto, N., Koba, A., Mercado, M., Shibata, F., Cooksey, K., Baird, A. & Ling, N. (1988). Complementary DNA cloning and sequencing of rat ovarian basic fibroblast growth factor and tissue distribution study of its mRNA. **Biochemical and Biophysical Research Communications** 157:256–262.

Sholley, M.M., Ferguson, G.P., Seibel, H.R., Montour, J.L. & Wilson, J.D. (1984). Mechanisms of neovascularization: vascular sprouting can occur without proliferation of endothelial cells. **Laboratory Investigation** 51:624–634.

Speir, E., Yi-Fu, Z., Lee, M., Shrivastav, S. & Casscells, W. (1988). Fibroblast growth factors are present in adult cardiac myocytes, *in vivo*. **Biochemical and Biophysical Research Communications** 157:1226–1340.

Taira, M., Yoshida, T., Miyagawa, K., Sakamoto, H., Terada, M. & Sugimura, T. (1987). cDNA sequence of human transforming gene *hst* and identification of the coding sequence required for transforming activity. **Proceedings of the National Academy of Sciences, USA** 84:2980–2984.

Wilkinson, D.G., Peters, G., Dickson, C. & McMahon, A.P. (1988). Expression of the FGF-related proto-oncogene *int-2* during gastrulation and neurulation in the mouse. **EMBO Journal** 7:691–695.

Zhan, X., Bates, B., Hu, X. & Goldfarb, M. (1988). The human *FGF-5* oncogene encodes a novel protein related to fibroblast growth factors. **Molecular and Cellular Biology** 8:3487–3495.

V Lymphokines and the endocrine system

The role of interleukin-1 in reproduction

M.L. POLAN, E.G. SCHNEIDER, A.W. WALSH, J.A. LOUKIDES, S. CARDING, M.P. DIAMOND AND K. BOTTOMLY

Department of Obstetrics and Gynecology, Section of Reproductive Endocrinology, Yale University School of Medicine, New Haven, CT 06510-8063, USA.

Keywords

Interleukin-1, estradiol, progesterone, peripheral monocytes, menstrual cycle, pregnancy, embryonic development.

Introduction

An interaction between the endocrine and immunologic systems has been assumed, but specific mechanisms have been difficult to document experimentally. However, recent evidence linking gonadal steroids with the production of the immune secretory product interleukin-1 (IL-1) has suggested a new, experimentally accessible interface between endocrinologic and immunologic phenomena. IL-1, a 17-kDa polypeptide produced by peripheral monocytes and tissue macrophages, is known to mediate a wide variety of inflammatory responses (Dinarello, 1984; Durum *et al.*, 1985). Important among these responses are the synthesis of collagenase and prostaglandin E_2 (PGE_2) (Mizel *et al.*, 1981), osteoclastic bone resorption (Gowen and Mundy, 1986), proliferation of lymphocytes, and the stimulation of other cytokines such as interleukin-2 (IL-2) (Stosic-Grujicic and Simic, 1982) and interleukin-6 (IL-6) previously termed INF-β2 (Wong and Clark, 1988). IL-1α (pI 5.0) and IL-1β (pI 7.0) bind to the same receptors and have the same spectrum of biologic activity (Hazuda *et al.*, 1988). Secretion of IL-1α predominates in human keratinocytes and mouse cell lines (Kupper *et al.*, 1986), while activated human macrophages secrete IL-1β and IL-1α in a ratio of 10 to 1 (March *et al.*, 1985). The human genes for both the α and β forms have been cloned (Auron *et al.*, 1984; March *et al.*, 1985) and cDNA probes are available for studies of levels of corresponding mRNAs.

Several lines of evidence suggest a direct interaction between gonadal steroids and IL-1. Early reports indicate that both estradiol (E_2) and progesterone stimulate macrophage phagocytosis and proliferation (Vernon-Roberts, 1969; Gotzos *et al.*, 1981). In 1984, Flynn showed that in-vitro production of IL-1 by monocytes derived from human placenta is modulated by physiologic amounts of both E_2 and progesterone. Dose–response curves demonstrated a stimulation of the production of IL-1 at low levels of both estrogen and progesterone, with suppression at higher concentrations of steroids. Recently, we have found a similar relationship between these gonadal steroids and secretion of aggregate bioactive IL-1 by cultured human peripheral monocytes (Polan *et al.*, 1988).

The bioactivity of IL-1 associated with peripheral monocytes as a function of the concentrations of estradiol and progesterone

IL-1 bioactivity in response to both E_2 and progesterone was measured in unstimulated peripheral monocytes from healthy male volunteers (Polan *et al.*, 1988). Macrophages were isolated by Ficoll centrifugation and adherence to tissue culture plates. After addition of E_2 and progesterone, cells were incubated for 48 hours and the conditioned medium was then dialyzed to remove steroids prior to measurement of secreted IL-1 bioactivity.

IL-1 bioactivity was measured in the thymocyte-proliferation assay using D10.G4.1 (D10), a murine helper T-cell clone. D10 cells are employed as responder cells, with either concanavalin A (Con A) or the clonotype-specific monoclonal antibody 3D3 as a co-stimulus, for the measurement of IL-1 activity via incorporation of [^{3}H]-thymidine, as described by Kaye and Janeway (1984). In all experiments, D10 cells were co-stimulated with 3D3 to initiate cell division (Polan *et al.*, 1988).

A dose–response curve for human monocyte IL-1 bioactivity as a function of the concentration of progesterone, after 48 hours of culture, was generated via incorporation of [^{3}H]-thymidine by D10 cells, as shown in Figure 1. Progesterone (10^{-9} mol/l) significantly ($p<0.05$ by the Newman–Keuls test) stimulated IL-1 activity above control levels without added steroid. Maximal stimulation of IL-1 activity was achieved with concentrations of progesterone ranging from 10^{-8} mol/l to 10^{-9} mol/l. There was a significant reduction in IL-1 activity at concentrations of progesterone above 10^{-7} mol/l ($p<0.05$).

Figure 2 shows a similar dose–response curve for IL-1 activity as a function of the concentration of E_2. A significant inhibition of IL-1 activity was observed at a concentration of E_2 of 10^{-7} mol/l ($p<0.05$). Thus, we have shown that IL-1 bioactivity associated with human peripheral monocytes is modulated by physiologic levels of gonadal steroids.

Levels of IL-1β mRNA as a function of the concentration of estradiol and progesterone

The initial studies described above document the secretion of IL-1 protein *in vitro* in response to various concentrations of gonadal steroids and suggest that these dose–response effects may have major clinical ramifications. We have investigated the molecular basis of this effect by examining levels of mRNA in peripheral human monocytes using an 800-base-pair cDNA probe for human IL-1β, which was generously provided by Dr Peter K.W. Harris of the Upjohn Company, Kalamazoo, MI.

Levels of IL-1β mRNA as a function of levels of gonadal steroids were examined. Human peripheral monocytes were isolated from healthy, normally cycling females by density-gradient centrifugation at 4°C using Sepracell-MN (Sepratech Corp., Oklahoma City, OK) to obtain a purified

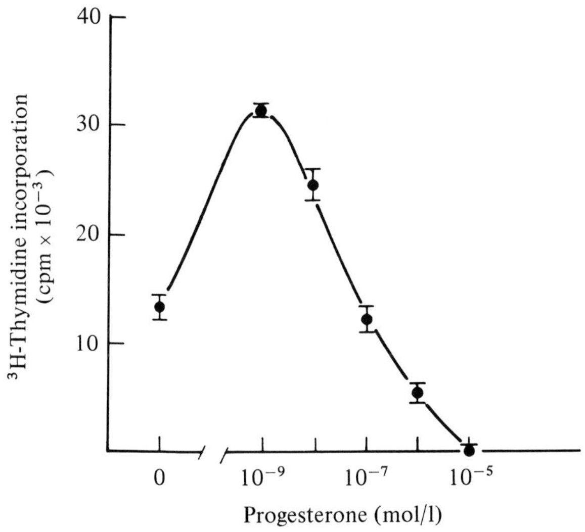

Fig. 1 Activity of IL-1 (±S.E.M.) from human peripheral monocytes incubated for 48 hours with increasing concentrations of added progesterone (0–10^{-5} mol/l). Levels of IL-1 were assayed by D10 thymocyte incorporation of [^{3}H]-thymidine (n = 3) (see text). Progesterone (10^{-9} mol/l) significantly ($p < 0.05$) stimulated production of IL-1 above control levels obtained without added steroid. Concentrations of progesterone $> 10^{-7}$ mol/l significantly inhibited production of IL-1 compared to lower concentrations (10^{-8}–10^{-9} mol/l) ($p < 0.01$, Newman–Keuls test).

population of monocytes (>85% monocytes). Cells were stimulated to produce IL-1 by treatment with lipopolysaccharide (LPS, 10 μg/ml), cultured for 6–8 hours, then centrifuged and washed. Total cellular RNA was isolated as described elsewhere (Chomczynski and Sacchi, 1987). Aliquots of 1–5 μg of RNA were denatured in glyoxal (Maniatis *et al.*, 1982), subjected to electrophoresis in a 1.3% agarose gel and subsequently transferred to a nylon filter (Zetabind Cuno Inc., Meriden, CT). Filters were then hybridized with ^{32}P-labeled cDNA, which had been synthesized using a random-primed DNA-Labelling Kit (Boehringer Mannheim, Mannheim, W. Germany).

A time course for production of IL-1β mRNA by peripheral monocytes stimulated with LPS is shown in Figure 3. Maximal amounts of the mRNA are present at 3–8 hours, with a significant decrease evident at 19 hours.

Northern blot analysis of dose–response curves for both progesterone (0–10^{-5} mol/l) and estradiol (0–10^{-5} mol/l) is shown in Figures 4 and 5. Autoradiographs were scanned on a Joyce-Loebl Chromoscan 3 densitometer (Malden, MA) and the amount of IL-1β mRNA as a fraction of the total RNA loaded on the gel was calculated and plotted against concentrations of

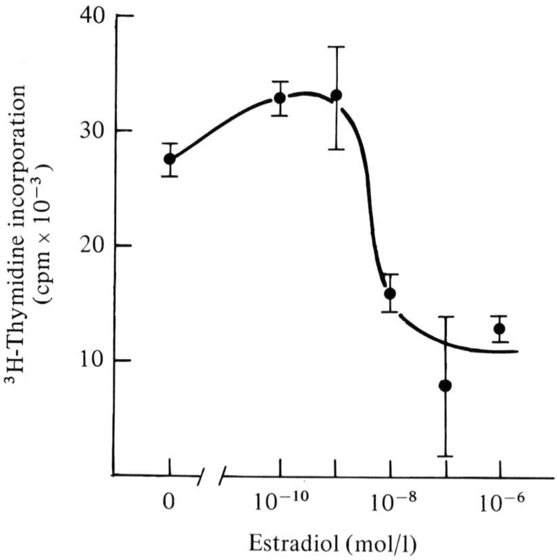

Fig. 2 Activity of IL-1 (±S.E.M.) from human peripheral monocytes incubated for 48 hours with increasing concentrations of added E_2 (0–10^{-6} mol/l). Levels of IL-1 were assayed by D10 thymocyte incorporation of [^{3}H]-thymidine (n = 3) (see text). E_2 at a concentration of 10^{-7} mol/l significantly inhibited production of IL-1 compared to lower concentrations (10^{-9}–10^{-10} mol/l) ($p < 0.05$, Newman–Keuls test).

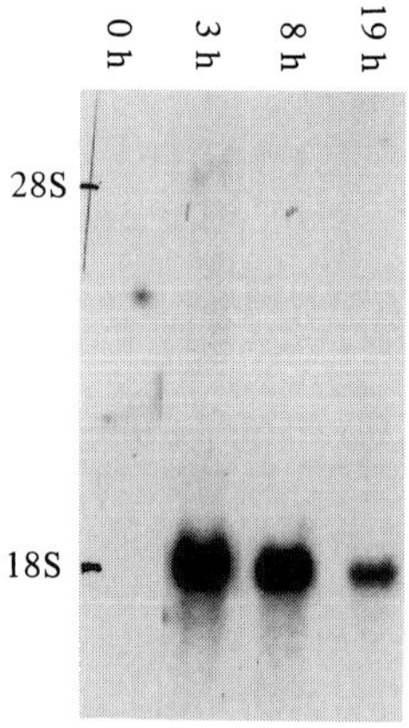

Fig. 3 Northern blot analysis of levels of human IL-1β mRNA in peripheral monocytes cultured with lipopolysaccharide for 0 to 19 hours.

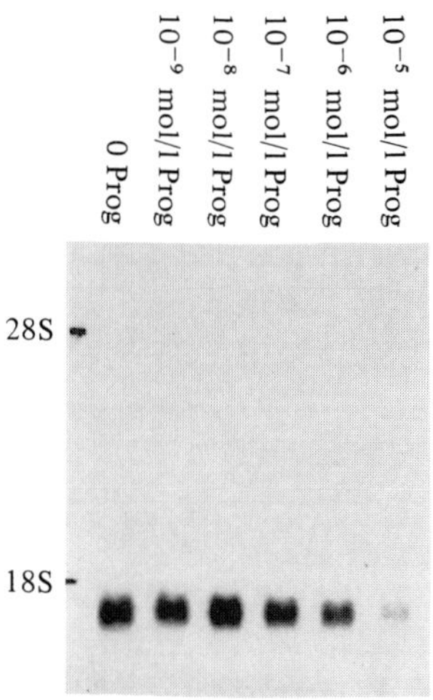

Fig. 4 Northern blot analysis of levels of IL-1β mRNA in human peripheral monocytes cultured for 7 hours with increasing concentrations of progesterone (0–10^{-5} mol/l).

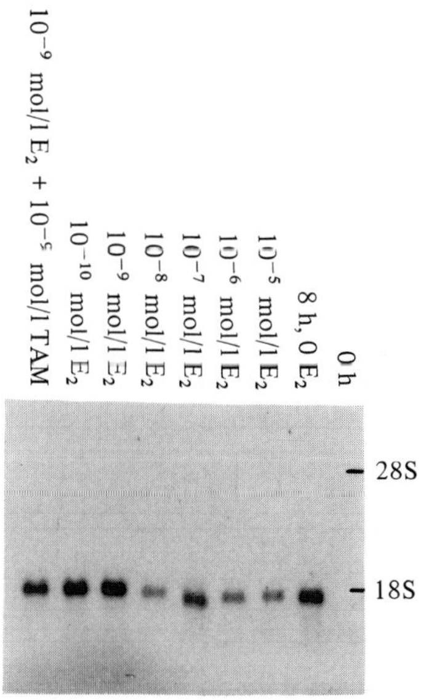

Fig. 5 Northern blot analysis of levels of IL-1β mRNA in human peripheral monocytes cultured for 7 hours with increasing concentrations of estradiol (0–10^{-5} mol/l). (TAM = tamoxifen.)

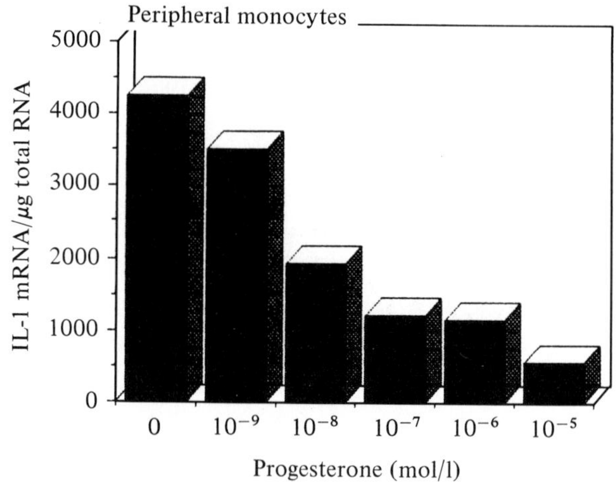

Fig. 6 Quantitative dose–response curve of levels of human IL-1β mRNA in cultured lipopolysaccharide-stimulated monoctyes, as a function of increasing concentrations of progesterone.

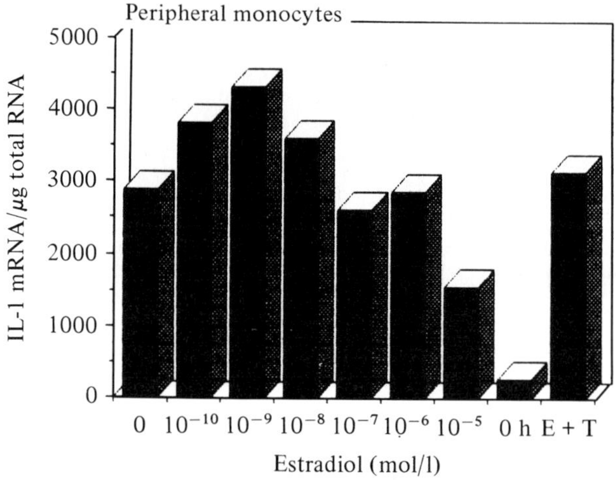

Fig. 7 Quantitative dose–response curve of levels of human IL-1β mRNA in cultured lipopolysaccharide-stimulated monocytes, as a function of increasing concentrations of estradiol. (T = tamoxifen.)

progesterone (Fig. 6) and E_2 (Fig. 7). In both cases, low concentrations of steroid (10^{-10}–10^{-9} mol/l) were associated with elevated levels of IL-1β mRNA and higher concentrations of steroid ($>10^{-7}$ mol/l) with decreased levels of IL-1β mRNA. Subsequent experiments using peritoneal macrophages isolated at the time of diagnostic laparoscopy (Fig. 8) also demonstrated an inverse relationship between levels of progesterone and IL-1β mRNA.

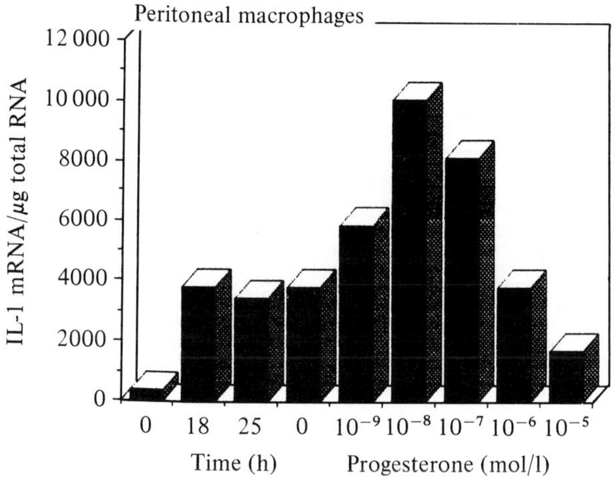

Fig. 8 Dose–response curve of levels of human IL-1β mRNA in lipopolysaccharide-stimulated human peritoneal macrophages cultured for 18 hours in the presence of increasing levels of progesterone.

Neither IL-1 nor IL-2 or any other product of activated human macrophages is toxic to early embryonic development in the mouse

Four-cell mouse embryos were harvested from oviducts of pregnant mare's serum gronadotropin (PMSG)-stimulated $B_6C_3F_1$/J female mice. Embryos were cultured with several preparations of purified IL-1 and IL-2 (Schneider *et al.*, submitted). As shown in Table 1 and Table 2, neither human recombinant IL-1α and IL-1β nor human or mouse recombinant IL-2 had any effect on mouse embryonic development to the blastocyst stage.

Although neither IL-1 nor IL-2 alone appeared toxic to mouse embryos, the possibility remained that the two interleukins together might have an effect on embryogenesis. Therefore, four-cell mouse embryos were incubated with preparations of both IL-1 and IL-2 at several different concentrations. None of the combinations of interleukins tested had any appreciable effect on embryogenesis.

However, these formulations were all recombinant preparations from *E. coli* and, therefore, the interleukins had not been subjected to any post-translational modifications which might have an effect on bioactivity. In addition, macrophages make products other than IL-1 which may play a role in embryo toxicity. To address these questions, human macrophages from peritoneal fluid were isolated, activated with LPS, and co-cultured with four-cell mouse embryos for 3–4 days. The results from five experiments with macrophages from five different patients (three control, and two with endometriosis) are summarized in Table 3 and show no appreciable effect of secretory products of peritoneal macrophages on mouse embryogenesis from

Table 1. *Effect of purified interleukin-1 on the development of mouse embryos*[a,b]

IL-1 preparation (U/ml)	Blastocysts (%) Control	Treated
hrIL-1α (Collaborative Research, Bedford, MA)		
1000	98 (54)	92 (37)
10000	93 (45)	92 (37)
hrIL-1β (Collaborative Research, Bedford, MA)		
100	91 (11)	92 (12)
1000	98 (41)	91 (22)
6000	94 (33)	94 (32)
10000	100 (20)	100 (10)
mrIL-1α (Hoffmann–La Roche, Nutley, NJ)		
100	91 (54)	86 (29)
1000	97 (34)	95 (19)
3000	83 (24)	100 (14)
30000	0 (10)	100 (10)
hrIL-1β (Genzyme, Boston, MA)		
100	93 (91)	88 (80)

[a]Purified recombinant IL-1 from several different sources was added to four-cell mouse embryos in Ham's F-10 that contained 1% BSA. The interleukin activity shown is the activity actually measured by the DlO bioassay. Numbers in parentheses refer to numbers of embryos in the experiments. mr, mouse recombinant; hr, human recombinant.
[b]Adapted and reprinted with permission from Schneider *et al.* (1989). **Biology of Reproduction** 40:825–834.

the four-cell to the blastocyst stage. Figure 9 shows representative samples of control mouse embryos and embryos co-cultured with the peritoneal macrophages from a patient with moderate endometriosis.

These experiments show that high concentrations of IL-1, IL-2 or secretory products from human macrophages do not interfere with the early stages of embryogenesis in the mouse. However, any effects on later stages of implantation and development remain to be analyzed.

IL-1 bioactivity as a function of gonadal steroids during the menstrual cycle and pregnancy

These studies were undertaken to explore the inverse relationship between secretion of IL-1 and gonadal steroids in young women during the menstrual

Table 2. *Effect of purified interleukin-2 on the development of mouse embryos*[a,b]

IL-2 preparation (U/ml)	Blastocysts	Control
hr1L-2 (AMGen, Thousand Oaks, CA)		
100	100 (37)	100 (10)
1000	97 (67)	95 (37)
10000	94 (56)	94 (37)
hr1L-2 (E.I. DuPont, Glenolden Labs, PA)		
100	91 (11)	92 (12)
1000	95 (62)	95 (41)
hrIL-2 (Collaborative Research, Bedford, MA)		
340	98 (40)	100 (18)

[a]Purified culture-derived or recombinant IL-2 from several different sources was added to four-cell mouse embryos in Ham's F-10 that contained 1% BSA. The interleukin activity shown is the activity actually measured by the bioassay. Numbers in parentheses refer to numbers of embryos in the experiments.
[b]Adapted and reprinted with permission from Schneider *et al.* (1989). **Biology of Reproduction** 40:825–834.

Table 3. *Table 3. Co-culture of mouse embryos with human pelvic macrophages*[a,b]

	IL-1 (U/ml)		Blastocysts (%)	
Patient Control	day 1	day 3	day 1	day 3
1 Control	7–9	n.d.[c]	100 (12)	100 (4)
2 Control	23–42	4–13	96 (28)	96 (15)
3 Control	15–20	1–2	86 (30)	70 (10)
4 Mild endometriosis	30–60	15–30	98 (56)	71 (7)
5 Moderate endometriosis	3420–8650	50–70	85 (55)	60 (5)

[a]Human pelvic macrophages were purified and co-cultured with four-cell mouse embryos for 3–4 days in Ham's F-10. Culture supernatants were changed daily, and IL-1 in these supernatants was measured by the D10 bioassay. Numbers in parentheses refer to numbers of embryos in the experiments.
[b]Reprinted with permission from Schneider *et al.* (1989). **Biology of Reproduction** 40:825–834.
[c]n.d., not determined.

cycle and pregnancy. We have examined the effect of physiologic levels of gonadal steroids on secretion of IL-1 by peripheral monocytes which were isolated before ovulation and during late luteal phase from women with human menopausal gonadotropin/human chorionic gonadotropin-stimulated cycles as well as during the mid-trimester and third trimester of pregnancy.

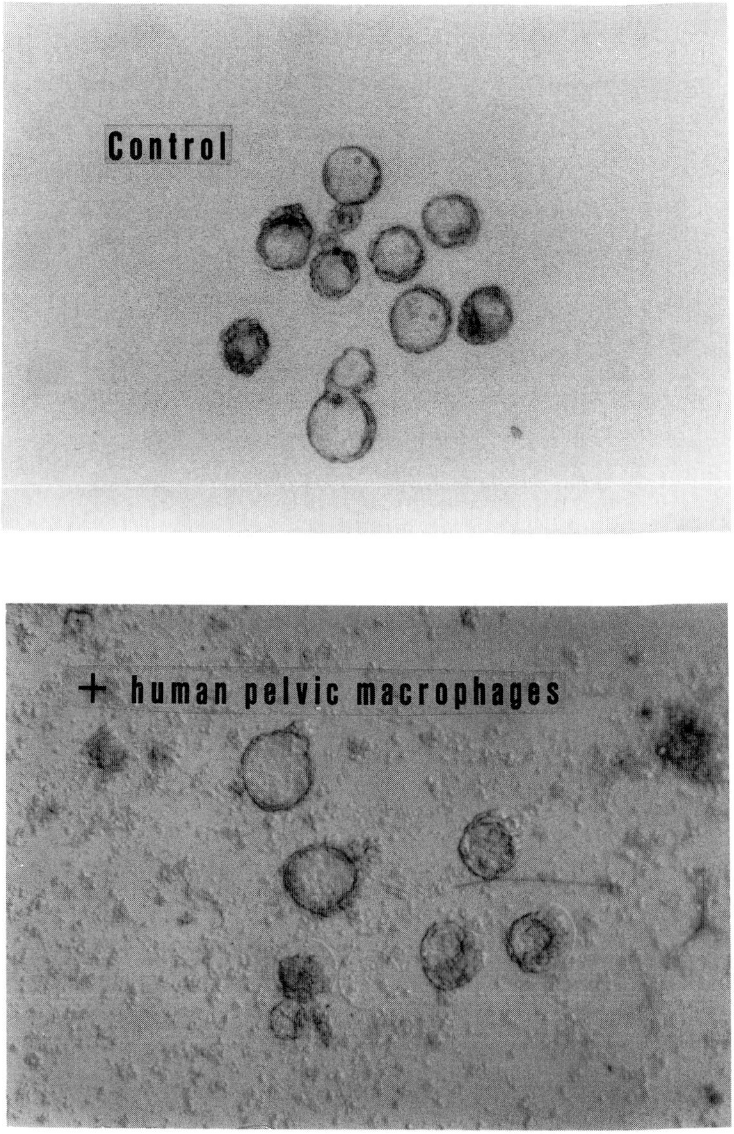

(a)

(b)

Fig. 9 Representative samples of control mouse embryos (a) and embryos co-cultured with peritoneal macrophages from a patient (no. 5 in Table 3) with moderate endometriosis (b). Reprinted with permission, from Schneider *et al.* (1989). **Biology of Reproduction** 40:825–834.

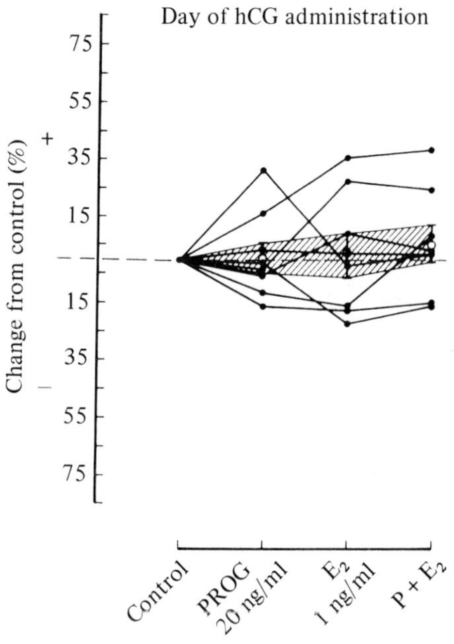

Fig. 10 Production of IL-1 by preovulatory peripheral monocytes, cultured in triplicate, 12 hours before administration of hCG with progesterone (20 ng/ml), estradiol (1 ng/ml) and both estradiol and progesterone, compared to production of IL-1 by control cultures. Data are expressed as percentage change in incorporation of [^{3}H]-thymidine compared to control cultures; shading represents the mean ± S.E.M. of values for the eight women.

We measured the production of IL-1 by cultures of preovulatory (n = 8) and late luteal phase (n = 8) peripheral monocytes incubated in the absence of exogenous steroids or in the presence of physiologic levels of progesterone and/or E_2. As shown in Figures 10 and 11, there was no consistent effect of gonadal steroids (Polan *et al.*, submitted).

Peripheral monocytes isolated from six women during the mid-trimester of pregnancy were cultured with physiologic levels of circulating E_2 (8 ng/ml), progesterone (60 ng/ml), or a combination of both steroids. Progesterone decreased production of IL-1 in cells from 4/6 women and a combination of both steroids decreased production of IL-1 in cells from 5/6 women. Results, expressed as the percent change from incorporation by control cultures and shown in Figure 12, revealed that levels of production of IL-1 in the presence of E_2 and in the presence of progesterone plus E_2 were lower than control levels (mean ± S.E.M. of −28.4 ± 20.6% and −33.5 ± 18.1%, respectively). Production of IL-1 by cells cultured in the presence of progesterone alone was

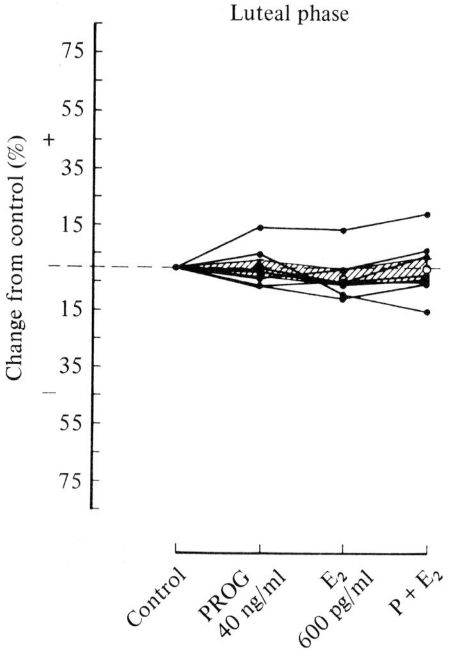

Fig. 11 Production of IL-1 by late-luteal peripheral monocytes, cultured in triplicate, 12 days after administration of hCG with progesterone (40 ng/ml), estradiol (600 pg/ml) and both estradiol and progesterone, compared to production of IL-1 by control cultures. Data are expressed as percentage change in incorporation of [^{3}H]-thymidine compared to control cultures; shading represents the mean ± S.E.M. of values for the eight women.

significantly ($p < 0.05$, Wilcoxon signed rank test) lower than that in control cells (mean ± S.E.M. of −25.5 ± 11.8%).

Peripheral monocytes isolated from the same six women during the third trimester of pregnancy were also cultured with physiologic concentrations of E_2 (12 ng/ml), progesterone (120 ng/ml) and a combination of both steroids. As seen in Figure 13, neither E_2, progesterone, nor a combination of the two steroids significantly altered the production of IL-1, as compared to control levels (mean ± S.E.M. of 2.3 ± 3.7%, 0.4 ± 4.1% and −5.5 ± 6.7%, respectively). Basal body temperatures were measured by four of the women for a week during the third trimester of pregnancy and, on all except one day, oral temperatures were ⩽98.0°F (37°C).

This study has provided the first demonstration that peripheral monocytes isolated during the mid-trimester of pregnancy respond to high but physiologic levels of gonadal steroids with an inhibition of secretion of IL-1.

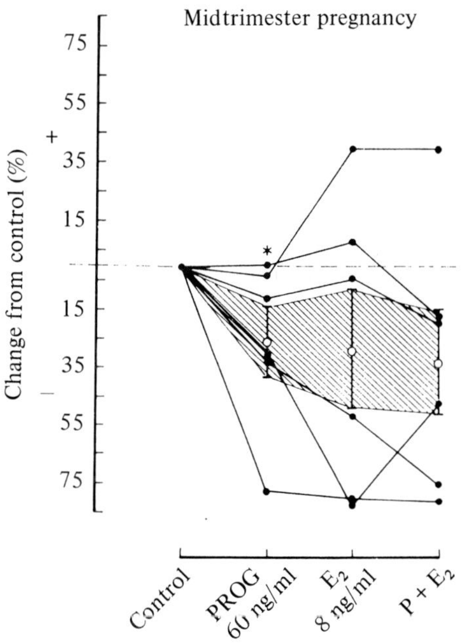

Fig. 12 Production of IL-1 by peripheral monocytes isolated from six women during the mid-trimester of pregnancy, cultured in triplicate with progesterone (60 ng/ml), estradiol (8 ng/ml) and both estradiol and progesterone, compared to production of IL-1 by control cultures. Data are expressed as percentage change in incorporation of [^{3}H]-thymidine compared to control cultures; shading represents the mean $\pm$S.E.M. of values for the six women. *Significant decrease in production of IL-1 in the presence of progesterone, 60 ng/ml. ($p < 0.05$ by Wilcoxon signed rank test.)

Preovulatory, late luteal phase, and third trimester monocytes do not. The absence of a response by preovulatory and late luteal phase monocytes is most probably due to low concentrations of gonadal steroids, which are insufficient to induce the inhibitory response. The absence of an effect during the third trimester of pregnancy is certainly not due to a paucity of steroids, but may result from the desensitization of the response in the face of repetitive stimulation (Gahring *et al.*, 1984).

Gahring and Daynes (1986) have described several mechanisms that are responsible for the eventual inability of animals to respond after chronic exposure to agents that stimulate production of IL-1. Such a desensitization phenomenon may occur in humans and may account for the inability of steroids to modulate the secretion of IL-1 during the third trimester of pregnancy. This hypothesis is strengthened by our observation that the

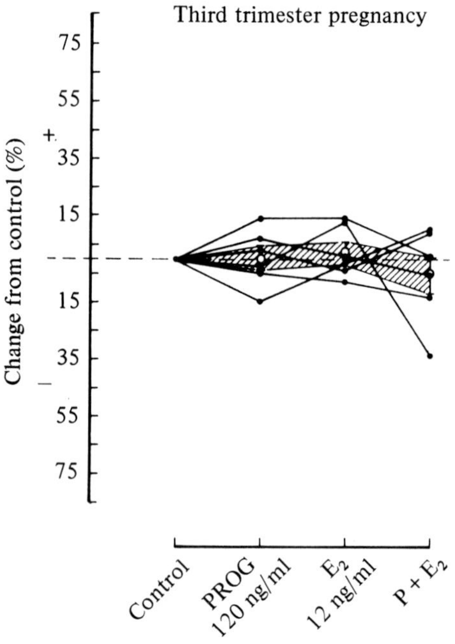

Fig. 13 Production of IL-1 by peripheral monocytes isolated from six women during the third trimester of pregnancy, cultured in triplicate with progesterone (120 ng/ml), estradiol (12 ng/ml), and both estradiol and progesterone, compared to production of IL-1 by control cultures. Data are expressed as percentage change in incorporation of [^{3}H]-thymidine compared to control cultures; shading represents the mean ± S.E.M. of values for the six women.

progesterone-induced elevation in basal body temperature during the luteal phase is absent during the third trimester of pregnancy. Since IL-1 is intimately related to the temperature response (Cannon and Dinarello, 1985), it may well be that regulatory mechanisms that control the secretion of monokines and/or the response of target organs are affected by prolonged exposure to steroids, with a resultant desensitization. Further studies are needed to determine the timing of the onset of modulation by steroids and the physiologic sequelae and reproductive impact of decreased secretion of IL-1 during pregnancy.

Discussion

IL-1 was initially thought to be identical to endogenous pyrogen (Duff and Durum, 1983), a postulate consistent with the observations of Cannon and Dinarello (1985), who documented a coordinated luteal elevation of both IL-1 and temperature. More recent evidence suggests that IL-1 may influence temperature indirectly by stimulating production of IL-6, and that IL-6 is the actual thermogenic factor (Nijsten *et al.*, 1987; Wong and Clark, 1988). However, monokines are clearly involved in the luteal increase in temperature, and the fact that exogenous progesterone can evoke an elevation of body temperature, in a manner similar to the postovulatory rise (Buxton and Atkinson, 1948), supports the hypothesis that gonadal steroids modulate the production of monokines.

We have shown that the bioactivity of IL-1 of peripheral monocytes is modulated by physiologic levels of E_2 and progesterone. More recent experiments using a cDNA probe for IL-β have confirmed that equivalent concentrations of these steroids modulate levels of IL-1β mRNA in peripheral monocytes (both E_2 and progesterone) and in pelvic macrophages (progesterone). In all cases, the relationship is an inverse one, with production of IL-1 being stimulated at low concentrations of steroids and decreasing as levels of steroids rise.

This inverse relationship has major ramifications for reproductive events. Although high concentrations of IL-1 and IL-2 do not appear to affect early embryonic development up to the blastocyst stage, subsequent peri-implantational and developmental stages may well be affected by fluctuations in levels of monokines. We have shown that the bioactivity of IL-1 is decreased in peripheral monocytes isolated from women during the mid-trimester of pregnancy. Decreased levels of IL-1 resulting from this interaction between the immune and endocrine systems may be important in protecting the fetus from attack by the maternal immune system. This modulation may be critical to the immunologic processes that allow embryonic implantation and survival in the fetus, since IL-1 stimulates the production of IL-2 (Stosic-Grujicic and Simic, 1982) which is necessary for the cytotoxic effect of T-cells (Domingo *et al.*, 1983). Several studies have demonstrated that pregnancy-associated steroids decrease the cytotoxicity of lymphocytes (Fizet *et al.*, 1983; Domingo *et al.*, 1985), and Domingo *et al.* (1985) showed that this decreased cytotoxicity is due to reduced production of IL-2. Decreased synthesis of IL-1 during pregnancy may result in an inhibition of both production of IL-1 and lymphocyte cytotoxicity, thus favoring embryonic implantation and fetal survival.

The second major clinical implication of this inverse relationship between levels of gonadal steroids and production of monokines involves the role of monokines in osteoporosis. Both IL-1 and tumor necrosis factor-α (TNF-α) have been shown to increase osteoclastic activity and bone turnover. Levels in peritoneal fluid of IL-1 are elevated in women with endometriosis (Fakih *et al.*, 1987), and cultures of peripheral monocytes and peritoneal macrophages have demonstrated significantly elevated production of IL-1 by monocytes from women with endometriosis (Parvizi *et al.*, 1988). The recent finding of concomitantly decreased bone mass in women with endometriosis (Comite *et al.*, 1987) raises the question of whether this bone loss may lead to the earlier development of symptomatic osteoporosis after menopause. More importantly, endometriosis is not the only clinical situation in which decreased bone density is associated with elevated production of IL-1. Recent evidence documents elevated rates of secretion of IL-1 by peripheral monocytes from patients with high-turnover idiopathic osteoporosis (Pacifici *et al.*, 1987). Peripheral monocytes from a subset of osteoporotic, menopausal women demonstrated significantly elevated rates of secretion of IL-1 which declined into the normal range with the administration of estrogen and progestin replacement therapy (Pacifici *et al.*, 1988).

Postmenopausal osteoporosis is a major public-health problem in the USA, accounting for more than 125 000 hip fractures annually, with their attendant morbidity and 20% mortality (Lane *et al.*, 1983). Although estrogen replacement therapy has been shown to prevent osteoporotic fractures (Weiss *et al.*, 1980), only recently has a direct receptor-mediated effect of estrogen been demonstrated in bone (Komm *et al.*, 1988; Eriksen *et al.*, 1988). Since we have demonstrated the ability of E_2 and progesterone to modulate both the bioactivity of IL-1 and levels of IL-1β mRNA in human peripheral monocytes, we hypothesize that this inverse relationship between the gonadal steroids and the production of monokines has important clinical ramifications in the etiology of postmenopausal osteoporosis.

This interface between the endocrine milieu and immunologic action is now amenable to experimental investigation. The spectrum of monokine-associated activities and the interrelationships involved in the induction of monokines have been revealed by use of the techniques of molecular biology. The interleukins IL-1α and IL-1β, as well as TNF-α, have been cloned and cDNA probes are available for studies of transcription and translation, using specific antibodies and bioassays. The recent demonstration that levels of immunologic monokines are modulated by E_2 and progesterone now offers us the possibility of investigating basic mechanisms of action of steroids and of elucidating significant clinical correlates of ovarian function.

Acknowledgements

We thank Joan Andrews for expert assistance in preparing the manuscript.

References

Auron, P.E., Webb, A.C., Rosenwasser, L.J., Mucci, S.F., Rich, A., Wolff, S.M. & Dinarello, C.A. (1984). Nucleotide sequence of human monocyte interleukin 1 precursor cDNA. **Proceedings of the National Academy of Sciences, USA** 81:7907.

Buxton, C.L. & Atkinson, W.B. (1948). Hormonal factors involved in the regulation of basal body temperature during the menstrual cycle and pregnancy. **Journal of Clinical Endocrinology and Metabolism** 8:544–549.

Cannon, J.G. & Dinarello, C.A. (1985). Increased plasma interleukin-1 activity in women after ovulation. **Science** 227:1247–1249.

Chomczynski, P. & Sacchi, N. (1987). Single-step method of RNA isolation by acid guanidinium thiocyanate-phenol-chloroform extraction. **Analytical Biochemistry** 162:156–159.

Comite, F., Jensen, P. & Hutchinson, K. (1987). Decreased bone mass in endometriosis. (Abstract 60) Presented at the 43rd Annual Meeting of the American Fertility Society, September 28–30.

Dinarello, C.A. (1984). Interleukin 1. **Reviews of Infectious Diseases** 6:51–95.

Domingo, C.G., Domenech, N., Aparicio, P. & Palomino, P. (1985). Human pregnancy serum inhibits proliferation of T8-depleted cells and their interleukin-2 synthesis in mixed lymphocyte cultures. **Journal of Reproductive Immunology** 8:97–110.

Duff, G.W. & Durum, S.K. (1983). The pyrogenic and mitogenic actions of interleukin-1 are related. **Nature** 304:449–451.

Durum, S.K., Schmidt, J.A. & Oppenheim, J.J. (1985). Interleukin 1: an immunological perspective. **Annual Review of Immunology** 3:263–288.

Eriksen, E.F., Colvard, D.S., Berg, N.J., Graham, M.L., Mann, K.G., Spelsberg, T.C. & Riggs, B.L. (1988). Evidence of estrogen receptors in normal human osteoblast-like cells. **Science** 241:84–86.

Fakih, M., Baggett, B., Holty, G., Tsang, K.Y., Lee, J.C. & Williamson, H.O. (1987). Interleukin-1: a possible role in the infertility associated with endometriosis. **Fertility and Sterility** 47:213–217.

Fizet, D., Bousquet, J., Piquet, Y. & Cabantous, F. (1983). Identification of a factor blocking a cellular cytotoxicity reaction in pregnant serum. **Clinical and Experimental Immunology** 52:648–654.

Flynn, A. (1984). Stimulation of interleukin-1 production from placental monocytes. **Lymphokine Research** 3:1–5.

Gahring, L., Baltz, M., Pepys, M.B. & Daynes, R. (1984). Effect of ultraviolet radiation on production of epidermal cell thymocyte-activating factor/interleukin 1 *in vivo* and *in vitro*. **Proceedings of the National Academy of Sciences, USA** 81:1198–1202.

Gahring, L.C. & Daynes, R.A. (1986). Desensitization of animals to the inflammatory effects of ultraviolet radiation is mediated through mechanisms which are distinct from those responsible for endotoxin tolerance. **Journal of Immunology** 136:2868–2873.

Gotzos, V., Cappelli-Gotzos, B. & Bovet, R. (1981). *In vitro* responses of proliferative and non-proliferative cells to high doses of 17β-estradiol: cytochemical study. **Acta Histochemica** 69:40–49.

Gowen, M. & Mundy, G.R. (1986). Actions of recombinant interleukin-1, interleukin-2 and interferon on bone resorption *in vitro*. **Journal of Immunology** 136:2478–2482.

Hazuda, D.J., Lee, J.C. & Young, P.R. (1988). The kinetics of interleukin 1 secretion from activated monocytes. **Journal of Biological Chemistry** 263:8473–8479.

Kaye, J. & Janeway, C.A. (1984). Induction of receptors for interleukin-2 requires T-cell-antigen:1a receptor crosslinking and interleukin-1. **Lymphokine Research** 3:175–181.

Komm, B.S., Terpening, C.M., Benz, D.J., Graeme, K.A., Gallegos, A., Korc, M., Greene, G.L., O'Malley, B.W. & Haussler, M.R. (1988). Estrogen binding, receptor mRNA, and biologic response in osteoblast-like osteosarcoma cells. **Science** 241:81–84.

Kupper, T.S., Ballard, D.W., Chua, A.O., McGuire, J.S., Flood, P.M., Horowitz,

M.C., Lightfoot, L. & Gubler, U. (1986). Human keratinocytes contain mRNA indistinguishable from monocyte IL-1α and β mRNA: keratinocyte 'epidermal cell derived thymocyte activating factor' (ETAF) is identical to interleukin 1. **Journal of Experimental Medicine** 164:2095–3000.

Lane, G., Whitehead, M.I. & Stevenson, J.C. (1983). How to diagnose and treat osteoporosis after menopause. **Contempory Obstetrics and Gynecology** Jan:38–53.

Maniatis, T., Fritsch, E.F. & Sambrook, J. (1982). **Molecular Cloning** Cold Spring Harbor Laboratory, p.200.

March, C.J., Mosely, B., Larsen, A., Cerretti, D.P., Braedt, G., Price, U., Gillis, S., Henney, C.S., Kronheim, S.R., Grabstein, K., Conlon, P.J., Hopp, T.P. & Cosman, D. (1985). Cloning, sequencing and expression of two distinct human interleukin complementary DNAs. **Nature** 315:641–647.

Mizel, S.B., Dayer, J.M., Krane, S.M. & Mergenhagen, S.E. (1981). Stimulation of rheumatoid synovial cell collagenase and prostaglandin production by partially purified lymphocyte-activating factor (interleukin 1). **Proceedings of the National Academy of Sciences, USA** 78:2474–2477.

Nijsten, M.W.N., Degroot, E.R., Ten Duis, H.J., Klasen, H.J., Hack, C.E. & Aarden, L.A. (1987). Serum levels of interleukin-6 and acute phase responses. **Lancet** 2:921.

Pacifici, R., Rifas, L., Teitelbaum, S., Slatopolsky, E., McCracken, R., Bergfeld, M., Lee, W., Avioli, L.V. & Peck, W.A. (1987). Spontaneous release of interleukin 1 from human blood monocytes reflects bone formation in idiopathic osteoporosis. **Proceedings of the National Academy of Sciences, USA** 84:4616–4620.

Pacifici, R., Rifas, L., Vered, I., McMurtry, C., McCracken, R., Avioli, L.V. & Peck, W.A. (1988). Interleukin-1 secretion from human blood monocytes in normal and osteoporotic women: effect of menopause and estrogen/progesterone treatment. **Journal of Bone Mineral Research** 3:S204.

Parvizi, S.T., Jensen, P., Decherney, A., Polan, M.L. & Comite, F. (1988). Elevated Interleukin-1 (IL-1) synthesis by peripheral monocytes in endometriosis. Abstract presented at the 35th Annual Meeting of the Society for Gynecologic Investigation, Baltimore, MD, March 17–20, p.284.

Polan, M.L., Daniele, A. & Kuo, A. (1988). Gonadal steroids modulate human monocyte interleukin-1 (IL-1) activity. **Fertility and Sterility** 49:964–968.

Polan, M.L., Kuo, A., Daniele, A. & Bottomly, K.. Gonadal steroids inhibit interleukin-1 (IL-1) secretion during mid-trimester pregnancy. **Journal of Clinical Endocrinology and Metabolism** (submitted).

Schneider, E.G., Armant, D.R., Kupper, T.S. & Polan, M.L. (1989). Absence of a direct effect of recombinant interleukins and cultured peritoneal macrophages on early embryonic development in the mouse. **Biology of Reproduction** 40:825–834.

Stosic-Grujicic, S. & Simic, M.M. (1982). Modulation of interleukin 1 production by activated macrophages: *in vitro* action of hydrocortisone, colchicine and cytochalasin B1. **Cellular Immunology** 69:235–247.

Vernon-Roberts, B. (1969). The effects of steroid hormones on macrophage activity. **International Review of Cytology** 25:131.

Weiss, N.S., Ure, C.L., Ballard, J.H., Williams, A.R. & Daling, J.R. (1980). Decreased risk of fractures of the hip and lower forearm with postmenopausal use of estrogen. **New England Journal of Medicine** 303:1195–1198.

Wong, G.G. & Clark, S.C. (1988) Multiple actions of interleukin 6 within a cytokine network. **Immunology Today** 9:137–139.

The role of peritoneal macrophages and their secretory products in endometriosis-associated infertility

J. HALME,[1] S. SPORN[2] AND S. HASKILL[3]

[1] *Department of Obstetrics and Gynecology, University of California at Los Angeles School of Medicine, Center for the Health Sciences, Los Angeles, CA 90024, USA;* [2] *Department of Microbiology and Immunology, University of North Carolina at Chapel Hill, USA;* [3] *Department of Obstetrics and Gynecology and Lineberger Cancer Research Center, University of North Carolina at Chapel Hill, USA.*

Keywords

Endometriosis, infertility, macrophages, monokines, growth factors, gene expression, regulatory genes, mediator genes.

Introduction

Endometriosis is a chronic, inflammatory condition in women of reproductive age which is characterized by the presence of ectopic lesions of endometrial tissue (Halme, 1985). Most commonly, lesions or implants are present in dependent areas of the peritoneal cavity. This endometrial tissue responds to fluctuations in circulating levels of estrogen and progesterone and undergoes changes that lead directly or indirectly to the symptoms of the disease, pain, and infertility.

Although an association exists between the presence of such implants and infertility, the basic pathophysiologic mechanism of reproductive failure has not been positively determined. Recently, studies of this mechanism have focused on the role of inflammatory macrophages and their secretory products (Halme *et al.*, 1983).

Macrophages in endometriosis

Ectopic endometriosis implants contain epithelial and stromal tissue that exhibits proliferative and secretory changes similar but not identical to those of the uterine endometrium. These implants also undergo menstruation *in situ*, and the sloughing off of endometrial tissue and bleeding lead to the attraction and influx of inflammatory cells, in particular monocyte macrophages, to the tissue. In fact, so-called hemosiderin-laden macrophages have long been a hallmark of the histology of endometriosis. Presumably this cyclic irritation by the implants leads to an accumulation of macrophages in the peritoneal cavity as well, and several investigators have documented an increase in the numbers of these cells in the peritoneal fluid of patients with endometriosis

Table 1. *Peritoneal macrophages in endometriosis*

Characteristics of a more mature population
acid phosphatase
myeloperoxidase
cell size
leucine-aminopeptidase
Functional properties
capping
internalization
phagocytosis of sperm

(Haney *et al.*, 1981; Halme *et al.*, 1982). Normal, regularly occurring stimuli in the human female peritoneal cavity that also attract monocytes include the ovulation-associated release of follicular contents and bleeding, retrograde menstruation, and presence of sperm after intercourse. In patients with endometriosis, the additional stimulus by the peritoneal–endometrial implants not only leads to an increase in the number of macrophages but also influences their differentiation.

Previous work from our laboratory has demonstrated that peritoneal macrophages in patients with endometriosis have the characteristics of more mature cells than macrophages from normal patients (Table 1). They exhibit higher levels of expression of acid phosphatase and, usually, lower levels of expression of myeloperoxidase (Halme *et al.*, 1984). The endometriosis-associated macrophages include a substantial subpopulation of large, mature-size macrophages and the average level of expression of leucine aminopeptidase is also increased (Halme *et al.*, 1987).

Some functional parameters of these macrophages have also been investigated. We have demonstrated that modulation of the capping and internalization functions of cell-surface antigen is active in endometriosis-associated macrophages to a much greater degree than in normal peritoneal macrophages (Halme *et al.*, 1987). There is also evidence from studies by other investigators to suggest that the rate of phagocytosis of sperm by peritoneal macrophages is increased in patients with endometriosis, and this increase has been suggested as a contributory mechanism in reproductive failure associated with endometriosis (Muscato *et al.*, 1982).

Macrophages are secretory cells and are capable of producing a wide variety of products. This secretory activity appears to be increased in patients with endometriosis. We have recently demonstrated that endometriosis-associated peritoneal macrophages often release a mitogenic competence activity *in vitro* that has many characteristics of platelet-derived growth factor (PDGF) (Halme *et al.*, 1988). In addition, Kauma *et al.* (1988) have demonstrated that

Table 2. *Peritoneal macrophages in endometriosis*

In vitro
macrophage-derived competence factor
fibronectin
In vivo
acid phosphatase
neutral protease
prostaglandins

endometriosis-associated macrophages, *in vitro*, are more likely to synthesize and release fibronectin, a high-molecular-weight protein which is important in adherence of cells to the extracellular matrix and in cell growth.

There is also a certain amount of indirect evidence for increased secretory activity by endometriosis-associated peritoneal macrophages (Table 2). We demonstrated early on in our research that there were increased levels of acid phosphatase and neutral protease activity in the peritoneal fluid of patients with endometriosis (Halme *et al.*, 1983). Variably elevated levels of prostaglandins have also been detected in the peritoneal fluid (see Syrop and Halme, 1987) and a preliminary report suggests that there are increased levels of interleukin-1 (IL-1) activity in the peritoneal fluid of these patients (Fakih *et al.*, 1987).

Expression of regulatory and monokine genes by peritoneal macrophages in patients with endometriosis

Very little is known about the molecular mechanisms that regulate the functions of human peritoneal macrophages. A great deal of the work on the molecular biology of the monocyte macrophage, in general, has focused on the regulation of expression of mRNA transcribed from proto-oncogenes and the genes for monokines, such as IL-1β and tumor necrosis factor α (TNFα) (Collart *et al.*, 1986). The expression of both lymphokines and the proto-oncogene *c-fos* is usually induced in response to inflammatory signals (Adams and Hamilton, 1984).

IL-1β and TNFα are important in the mediation of host responses to inflammation (Le and Vilcek, 1987; Table 3). They exert many common effects on cells involved in inflammation, and these effects include functional activation of lymphocytes, neutrophils, endothelial cells, and macrophages. TNFα, in addition, has pronounced cytotoxic effects on tumor cells.

Although the precise role of *c-fos* is not known, it has been shown to be one of the earliest genes expressed (Verma and Sassone-Corsi, 1987) and has been implicated as a regulatory gene. There is evidence that *c-fos* is involved in the

Table 3. *Biologic activities of IL-1β* and TNFα[a]

	IL-1β	TNFα
T-cell activation	+	+
Cytotoxicity	±	+
Pyrogenicity	+	+
Neutrophil activation	+	+
Endothelial activation	+	+
Mitogenic to fibroblasts	+	+

[a]See Le and Vilcek (1987).

attainment of competence for cell division (Greenberg and Ziff, 1984), differentiation (Muller and Wagner, 1984), and early events in signal transduction mechanisms (Verma and Sassone-Corsi, 1987).

We have examined the correlation between expression of mRNA for IL-1β, TNFα, and *c-fos* in human peritoneal macrophages and the presence or absence of the inflammatory state associated with endometriosis.

Materials and methods

We obtained fresh peritoneal macrophages from patients who were undergoing laparoscopy either for tubal ligation or evaluation of infertility. As controls, peripheral monocytes were obtained from platelet phoresis and separated by centrifugation in Percoll. Peritoneal macrophages were sedimented in Ficoll–Hypaque and part of the sample was subjected to evaluation of cell size by flow cytometry, as described earlier (Halme *et al.*, 1987). Total RNA was isolated by the guanidine isothiocyanate–caesium chloride technique (Chirgwin *et al.*, 1979), subjected to electrophoresis on 1% agarose gels, blotted by Northern transfer onto nitrocellulose, and hybridized to oligonucleotide probes for TNFα, IL-1β, and β actin (Cetus Corporation). cDNA probes for *c-fos* and HLA-DR were employed (Das *et al.*, 1983).

Results

The mean total number of peritoneal macrophages in patients who had normal pelvic anatomy was $3.4 \times 10^6 \pm 1.45$. In patients with endometriosis, the number was significantly higher, being $34.6 \times 10^6 \pm 10.3$. The proportion of large cells was approximately 10% in populations of peritoneal macrophages from normal women. By contrast, the endometriosis-associated peritoneal macrophages exhibited a distinct subpopulation of large-size macrophages which comprised an average of 43% of the total number of cells. These results are in agreement with our previous data on the distribution of sizes of human peritoneal macrophages (Halme *et al.*, 1987).

Northern blot analyses were performed to examine the levels of mRNA for IL-1β, TNFα, and HLA-DR in blood monocytes, in a pooled sample of macrophages from four normal women and in four individual samples of endometriosis-associated peritoneal macrophages. mRNAs for IL-1β and TNFα were expressed at low levels in freshly isolated blood monocytes and were expressed at high levels after activation of the cells by adherence to the plastic substratum. Normal peritoneal macrophages expressed zero or low levels of mRNA for IL-1β and TNFα. This result is indicative of a non-activated state, as is the case with fresh monocytes. However, the endometriosis-associated peritoneal macrophages expressed much higher levels of mRNA for IL-1β and TNFα in three out of four cases. The increased expression of these mRNAs may reflect the inflammatory situation present in the peritoneal cavity of patients with endometriosis.

We have previously demonstrated that levels of the major histocompatibility antigen HLA-DR on the cell surface were tenfold higher in the case of both endometriosis-associated and normal peritoneal macrophages than in the case of fresh monocytes (Halme *et al.*, 1987). This difference was also reflected in the level of HLA-DR mRNA in these cells.

Expression of *c-fos* mRNA has been associated with stage-specific differentiation in the development of cells. The pool of normal peritoneal macrophages expressed the mRNA for *c-fos* at lower levels than the pool of fresh monocytes, whereas the endometriosis-associated macrophages expressed much higher levels of *c-fos* mRNA in all four cases examined.

Previous studies have shown that levels of *c-fos* mRNA are responsive to signals that induce proliferation, and *c-fos* may exert an influence on differentiation. At present, it appears that *c-fos* is constitutively expressed in the peritoneal macrophages associated with endometriosis, perhaps as a result of chronic stimulation of these cells, which leads to a differentiated inflammatory state.

In order to put our results in perspective, we have summarized some of the features of monocyte and macrophage populations (Table 4). There appears to be a progression of maturation or development of the inflammatory response. Monocytes represent the least differentiated type of cell, while normal peritoneal macrophages represent an intermediate stage of development and manifest increased expression of HLA-DR antigen. Endometriosis-associated peritoneal macrophages represent a mature, differentiated population of inflammatory cells expressing both regulatory and mediator genes or genes for monokines. The monocytes activated by a 30-minute incubation on a plastic substratum demonstrate the turning on of inflammatory genes without an increase in the size of the cells.

Table 4. *Summary of characteristics of monocytes and macrophages*

		mRNA expression			
	Increase in cell size	HLA-DR	IL-1β	TNFα	c-fos
Fresh monocytes	− − −	+	−	+/−	+/−
Monocytes after 30-min adherence to plastic	− − −	+	+ +	+ +	+ + +
Normal peritoneal macrophages	+/−	+ + +	−	−	+/−
Endometriosis-associated peritoneal macrophages	+ +	+ + +	+ +	+ +	+ + +

Discussion

We have identified the mRNAs for TNFα and IL-1β in cells from patients with endometriosis. Expression of mRNA does not necessarily mean that the translated protein is being produced or secreted. However, preliminary studies have identified the presence of the relevant activities in the peritoneal fluid of patients with endometriosis, suggesting that local secretion of these mediators could be responsible for the subfertility associated with endometriosis (Fakih *et al.*, 1987).

Indeed, direct experiments have documented that purified or recombinant IL-1β, TNFα, and other products of macrophages can have effects on reproductive processes. Conversely, endometriosis-associated peritoneal fluid has been found to inhibit several of the steps involved in reproductive function (Table 5).

One of the suggested mechanisms whereby cytokines or secretory products of endometriosis-associated, peritoneal inflammatory cells might affect fecundity involves an adverse effect on sperm motility. Oak *et al.* (1985) observed a significant reduction in the percentage of motile sperm when normal sperm were incubated with peritoneal fluid from patients with endometriosis, as compared with sperm incubated in fluid obtained from fertile women. The reduction in motility was positively correlated with the volume of peritoneal fluid *in vivo*. In similar experiments, using purified lymphokines and monokines, Hill *et al.* (1987a) detected significant effects on motility when sperm were incubated with relatively high concentrations of recombinant TNFα, or of lymphokine or interferon gamma (Hill *et al.*, 1987). IL-1β did not exert an antimotility effect in their experiments.

Several studies have addressed the question of whether peritoneal fluid or secretory products from leukocytes of patients with endometriosis can interfere with the interaction between the gametes. Chacho *et al.* (1986) incubated normal human sperm with zona-free hamster eggs in the presence of medium conditioned with peritoneal macrophages taken from patients with

Table 5. *Aspects of the reproductive process that were adversely affected by lymphokines and by peritoneal fluid from women with endometriosis*

Motility of sperm
Penetration of sperm
Capture of ovum
Early development of conceptus
Implantation

and without endometriosis. They noted a significant reduction in the percentage of successful penetrations and in the penetration index in both groups. They further demonstrated dose dependency and the heat stability of the active factor and found that it was released both from heat-killed and from viable macrophages (Chacho *et al.*, 1987). Sueldo *et al.* (1987) studied the effect of peritoneal fluid from patients with endometriosis on the interaction of murine gametes *in vitro*. Fertilization of mouse ova was adversely affected to a significantly higher degree in the presence of peritoneal fluid from patients with endometriosis than in the presence of peritoneal fluid from control patients. The factor involved appeared to be filterable and heat labile. These studies support the hypothesis that products secreted by macrophages are capable of adversely affecting the interaction between gametes.

A third suggested mechanism whereby factors in peritoneal fluid might adversely influence reproduction comes from studies by Suginami *et al.* (1986). They incubated oviductal fimbriae from golden hamsters with peritoneal fluid from human patients and determined the ability of the fimbriae to capture mouse oocytes–cumulus complexes. They detected a factor that inhibited fimbrial ability to capture ova in peritoneal fluid from patients with endometriosis but not in peritoneal fluid from other patients. This ovum-capture inhibitor was soluble in water and, on the basis of gel filtration, had an apparent molecular weight of greater than 100 kDa.

Two lines of indirect evidence exist to support the idea that factors secreted by macrophages may exert an adverse effect on fecundity by affecting the early development of the conceptus. Morcos *et al.* (1985) studied the effect of peritoneal fluid on the cleavage of two-cell mouse embryos *in vitro*. They found that heat-inactivated peritoneal fluid from patients with endometriosis was more toxic to mouse embryos than a similar concentration of peritoneal fluid from patients without endometriosis. Fakih *et al.* (1987) detected IL-1β activity in peritoneal fluid and macrophage-conditioned medium derived from seven patients with mild endometriosis, while no activity was similarly associated with fluid and cells from seven fertile patients. They demonstrated that recombinant IL-1 adversely affected the growth of mouse embryos *in vitro*. Hill *et al.* (1987b) demonstrated that IL-2 (B-cell growth factor) and interferon gamma, the two lymphokines, significantly arrested mouse embryonic development over a wide range of concentrations (Hahn *et al.*, 1986). The monokines, IL-1 and TNF, only exerted an effect at very high concentrations. These results indicate that products of activated lymphocytes and macrophages can have detrimental effects on preimplantation embryos. Hahn *et al.* (1986) found that the rate of implantation was significantly reduced in rabbits with surgically induced endometriosis. In addition, when they injected peritoneal fluid from animals with endometriosis into control animals prior to artificial insemination, a significant reduction in the number of normal fetuses was observed. These studies suggest that, at least in rabbits that have endometriosis and also perhaps in the human, the disease may be associated with a factor in the peritoneal fluid that either prevents implantation or induces early spontaneous abortions.

In summary, several lines of evidence exist to suggest the abnormal maturation or activation of peritoneal macrophages in patients with mild endometriosis. Both direct and indirect support has been accumulating for the hypothesis that secretory products of these cells may then play an important role in the development of subfertility in endometriosis by a variety of mechanisms, including adverse affects on gamete survival, the interaction of gametes, and early embryonic development.

The possibility of a regulatory mechanism that exists to prevent development of an inflammatory response and the resulting negative effects in the normal peritoneal cavity should be considered. The recent work of Polan *et al.* (1988) adds the interesting aspect of hormonal regulation of macrophage secretory activity.

Since high concentrations of sex steroids appear to have a suppressive effect on the release of monokines, they may be involved in the natural prevention of the development of an inflammatory response. All these investigations form a basis on which future studies will most certainly be able to build as we attempt to define still further the role of inflammatory cells and their secretory products in endometriosis. They also provide a potential for future intervention to improve fertility by use of products such as specific inhibitors of the differentiation of macrophages or inhibitors of their secretory products.

References

Adams, D.O. & Hamilton, T.A. (1984). The cell biology of macrophage activation. **Annual Review of Immunology** 2:283–318.

Chacho, K.J., Andresen, P.J. & Scommegna, A. (1987). The effect of peritoneal macrophage incubates on the spermatozoa assay. **Fertility and Sterility** 48:694–696

Chacho, K.J., Chacho, M.S., Andresen, P.J. & Scommegna, A. (1986). Peritoneal fluid in patients with and without endometriosis: prostanoids and macrophages and their effect on the spermatozoa penetration assay. **American Journal of Obstetrics and Gynecology** 154:1290–1299.

Chirgwin, J.M., Prezybyla, A.E., MacDonald, R.J. & Rutter, W.J. (1979). Isolation of biologically active ribonucleic acid from sources enriched in ribonuclease. **Biochemistry** 18:5294–5299.

Collart, M.A., Belin, D., Vassalli, J.-D., de Kossodo, S. & Vassalli, P. (1986). Gamma-interferon enhances macrophage transcription of the tumor necrosis factor/cachectin, interleukin 1 and urokinase genes, which are controlled by short-lived repressors. **Journal of Experimental Medicine** 164:2113–2118.

Das, H.K., Lawrance, S.K. & Weissman, S.M. (1983). Structure and nucleotide sequence of the heavy chain gene of HLA-DR. **Proceedings of the National Academy of Sciences, USA** 80:354–357.

Distel, R.J., Ro, H.-S., Rosen, B.S., Groves, D.L. & Spiegelman, B.M. (1987). Nucleoprotein complexes that regulate gene expression in adipocyte differentiation: direct participation of *c-fos*. **Cell** 49:835–844.

Fakih, H., Baggett, B., Holtz, G., Tsang, K.-Y., Lee, J.C. & Williamson, H.O. (1987). Interleukin-1: a possible role in the infertility associated with endometriosis. **Fertility and Sterility** 47:213–217.

Greenberg, M.E. & Ziff, E.B. (1984). Stimulation of 3T3 cells induces transcription of the *c-fos* proto-oncogene. **Nature** 311:433–438.

Hahn, D.W., Carraher, R.P., Foldesy, R.G. & McGuire, J.L. (1986). Experimental evidence for failure to implant as a mechanism of infertility associated with endometriosis. **American Journal of Obstetrics and Gynecology** 155:1109–1113.

Halme, J. (1985). Basic research in endometriosis. **Obstetrics and Gynecology Annual** 14:288–309.

Halme, J., Becker, S., Hammond, M.G. & Raj, S. (1982). Pelvic macrophages in normal and infertile women: the role of patent tubes. **American Journal of Obstetrics and Gynecology** 142:890–895.

Halme, J., Becker, S., Hammond, M.G., Raj, M.H.G. & Raj, S. (1983). Increased activation of pelvic macrophages in infertile women with mild endometriosis. **American Journal of Obstetrics and Gynecology** 145:333–337.

Halme, J., Becker, S. & Haskill, S. (1987). Altered maturation and function of peritoneal macrophages: possible role in pathogenesis of endometriosis. **American Journal of Obstetrics and Gynecology** 156:783–789.

Halme, J., Becker, S. & Wing, R. (1984). Accentuated cyclic activation of peritoneal macrophages in patients with endometriosis. **American Journal of Obstetrics and Gynecology** 148:85–90.

Halme, J., White, C., Kauma, S., Estes, J. & Haskill, S. (1988). Peritoneal macrophages from patients with endometriosis release growth factor activity *in vitro*. **Journal of Clinical Endocrinology and Metabolism** 66:1044–1049.

Haney, A.F., Muscata, J.J. & Weinberg, J.B. (1981). Peritoneal fluid cell populations in infertility patients. **Fertility and Sterility** 35:696–698.

Hill, J.A., Haimovici, F. & Anderson, D.I. (1987a). Products of activated lymphocytes and macrophages inhibit mouse embryo development *in vitro*. **Journal of Immunology** 139:2250–2254.

Hill, J.A., Haimovici, F., Politch, J.A. & Anderson, D.J. (1987b). Effects of soluble products of activated lymphocytes and macrophages (lymphokines and monokines) or human sperm motion parameters. **Fertility and Sterility** 47:460–465.

Kauma, S., Clark, M.R., White, C. & Halme, J. (1988). Production of fibronectin by peritoneal macrophages and concentration of fibronectin in peritoneal fluid from patients with or without endometriosis. **Obstetrics and Gynecology** 72:13–18.

Le, J. & Vilcek, J. (1987). Biology of disease. Tumor necrosis factor and interleukin 1: cytokines with multiple overlapping biological activities. **Laboratory Investigation** 56:234–248.

Morcos, R.N., Gibbons, W.E. & Findley, W.E. (1985). Effect of peritoneal fluid on *in vitro* cleavage of 2-cell mouse embryos: possible role in infertility associated with endometriosis. **Fertility and Sterility** 44:678–683.

Muller, R. & Wagner, E.F. (1984). Differentiation of F9 teratocarcinoma stem cells after transfer of *c-fos* proto-oncogenes. **Nature** 311:438–442.

Muscato, J.J., Haney, A.F. & Weinberg, J.B. (1982). Sperm phagocytosis by human peritoneal macrophages: a possible cause of infertility in endometriosis. **American Journal of Obstetrics and Gynecology** 144:503–510.

Oak, M.K., Chantler, E.N., Williams, C.A. & Elstein, M. (1985). Sperm survival studies in peritoneal fluid from infertile women with endometriosis and unexplained infertility. **Clinical Reproduction and Fertility** 3:297–303.

Polan, M.L., Daniele, A. & Kuo, A. (1988). Gonadal steroids modulate human monocyte interleukin-1 (IL-1) activity. **Fertility and Sterility** 49:964–968.

Sueldo, C.E., Lambert, H., Steinleitner, A., Rathwick, G. & Swanson, J. (1987). The effect of peritoneal fluid from patients with endometriosis on murine sperm–oocyte interaction. **Fertility and Sterility** 48:697–699.

Suginami, H., Yano, K., Watanabe, K. & Matsuura, S. (1986). A factor inhibiting ovum capture by the oviductal fimbriae present in endometriosis peritoneal fluid. **Fertility and Sterility** 46:1140–1146.

Syrop, C.H. & Halme, J. (1987). Peritoneal fluid environment and infertility. **Fertility and Sterility** 48:1–9.

Verma, I.M. & Sassone-Corsi, P. (1987). Proto-oncogene *fos*: complex but versatile regulation. **Cell** 51:513–514.

VI New leads for fertility regulation research: summary of the symposium

Summary: Focus on growth regulatory factors for new leads in fertility regulation research

E. DICZFALUSY, J. FINDLAY, P. VAN LOOK AND G. WAITES

The main purpose of this symposium was to review current knowledge on the molecular biology of growth regulatory factors – particularly their role in reproduction – in order to identify potential leads for developing new methods for the regulation of fertility.

The evidence presented at the symposium confirmed that a number of these growth factors and related substances influence (by both autocrine and paracrine means) gonadal function in humans as well as in animals. However, our understanding of the biology of these substances is still largely incomplete, and the physiological relevance of the results of experiments *in vitro* is largely unknown. As a result, the potential of this field to provide new leads in the development of novel approaches to fertility regulation cannot be fully assessed as yet. However, the data presented during the symposium gave an indication of the problems that are likely to be encountered. The first problem relates to the ubiquitous nature of these substances and to the fact that few of them are specifically and exclusively involved in reproductive function, making them not particularly suitable targets for 'contraceptive attack'. Substances whose effects are limited to the reproductive tissues only are generally better and easier targets.

Secondly, because most of these factors appear to exert primarily a local regulatory role through paracrine or autocrine mechanisms, it may be difficult to achieve effective local concentrations of exogenous agents administered to influence their actions.

Thirdly, the peptide nature of these substances and the structural homology that exists between some of them (e.g. among the members of the transforming growth factor-β family, which includes the inhibins, activins, Mullerian inhibiting substance, etc.) are likely to limit their potential use in fertility regulation. Peptide agonists or antagonists could be costly to produce, they would require the development of specifically dedicated delivery systems and they might induce an immune response.

Four promising areas of research were none the less identified. The first relates to the process of meiosis, which is a unique attribute of the gonads and, thus, offers possibilities for the design of agents that could influence reproductive function in a selective and specific manner. Evidence presented at the symposium suggests that, during the course of meiosis, certain proteins are present that are not found during mitosis. The control and function of these proteins, which include, for example, the product of the expression of the *c-mos* proto-oncogene, deserve further study.

A second group of possible targets consists of the factors that control angiogenesis in the ovary and the endometrium. Although the formation of new blood vessels occurs at various times in different tissues of the body, the process of angiogenesis in the ovary and the endometrium is unique since it follows a cyclical pattern linked to the menstrual cycle.

The third area identified for further research relates to the interaction between the reproductive and the immune systems. There is a growing body of evidence to support the notion that interleukins exert effects on the reproductive tissues in addition to their immunological functions. For example, it has been demonstrated that interleukin-1, which is produced by macrophages located in the reproductive organs, is capable of, *inter alia*, inducing the production of prostaglandins. Interleukins have also been reported to be involved in spermiogenesis, sperm motility, fertilization, development of the embryo, and pituitary function. Since the immune system appears to have effects on reproductive function, and since infection by human immunodeficiency virus (HIV) affects the immune system, further research on the molecular biology of the reproductive and immune systems will be relevant also in the context of the possible interaction between hormonal contraceptives and HIV infection.

Fourthly, interference with the binding sites of certain receptors may be a fruitful area for further study, as demonstrated by the recent development of antiprogestins. Although the design of agents capable of binding to the cellular receptors for endogenous peptides or proteins would seem more complicated than the synthetic blockers of receptors for steroids, more detailed knowledge about how the conformation of receptors may permit the design of simple, organic molecules with affinity for the receptors. In this regard, the receptor for follicle-stimulating hormone was considered to offer the most promise because of its specificity and its relevance to the regulation of fertility.

The study of local regulatory agents requires in-vitro model systems. Two techniques of particular importance were discussed at the symposium: the methods of determining stage of spermatogenesis coupled with gene-related events, and new techniques of cell culture which provide a more appropriate environment and allow polarity of cells. A particular challenge remaining is to devise methods of testing the physiological relevance of growth factors *in vivo*.

Index

Note: abbreviations used are explained on pages xix–xxii.